Principles of Skin Care

A Guide for Nurses and Other Health Care Professionals

Rebecca Penzer RN, BSc(Hons), PGDipEd, MSc

*Community Dermatology Nurse Specialist, Norfolk Community Health and Care
Dermatology Nurse Specialist, Queen Elizabeth Hospital, King's Lynn
Deputy Chair, International Skin Care Nursing Group*

Steven J. Ersser RGN, BSc (Hons), PhD (Lond), CertTHEd

*Professor of Nursing Development & Skin Care Research
Director, Centre for Wellbeing & Quality of Life
School of Health & Social Care
Bournemouth University, UK
Chair, International Skin Care Nursing Advisory Board*

With contributions from:

Julie Van Onselen BA(Hons), DipN, DipMar, RGN, RSCN, ENB 998, N25(DermN)

JVO Consultancy-education in dermatology and Dermatology Nurse, Oxon PCT

Rachel Duncan MPhil, BN (Hons), PGCE, ENB 237, RGN

*Macmillan Clinical Nurse Specialist – Skin Cancer
St Helens and Knowsley Teaching Hospitals NHS Trust*

Jean Robinson RGN, RSCN, MA

*Clinical Nurse Specialist Children's Dermatology
Barts and The London NHS Trust*

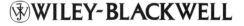

WILEY-BLACKWELL

A John Wiley & Sons, Ltd., Publication

Registered office
John Wiley & Sons Ltd, The Atrium, Southern Gate, Chichester, West Sussex, PO19 8SQ, United Kingdom

Editorial offices
9600 Garsington Road, Oxford, OX4 2DQ, United Kingdom
2121 State Avenue, Ames, Iowa 50014-8300, USA

For details of our global editorial offices, for customer services and for information about
how to apply for permission to reuse the copyright material in this book please see our website
at www.wiley.com/wiley-blackwell.

Library of Congress Cataloging-in-Publication Data

Penzer, Rebecca.
    Principles of skin care : a guide for nurses and other health care professionals / Rebecca Penzer, Steven J.
  Ersser ; with contributions from Julie Van Onselen, Rachel Duncan, Jean Robinson.
       p. ; cm.
    Includes bibliographical references and index.
    ISBN 978-1-4051-7087-1 (pbk. : alk. paper)
      1. Dermatologic nursing.   2. Skin—Care and hygiene.   I. Ersser, Steven.   II. Title.
  [DNLM: 1. Skin Diseases—nursing.   2. Skin Care—nursing. WY 154.5 P419p 2010]
    RL125.P46 2010
    616.50231—dc22

                                                                                        2009033608

A catalogue record for this book is available from the British Library.

Set in 10/12 pt Sabon by MPS Limited, A Macmillan Company
Printed and bound in Malaysia by KHL Printing Co Sdn Bhd

1   2010

Contents

Acknowledgements

We would like to thank the following people for their help and support in writing this book: Dr David Paige, Dr Mike Cork, Professor Eugene Healy, Professor Terence Ryan, Dave Roberts, Dr Elizabeth Norton, Andrew Kerr and Alison Jackson. Thanks also to the Wessex Cancer Trust.

Introduction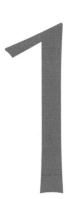

Rebecca Penzer

Perhaps more than any other organ of the body, the skin is multidimensional; in the totality of human experience the skin is key. It is a physical presence and Chapter 2 of this book considers in some depth the biology of the skin. But the skin goes way beyond this. It has emotional and psychological importance, it can affect whether we are discriminated against, or not, it is a sexual organ, it is a work of art (and a canvass for works of art), it is used to determine social acceptability, it is a tool to market everything from the obvious (make-up) to the less obvious (sanitary towels) and we use and abuse it in the pursuit of youth and beauty.

This introductory chapter to 'Principles of Skin Care: A Guide for Nurses and Other Health Care Professionals' is a light hearted look at the skin and what it means to us as humans. It is how-ever, a significant chapter. To be able to care for patients who have dysfunctional skin, it is key to understand what is meant by skin health. Whilst much of the rest of this book is dedicated to describing what happens when the skin is no longer healthy, there is a recurrent theme of using nursing skills to promote skin health and prevent disease.

Thus, this chapter looks to answer the questions about what is skin and what is the human experience of skin, through a cultural lens. The multifaceted concept of skin health is introduced and will be revisited as a key topic throughout the book. Finally a summary of the contents of the book will be given.

What is skin?

The basic definition of skin both in a medical and English dictionary describes it as the external layer of the body. But this description is really wholly inadequate. It infers that the skin is an inert envelope that contains the bones, muscles, organs and blood that allow us to exist. Whilst the skin is our external covering that holds us together, it is far from inert. To express it crea-tively, the skin is a combination of a lunar land-scape, a zoological and botanical haven in which there is the potential for an immunological party. Expressed more traditionally, the surface of the skin is a rough, undulating environment with skin cells desquamating all the time. It is covered with bacteria and fungus that live in harmony with us and protect us from invading pathogens. In a normal state the immune system within the skin is quiet and relatively inactive, but if the skin is challenged in any way, a range of immunological cascades are set in motion. In some conditions such as psoriasis these immunological changes are not within a normal range and cause severe inflammation and hyperproliferation of skin cells.

Defining the skin as our external surface is also limited because it does not include our internal skin surfaces such as the mouth or the vagina. And of course the scope of the term dermatology goes beyond what is traditionally described as skin to an interest in both hair and nails, commonly thought of as skin appendages which are constructed of the same basic building blocks as skin itself.

Understanding of the science of skin is constantly expanding. Of key importance in improving understanding of skin and how it functions, is research. Important areas of biological scientific research include how the immune system within the skin functions and how genetic make-up influences the expression of skin disease and how humans respond to treatment. But to truly understand 'What is skin' we must gain insights that go beyond comprehending physical function. Research can also help to uncover some of the psychological and social impacts of experiencing skin disease. For example what affects how people cope with a chronic condition and how quality of life might be affected?

What is skin for the lay person? The way the skin looks plays an important role and the aesthetics of the skin are considered shortly, but the skin has also influenced our language in all sorts of colourful ways. Skin can probably win the prize for the organ most used in common parlance and slang! Table 1.1 gives some examples. This reflects the cultural and symbolic importance of skin as an integral part of our language.

Skin health

Introduction

Simply put, healthy skin is skin that is not diseased. However, this might be thought of as a somewhat limited interpretation of the concept. An alternative view is that healthy skin is skin which fulfils all its physical, psychological and social functions. This view incorporates a wider conception of skin health which goes beyond the physical and embraces psychological, social and quality of life issues. This book aims to embrace this wider concept of skin health and to emphasise how nursing skills can be used to meet all those patient needs. This section will specifically look at areas relating to skin health which do not 'belong' in any other part of this book, but none-the-less warrant attention.

Display, decoration and adornment

The way the skin is displayed (used as an organ of display) is significantly affected by social and cultural influences. Throughout history humans have felt compelled to change their skin in ways that are rarely good for its physical health.

Table 1.1 The use of the skin concept in common parlance.

Saying	Meaning
By the skin of one's teeth	By a narrow margin
Get under someone's skin	To irritate or provoke someone
No skin off someone's nose	No disadvantage to someone
Skin and bone	Very thin
Skin-up	Roll a joint
Skin deep	Superficial
Skin-flick	A film of adult nature involving nudity
Skinful	A large amount to drink
Skin game	A swindling game or trick
Skin and blister	Sister (Cockney rhyming slang)
Have a thick skin	To be unbothered by things
Save ones skin	To avoid harm especially escaping death

However, adornment, decoration and display have other important sociological implications indicating belonging to group and tribes or conversely to show rebellion and individuality.

Signals given through the skin can indicate a wide range of social norms and values. The obvious ones include religious observance reflected by the amount of skin and hair covered and by what types of garments are worn. Clothing and adornments vitally allow humans to fit into their own social system and indicate a sense of belonging. The social norms in relation to displaying the skin are time dependent. Thus a British woman living in Victorian times might have felt it disgraceful to expose her ankles, whereas in the 21st century this is not generally considered scandalous behaviour! Piercing and tattooing give a wide range of social signals including membership of certain groups. However, once again, in the 21st century these rules too are becoming more blurred and less strictly adhered to with a wide cross section of society choosing to have tattoos and various body piercings.

As with other organs of the body, humans are prone to abuse their skin. Fair skinned people aim for the perfect sun-tan and in the process of getting to this point put themselves at risk of both malignant and non-malignant skin cancers. It is becoming an increasingly common practice for people with darker skins to want to lighten them. This is done through a number of unregulated mechanisms including the use of potent topical steroids, which cause a range of other health problems, as well as the desired skin lightening. Depending on the extent and time frame of steroid use, these effects may also become systemic.

Abuse and discrimination

Whatever the context of skin decoration and skin adornment, it is usually done in order to make a personal statement. However there are instances when skin marking and/or skin alteration is abusive and detrimental to personal health. For example, the tattooing of numbers onto the arms of prisoners in concentration camps was designed to dehumanise and depersonalise people. Individuals became a number rather than a name. Female genital mutilation is another example of a practice which is abusive. Whilst some people within cultural groups accept the practice as part of becoming a woman, it is widely condemned as an abusive, dangerous and unnecessary practice.

The course of human history is littered with tragedies of discriminatory behaviour brought on by false judgements made because of the colour of the skin. Discriminatory behaviour due to skin colour is now illegal in many parts of the world and the last 20 years have witnessed massively significant events in the quest for racial equality. The ending of apartheid in South Africa and the election of an African American as President of the United States of America are two examples of this. But discriminatory behaviour because of skin colour does still exist. A recent Health Care Commission highlighted that many Trust institutions within the British National Health Service were still not meeting their obligations as equal opportunities employers. It states that although ethnic minority groups make up 16% of the workforce only 10% are in senior management positions and 1% in a chief executive position (Commission for Healthcare Audit and Inspection, 2009).

For one group of people racism, ignorance and misunderstanding because of the colour of their skin, remains life threatening. There are a significant number of people living with albinism in East Africa. Albinism is a genetically inherited condition where the pigment of the skin, hair and eyes is either reduced or missing altogether. Whilst albinism does occur in the Caucasian population, it is more prevalent and more noticeable in black Americans. Some estimates put the number of those with albinism at 1 in 4000 in Tanzania, whilst the figures for the European population is more like 1 in 20,000 (Smith, 2008). Life for an African with albinism is curtailed due to hugely increased risk of skin cancer; however recent urbanisation of the population has led to an increase in murder and mutilation. It is thought that possessing a body part of someone who has albinism acts as a magic charm, which can lead to instant wealth (Smith, 2008).

Environment

As the skin is in constant contact with its surroundings, the environment is an important consideration when thinking about skin health. The immediate, local environment has a biological impact, thus if it is cold the skin responds with goose bumps, if it is hot it will sweat. A hot dry environment particularly one found in overheated homes can cause the skin to become very dry and itchy, particularly in the elderly. This section will look at the impact that environmental changes at a global level may have on the skin and touch on diseases related to poverty.

Environmental changes

It is difficult to prove categorically that any long-term, global environmental changes have a direct impact on skin health. There are many confounding factors to consider, and it is therefore virtually impossible to make a direct link between degradation of the environment and changes in skin health. For example, there is no doubt that our earth has less ozone protection than it did, which means that we are less well protected from UV radiation than in previous centuries (Earth Observatory, 2009). How much the increase in skin cancers can be attributed to this and how much can be attributed to behaviour change (e.g. more exposure to UV radiation due to increased number of holidays in sunny climates) is difficult to say. However the Earth Observatory report quotes the United Nations Environment programme as saying that a sustained decrease of 1% in the ozone layer will ultimately lead to a 2–3% increase in skin cancer.

For atopic eczema, there would appear to be an upward trend over the last 30–40 years with an increasing prevalence of the disease (Williams, 1997). This trend seems to affect urban populations more than rural (Sherriff *et al.*, 2002). This may be attributable to the hygiene hypothesis (see Box 1.1), but this theory is not agreed upon by all practitioners.

Box 1.1   Hygiene hypothesis

This theory was first proposed in 1989 by a public health physician. He suggested that the rising levels of hay fever and other atopic conditions may be attributed to better living conditions. The fact that young children were exposed to fewer infections due to increased household cleanliness and decreased family size, meant they were more susceptible to developing atopic diseases including eczema. The theory behind this is an immunological one; by challenging a child's immune system with infective processes it is less likely to 'produce' atopic symptoms (Strachan, 2000). This is explored further in Chapter 9.

Diseases of poverty

Skin diseases of poverty are usually related to infective processes or infestations. Poor living environments, lack of access to clean water and hot climatic conditions all lead to increased likelihood of infections or infestations of the skin. Specific examples include scabies, which in resource poor countries, where people live in very close proximity to one another, affect significant proportions of the population, especially children. Fungal and bacterial infections are more likely when there is lack of clean washing water, when wounds cannot be properly dressed and when people may be immunocompromised through poor diet or HIV infection. Vector borne diseases for example those carried by a mosquito, are more common in tropical areas where disease carrying mosquitoes thrive. An example of such a disease is lymphatic filariasis (described in Box 1.2) which can cause lymphoedema, hydrocoele and significant skin changes. It is important because of the scale of the problem (1.3 billion people around the world are at risk of contracting the disease and 120 million are infected) and because of the serious impact that it has on quality of life and economic stability (Global Alliance for the Elimination of Lymphatic Filariasis, 2004).

Box 1.2   Lymphatic filariasis

Lymphatic filariasis is a mosquito borne disease in which parasites known as filarial worms damage the lymphatic system. Small microfilariae are transmitted from mosquitoes to humans when the insect takes a blood meal. The microscopic parasites grow into worms which can reach 10 cm in length. These live in 'nests' in the lymphatic system causing significant damage. As a result lymphatic function is affected causing swelling and compromised skin function which, over time, can lead to elephantiasis. As a result of these huge limbs and grotesque skin changes, many people experience significant morbidity and disability. Working can become difficult or impossible. Undertaking activities of daily living is a challenge. Many people are ostracised from their communities and feel socially unacceptable. The good news, however, is that the disease can be eliminated through distribution of anti-parasitic drugs. This alongside a programme of managing the morbidity caused by lymphoedema and skin changes is a global health programme. For more details see www.filariasis.org.

Cosmetic

If we accept that skin is healthy only if the individual is content with the way their skin looks, feels and functions, cosmetic and aesthetic considerations become part of skin health.

Currently in the UK cosmetic dermatology remains a relatively small proportion of a dermatologist's work and most of what is done is as part of private practice. However in other countries, for example the United States of America, office-based dermatologists provide extensive cosmetic services with nurses providing significant support and education to patients and technical assistance to their medical colleagues. For many the march towards dermatologists doing more cosmetic work is an inevitable part of the modern age. If we accept the fact that skin health includes the psychological well-being which comes as part of feeling good about oneself, this shift may seem acceptable. However, in a national health service with limited resources, providing cosmetic care within that system is generally considered inappropriate. Indeed when dermatologists' skills are at a premium in order to manage chronic skin disease and skin cancer, it may be considered immoral to use those skills for non-dermatological disease procedures.

It can be a challenge to determine when a skin problem is 'purely cosmetic' and when it is a dermatological disease requiring treatment. For example, removal of a skin tag (which is harmless to physical health) may be seen as a cosmetic procedure and therefore not a treatment to be carried out as part of a national (public) health service. However, if the skin tag is exactly in a position which catches on a bra-strap and causes pain and discomfort each day, a case may be made for its removal. Likewise a skin tag on the neck may cause acute embarrassment and psychological damage for an individual and thus seeing its removal as part of a treatment process, is a relevant approach. The first example may seem more clear cut, but that is because priorities in health care are usually given to problems that give physical rather than emotional pain. It is easy to see that the line between cosmesis and treatment is blurred and often fraught with controversy.

The beauty industry focuses on the attributes of young looking skin and works hard to persuade a youth oriented world that those attributes are positive and desirable. These messages are so effective that individuals will go to considerable lengths to achieve younger looking skin. Table 1.2 gives some examples of beauty treatments with their intended outcomes, methods of working and possible side effects. In general youth enhancing treatments aim to reduce signs of ageing by smoothing and/or filling wrinkles and improving texture and colouring. Any nurses interested in working in the field of aesthetics would do well to read the latest Royal College of Nursing Guidance (2008) (Royal College of Nursing, 2008).

Table 1.2 Examples of cosmetic procedures.

Type of treatment	How it works	Outcome	Possible side effects
Botulinum toxin	The toxin botulinum is produced by the bacteria *Clostridium botulinum*. A purified formulation of the toxin (tradename Botox) can be injected into facial muscles and cause paralysis by preventing the release of acetylcholine from motor nerve endings. It also controls sweating by blocking sympathetic nerve fibres.	It is used particularly on the face to reduce frown lines and crows feet. The muscle paralysis means that the skin looks smoother. The effect will last for several weeks and individuals may opt to have treatments every 3–6 months.	Bruising at the injection site; Eyelid droop if the botulinum toxin tracks down into the eyelid muscle. Headache.
Exfoliation	Physically removing the outermost layer of dead keratinocytes using a rough substance, either a cleanser or a rough cloth/sponge. This is a mild non-invasive treatment, easily carried out at home.	The skin will appear 'brighter' and smoother.	Soreness and discomfort especially for people who have very sensitive skin.
Fillers	A filler smoothes out the skin surface, usually by the injection of a substance into the skin. Substances such as collagen and hyaluronic acid are injectable and need to be redone to maintain effect as they are absorbed into the body over time.	The skin will appear smoother. It can be used to reduce facial lines and can also be used on depressed acne scars	Numbness; Allergic reactions; Bleeding and bruising.
Laser resurfacing	There are different methods of laser resurfacing. Non-ablative methods have fewer unwanted side effects and treat only the dermis without affecting the epidermis. Ablative methods are more effective but associated with more risk and a longer recovery time	The skin is rejuvenated with fewer wrinkles, lines and blemishes. It may also be helpful in removing scars.	Few side effects are associated with non-ablative methods. Ablative methods are likely to lead to erythema, swelling, soreness and potential for infection.
Microdermabrasion	A type of exfoliation using a variety of techniques including 'crystal' and 'diamond' microdermabrasion. Often carried out in spas but increasingly marketed to the home environment.	As with exfoliation. Often a series of treatments will be recommended.	As with exfoliation above.

(continued)

Table 1.2 (*continued*)

Type of treatment	How it works	Outcome	Possible side effects
Peels	Chemicals are applied to the skin surface to remove the top layers of skin, the extent of epidermal removal depends on the strength of the peel.	Smoothes the skin surface and also improves skin tone. It may also be helpful in treating mild acne scarring	A mild peel is described as being like sunburn and may cause skin scaling; a more severe peel will lead to blistering, swelling and considerable discomfort and possible skin infection. May lead to scarring.
Retinol	Creams containing retinol or pro-retinol (a form of vitamin A) are thought to increase levels of glycosaminoglycan and procollagen. This leads to greater skin strength and a reduction in the appearance of ageing.	Reduces fine lines and wrinkles.	Skin redness and soreness; increased sensitivity to sun exposure.
Thread face-lift	Threads with small 'teeth' on them are passed through subcutaneous fat just below the skin, with a needle. The threads are then pulled tight and secured with a suture.	Sagging or wrinkled skin is smoothed out, but it will not change the shape of the face. The change is permanent but the skin continues to age so the effect lasts for about 5 years.	Possible bruising; infection is a risk. If not carried out well facial asymmetry may result.

What is in this book

This book is split into two broad sections: 'Fundamental principles of managing the skin' and 'Principles of illness management'. In the first section, some of the core nursing issues that are relevant across the board of dermatological care are addressed. In order to be able to address the health needs of patients with dermatological conditions, the authors feel that it is important to get to grips with these fundamental issues. Thus Chapter 2 provides an in-depth look at the biology of the skin and its appendages. It is difficult to understand, never mind to explain to patients, what is going wrong with their skin without this core knowledge. Whichever field of nursing is being discussed, planning care is a critical nursing activity. Chapter 3 looks at the process of patient assessment, planning care and monitoring interventions. As nursing roles

develop, increasing numbers of practitioners will be independent prescribers and this is also explored in this chapter.

In this introductory chapter there is a focus on the importance of skin health. Chapter 4 takes a generic look at what happens when the skin becomes vulnerable and fails, in other words skin health is compromised. It provides an in-depth examination of the nursing activities needed to prevent skin break down and thus promote skin health.

Emollient therapy remains one of the mainstays of chronic skin disease management. It is important for both preventive care and treatment and as such could perhaps have been placed in either section of this book. However, as a generic topic which is relevant across so many disease areas emollient therapy warranted its own chapter. In Chapter 5, detailed examination is given to how emollients work and how they should be used.

Uniquely this text book has chosen to devote two chapters to topics which are often touched upon in dermatology but rarely given a significant amount of attention. Chapter 6 looks at the psychological and social impacts of skin disease emphasising the nursing role in helping patients with the mental difficulties that skin diseases can impose. Chapter 7 takes some of the themes from Chapter 6 and develops them specifically to consider how nurses can help patients to improve their adherence with treatment. In both chapters, theories are related to practice to enable the practitioner to develop their skills in the most useful way.

The second section will be more familiar to most readers in that it covers the dermatological conditions most commonly seen in practice: Chapter 8 psoriasis, Chapter 9 eczema, Chapter 10 acne, Chapter 11 skin cancer, Chapter 12 infective disorders and Chapter 13 more uncommon skin conditions. In each chapter pathological processes have been considered in some detail and then treatments and nursing interventions. Evidence has been widely used, particularly systematic reviews when they are available. Whilst most of the conditions in Chapter 13 are indeed more uncommon, some of them are not that uncommon but they do not fit into any of the other chapters so they need to appear here!

Before concluding it is important to mention clinical images. Throughout the text the authors have attempted to provide clinical images that help to illustrate disease appearance and distribution. However, we would strongly recommend that you supplement these pictures by looking at websites that provide an excellent array of visual resources (see Box 1.3)

> **Box 1.3 Websites for dermatology images**
>
> www.dermnet.com
> www.dermatlas.org
> www.dermnetnz.org
> www.dermis.net

Conclusion

The authors have aimed to create a book which helps nurses and other health care practitioners to practice in a way that is as evidence-based as possible. We also hope that this book helps to develop practitioners who work with compassion, recognising that patients with skin disease are often affected in many dimensions of their lives. This may be through physical discomfort, psychological pain or social exclusion. Whatever the impact on individual patients, nurses who understand skin disease are well placed to alleviate suffering. This may be through direct intervention to treat a disease condition or through health promotion to improve skin health and prevent skin disease.

References

Commission for Healthcare Audit and Inspection (2009). *Tackling the Challenge: Promoting Race Equality in the NHS in England*. London: The Healthcare Commission.

Earth Observatory (2009). *Ultraviolet Radiation: How it Affects Life on Earth*. NASA. http://earthobservatory.nasa.gov/Features/UVB/uvb_radiation2.php last accessed 24/11/09

Global Alliance for the Elimination of Lymphatic Filariasis (2004). A Future Free of LF. Retrieved 15 April 2009, from www.filariasis.org.

Royal College of Nursing (2008). *Aesthetic Nursing: RCN Guidance on Best Practice*. London: Royal College of Nursing.

Sherriff, A., J. Golding, ALSPAC study team *et al.* (2002). Hygiene levels in a contemporary population cohort are associated with wheezing and atopic eczema in preschool infants. *Archives of Disabled Child*, 87: 26–29.

Smith, A. (2008). Albino Africans live in fear after witch-doctor butchery. *The Observer*, 35. http://www.guardian.co.uk/world/2008/nov/16/tanzania-humanrights last accessed 24/11/09

Strachan, D. (2000). Family size, infection and atopy: The first decade of the "hygiene hypothesis". *Thorax* 55(Suppl 1): S2–S10.

Williams, H.C. (1997). *Dermatology Health Care Needs Assessment*. Oxford: Radcliffe Medical Press.

Part 1

Fundamental principles of managing the skin

Biology of the skin

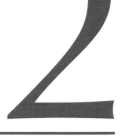

Rebecca Penzer

Introduction

The skin is the largest organ of the body weighing between 2 and 4.5 kg (16% of body weight) and covering approximately 2 m² (Tortora and Derrickson, 2006). The skin is between 1 and 2 mm thick, depending on the part of the body that is being considered. It is dynamic and changing, capable of healing itself and responding to the external environment in such a way that ensures human survival. Like all other organs, the skin is capable of failure, the results of which can be physically and psychologically debilitating and potentially lethal.

To understand how to care for the skin, it is necessary to have an understanding of skin biology. Therefore this chapter will cover:

- Skin structure and function;
- Skin changes from pre-birth to old age;
- Ethnic differences.

Skin structure

The skin is composed of two main layers (Figure 2.1). The epidermis is the outer layer which comes into contact with the external environment. It is considerably thinner than the dermis, approximately 10% of total skin thickness. The dermis is the powerhouse of the skin, providing the supportive structures to allow the epidermis to function.

Epidermis

The epidermis, which forms the top layer of skin, is constantly shedding millions of dead

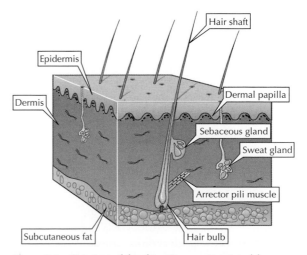

Figure 2.1 Structure of the skin. (Source: Reprinted from Graham-Brown and Burns, 2006.)

cells. It is estimated that normal skin sheds at a rate of a million cells every 40 minutes (Hinchcliffe *et al.*, 1999) which equates to around 18 kg over a lifetime (Marieb and Hoehn, 2007). This process of skin cell shedding is known as desquamation. As skin cells are shed, new cells are constantly pushing up from underneath to replace them. If cells develop too quickly, the skin becomes piled up and thickened (as in skin diseases such as psoriasis) and if too slowly, the skin will be thin and atrophied (as occurs in old age). The normal transit time for epidermal cells (i.e. the time they take to move from the bottom layer of the epidermis to the top layer) is around 35 days. Epidermal thickness varies over the surface of the skin and can be thought of as either 'thick' skin or 'thin' skin. Thick skin occurs on the palms and soles and has neither hair follicles nor sebaceous glands but does have sweat glands. In these areas, the epidermis is between 400 and 600 μm. Thin skin, which covers the rest of the body, has hair follicles, sebaceous glands and sweat glands and is between 75 and 150 μm thick.

Ninety percent of epidermal cells are keratinocytes which are thought of as the building blocks of the epidermis. They start off as actively dividing cells and by the time they reach the skin surface they are anucleate bundles of keratin known as corneocytes. Keratin is synthesised within the keratinocytes from amino acids, particularly cysteine which allows for disulphide bond cross-linking which gives added strength to the skin. This is particularly predominant in hair and nails. Keratin is the same basic building block that is found in hair and nails in humans and horns, claws, hoofs and feathers in animals and birds.

Other epidermal cells include melanocytes (around 8% of total number of cells) and Langerhans cells (Figure 2.2).

Basal layer

Also known as the stratum basale or stratum germinativum, this is a single layer of columnar-shaped keratinocytes, some of which are stem cells undergoing constant cell division to produce new keratinocytes (Tortora and

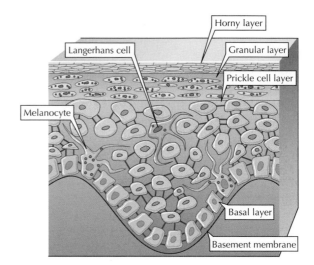

Figure 2.2   Layers of the epidermis. (Source: Reprinted from Graham-Brown and Burns, 2006.)

Derrickson, 2006). Each active basal cell divides every 4 days to produce daughter cells which then go on to differentiate and mature. These basal cells are 'power-houses' of activity containing various cellular structures which allow them to replicate effectively. Each cell has a large nucleus made up of cytoplasm containing ribosomes, which are attached to rough endoplasmic reticulum, a small Golgi complex and a few mitochondria (Table 2.1).

Table 2.1   Structures seen within basal cells.

Cell structure	Activity
Ribosomes	Sites of protein synthesis
Rough endoplasmic reticulum	A network of channels that serves as intracellular transportation, supporting, packaging and transporting molecules
Golgi complex	Modifies, sorts, packages and transports proteins received from the endoplasmic reticulum
Mitochondria	Produce adenosine triphosphate (ATP), crucial for energy production

The basal layer also includes the melanocytes, responsible for producing melanin which gives colour to skin and hair and protection from ultraviolet (UV) radiation. The production of melanin is under genetic control and is regulated by melanocyte stimulating hormone (MSH) secreted from the anterior lobe of the pituitary gland. Clinically, it is interesting to note that MSH is very similar in structure to adrenocorticotrophic hormone (ACTH). People with increased ACTH secretion, for example in Addison's disease, show increased pigmentation in sun-exposed sites and where they experience mild trauma (Hinchcliffe *et al.*, 1999) because ACTH acts as MSH.

The production of melanin occurs within organelles known as melanosomes, in the cytoplasm of the melanocytes. Within these melanosomes, the amino acid tyrosine is converted into melanin in the presence of the enzyme tyrosinase. From here it is transferred into the cytoplasm of the surrounding keratinocytes. Variations in hair pigment are caused by biochemical differences in the melanin produced in blondes, brunettes and redheads. The racial differences in skin pigment can be explained by the fact that in Caucasians, melanosomes are grouped in complexes which degenerate as the keratinocytes move towards the surface of the skin. In darker skinned people the skin contains the same number of melanocytes, but the melanosomes are larger, remain separate and persist throughout the thickness of the epidermis (Graham-Brown and Burns, 1996). The quantity of melanin found in keratinocytes depends to a large extent on genetic make-up and the environment, that is how much UV exposure someone is subjected to.

Finally, the epidermis contains specialised cells called Merkell cells. At the interface of the epidermis and dermis, the flattened process of a sensory neuron comes into contact with the tactile disc of the Merkell cells thus detecting certain aspects of touch and sensation.

Prickle cell layer (stratum spinosum)

As keratinocytes mature and differentiate, they go through the transition to the prickle cell layer where the cells become interlocked by a network of desmosomes. Desmosomes are designed specifically to hold cells together and as such are important structures which give the resilience to the skin. They consist of a plaque on either side of the plasma membrane (where a plaque is a dense layer of protein). On one side of this plaque, extending into the intracellular space, are glycoproteins known as cadherins which attach to one another. On the other side of the plaque, filaments consisting of keratin (known as tonofilaments), stretch from one side of the cell to the other where they attach to other desmosomes (Figure 2.3). This provides the cell with structural stability. The cells in this layer are so called because when they are fixed and observed under a microscope, the cells pull slightly away from each other so that the desmosomes can be seen stretching across the intracellular space giving the cells a prickle-like appearance.

The prickle cell layer of the epidermis is between 8 and 10 layers thick. Keratohyalin granules are present in the keratinocytes and they contain a substance which combines with intermediate filaments of the cytoskeleton converting them to keratin; these also contribute to the resilience of the skin. Also in this section of the skin, lipid-filled membrane coating bodies start to develop.

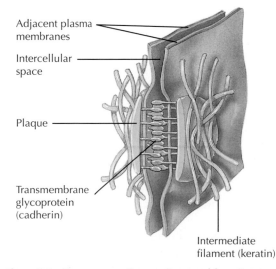

Figure 2.3 Desmosome. (Source: Reprinted from Tortora and Derrickson, 2006.)

Langerhans cells are present in the prickle layer. These cells are highly specialised dendritic cells which are an important part of the immune system, located within the skin. They are called dendritic cells because the surface membrane is folded in a similar way to the dendrites of the nervous system. This is so that the Langerhans cells can have maximum surface area to allow interaction with other cells. As immature cells, they are highly endocytotic (i.e. their plasma membrane invaginates producing an intracellular vesicle which surrounds the ingested material). However, as the Langerhans cells differentiate they have an increased capacity to migrate to T-cell areas and to function as antigen-presenting cells (Roitt and Delves, 2001). Mature Langerhans cells are covered in molecules known as major histocompatibility complex molecules, class II. These are adept at presenting the pieces of antigen protein to T-cells, which are then destroyed (Lydyard *et al.*, 2000).

Granular layer (stratum granulosum)

Also called the stratum granulosum, this is the part of the epidermis where there is high lyso-somal activity. Lysosomes are organelles which contain enzymes that digest the cell contents causing the cell nuclei to disintegrate. At this stage the keratohyalin granules become more prominent within the cell and the lipid-filled membrane coating vesicles, which have been produced in both the granular and prickle cell layers, start to undergo exocytosis extruding the glycolipid over the keratinocyte membranes, thus helping to lubricate and waterproof the skin. These lipids include 40% ceramides, the rest being comprised of fatty acids, cholesterol and cholesterol sulphate. Langerhans cells continue to be present in the granular layer.

Horny layer (stratum corneum)

The horny layer or stratum corneum is the outer layer that interfaces with the environment. It is vital that it is capable of keeping out unwanted allergens and pathogens and retaining moisture by preventing water loss by evaporation. The cells of this outer layer are fibrous, tough bundles of keratin known as corneocytes. Filaggrin,

a protein, which is also seen in the cells at this point, binds with keratin to help provide an effective skin barrier. Recent research has shown that the correct functioning of filaggrin is essential for effective barrier function of the skin. Examining the genetic make-up of people who suffer from icthyosis and atopic eczema shows loss of function mutations for filaggrin which may explain why the barrier function is compromised in these individuals (Hoffjan and Stemmler, 2007).

The horny layer contains a number of substances known as natural moisturising factors (NMF). These substances which include lactic acid, pyrrolidonecarboxylic acid and urea are water loving. They attract and hold water thus helping to maintain the hydration of the horny layer. Around 15% of the stratum corneum is water, if this falls below 10% the skin will become dry. The lipids, which were produced in the prickle and granular layers, continue to be present in the horny layer. They form what is known as a lipid bilayer which helps to further fortify the barrier function of the skin.

In order to ensure the effective barrier function of the skin, all these mechanisms need to be in place.

(1) *Keratin and filaggrin*: to maintain a tough barrier to keep out allergens and pathogens;
(2) *NMF*: to attract and retain moisture;
(3) *Lipids*: to lubricate and waterproof the skin as well as helping to trap the moisture in the stratum corneum.

Basement membrane zone

This is a specialised area of the skin consisting of a number of different layers and structures which ensure that the dermis and the epidermis are held together. Hemidesmosomes anchor keratinocytes to the basement membrane. These are similar to desmosomes but only have one plaque attached to the glycoprotein integrin outside the plasma membrane and attached to laminin in the basal lamina (lamina lucida) (Figure 2.4). The corrugated shape of the basement membrane zone helps to ensure that the

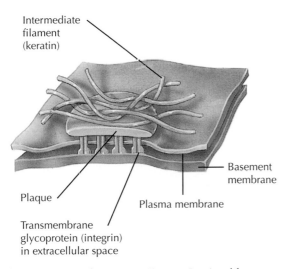

Figure 2.4 Hemidesmosome. (Source: Reprinted from Tortora and Derrickson, 2006.)

rete ridges of the epidermis interdigitate with the dermal papillae providing further stability.

The effectiveness with which the two layers of the skin hold together can be compromised in some genetically inherited disorders, for example epidermolysis bullosa, or by diseases that develop later in life, for example bullous pemphigoid (see Chapter 13 for further details).

Dermis

Lying between the epidermis and the subcutaneous fat, the dermis is the support system for the epidermis, providing it with nutrients and oxygen and removing waste products. It consists largely of connective tissue.

Connective tissue consists of a ground substance with protein fibres distributed throughout it. The ground substance contains water and a mixture of large organic molecules which are a combination of polysaccharides (complex carbohydrates) and proteins. The most common type of polysaccharides in connective tissue is glycosaminoglycans (GAGS). These help to trap moisture, making the ground substance more jelly-like and viscous. GAGS include hyaluronic acid which binds cells together, lubricates joints and shapes the eyeball.

This ground substance plays an important role in providing bulk for the dermis which acts as a shock absorber and a lubricant between the collagen and elastin (protein) fibres when the skin moves. Due to its high viscosity, hormones, waste products and nutrients may pass through it; however, it is difficult for bacteria to move through.

The protein component of the dermis is largely made up of collagen and elastin. Fibroblasts, which are found extensively throughout the dermis, are responsible for the production of collagen and elastin. The fibres that make up collagen are tough and resist stretching but they are flexible and as such they give structural strength to the skin. Bundles of collagen lie parallel to one another throughout the dermis forming cleavage or tension lines (Figure 2.5). Surgical incisions that are made parallel to these lines are much less likely to gape and will heal more effectively, than those that are made across tension

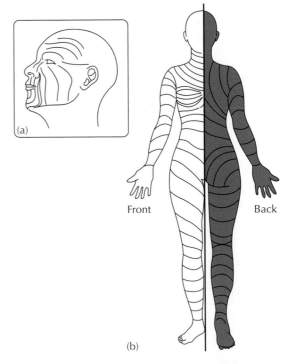

Figure 2.5 Relaxed skin tension lines. On the head and neck (a) these are readily identified by following the existing wrinkle or skin-crease lines. On the limbs the lines tend to run obliquely around rather than along the limb (b).

lines. Collagen also has a strong water binding capability helping to maintain hydration in the dermis. Twenty-five percent of the body's protein is collagen.

Elastic fibres, which are thinner than the collagenous fibres, are made of a stretchy, coiled protein called elastin. These springy fibres allow the skin to return to its normal shape after being stretched.

The dermis also contains tissue mast cells containing vasoactive chemicals (e.g. histamine); these are involved in moderating the immune and inflammatory responses in the skin and are found near hair follicles and blood vessels. Macrophages and histocytes are also present, which are phagocytic and engulf particulate matter. Blood vessels and cutaneous lymphatics run through the dermis, as do a number of nerve bundles and sensory receptors.

There are two distinct layers to the dermis, the papillary and the reticular.

At the interface with the epidermis, the papillary layer is approximately 1/5th of the total thickness of the dermis. It is the less dense of the two layers and contains thin elastic fibres. It also carries the blood vessels and nerve endings that supply the epidermis. This layer is thrown into 'peg like' projections known as dermal papillae which interlock with the rete pegs of the epidermis. Some of the dermal papillae contain capillary loops and others contain nerve endings and touch receptors such as Meissner's corpuscles. The human fingerprint, unique to each of us, is created by dermal papillae lying on dermal ridges, thus producing epidermal ridges that create a print when in contact with a surface. Usefully, the epidermal ridges on palms and soles increase friction and allow for a better grip.

The denser reticular layer makes up the bulk of the dermis. It is packed with collagen and coarse elastic fibres that give the dermis its strength and flexibility.

Ethnic differences in skin structure

There is little consensus about differences in skin structure between ethnic groups. It is commonly thought that Afro-Caribbean skin is drier than Caucasian skin. Researchers differ in their views on this. Wesley and Maibach (2003) found that there was greater transepidermal water loss in black skin whereas Grimes *et al.* (2004) found that there was no difference. Both authors agreed, however, that there was no difference in the water content of the epidermis. One explanation as to why it is commonly thought that black skin is drier than white skin is that when skin cells shed, they are more noticeable against black skin than white, giving an 'ashy' tone to the skin. What does seem to be true is that desquamation is greater in black skin than white skin (up to 2.5 times) (Wesley and Maibach, 2003).

There is debate, also, around whether black skin has a higher pH than white skin. Wesley and Maibach (2003) arguing it is the case and Grimes *et al.* (2004) that it is not. One suggested mechanism for a higher skin pH in people with black skin is that they have more active apocrine glands, the secretions from these may explain a more acidic skin pH.

Whilst keloid scarring occurs in all racial groups, it is more common in those of Afro-Caribbean descent. Afro-Caribbean men are more likely to suffer from ingrown hairs following shaving. The hair follicle is curved and as the hair (which has been made pointy by shaving) grows, it is more likely to grow back into the skin, thus causing an inflammatory reaction; this may be misdiagnosed as acne. It is known as pseudofolliculitis barbae. Post-inflammatory and/or post-traumatic hyperpigmentation is more commonly seen in darker skins. This will usually fade, but may be the source of considerable concern.

Subcutis

Lying beneath the dermis, this layer of fat provides padding and insulation. It varies in its thickness across the body, and this varies depending on the sex of an individual. Women tend to have thicker fat layers around the hips and bottom whereas men tend to develop it around their abdomen.

Appendageal structures

Whilst these emerge from the skin through the epidermis and are considered epidermal appendages, most of them lie within the dermis or the subcutis. As such they include hair, nails, sebaceous and sweat glands.

Hair

The surface of the skin is virtually completely covered by invaginations of the epidermis, known as hair follicles. An invagination can be described as the folding of something so that an external surface becomes an internal surface. Thus in the case of the epidermis, the surface of a hair follicle is covered in the same cells as the surface of the external skin. Out of the follicle a keratin tube grows known as hair. The only parts of the skin surface that are not covered in hair are the lips, the palms of the hands and the soles of the feet – these parts of the skin are described as glabrous. For our early ancestors hair was vital for protection and for insulation. Now, as we have evolved into relatively hair-free beings, hair is much more about display, representation of cultural norms and sexual attraction. Hair does still offer some element of insulation and protection for the scalp, but clothing now provides most of the warmth and protection for the body.

Hair growth

Hair growth occurs in three phases. The active growth phase, known as anagen, is usually about 3 years for head hair (although it can be up to 9 years – see later). This allows the hair on the head to grow to some considerable length; pubic and eyebrow hair have shorter growth phases (usually around a month). This means they fall out before they get very long. The resting phase, known as catagen, is when the hair sits in the follicle but is not actively growing and is followed by telogen when the hair is shed. It is normal for an individual to shed 70–80 hairs a day. When removing terminal hairs by plucking or waxing, the phase that the hair is in will effect, how hard the hair is to remove and how long it will take to grow back. Thus if the hair is

in catagen or telogen it will come out relatively easily, but the growth phase starts again relatively quickly. If the hair is plucked during anagen, it is harder to remove but will take longer to grow back.

Types of hair

There are three different types of hair, terminal, vellus and lanugo. Lanugo hairs are present *in utero* but are shed in early childhood. Vellus hairs are the fine downy hairs that cover most of the body, particularly in women and children. Terminal hairs are generally much coarser and thicker and include those which cover the scalp, beard, chest hair and pubic areas. The quantity and texture of hair is determined largely by genetic make-up, but hormonal changes can also influence hair growth and hair loss.

Terminal hair shape varies depending on the ethnic origin of an individual. In terms of hair type, three ethnic groups can be considered: black (Afro-Caribbean), Caucasian and Indo-Chinese.

- *Afro-Caribbean*: when cut in cross-section, the hair is thin and a flattish oval in shape. The hair is twisted and curly causing it to become easily tangled and broken. The pigments within black hair are a combination of black and red, with around 40% of black women having near black hair, 50% black/brown hair and around 10% having auburn shades.
- *Caucasian*: a cross-section shows a slightly fatter oval shape than for black hair, generally being fine textured and varying from wavy to straight. It is the only ethnic group with a wide variety of pigment varying from white blonde to reds to black.
- *Indo-Chinese*: the cross-section shows an almost perfectly round shape and the hair is generally straight or very slightly wavy. It is a very strong type of hair with a great capacity for growth. The anagen phase can be twice as long as that of other hair types and the shedding rates less. This means that head hair can grow to the waist or below (Kingsley, 2003).

The basic structure of the hair is the same regardless of ethnic variations. It starts growth

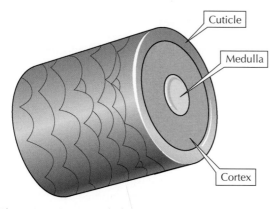

Figure 2.6   Structure of a hair. (Source: Reprinted from Graham-Brown and Burns, 2006.)

from the dermal papilla at the base of the hair shaft, where the keratinocytes divide, differentiate and gradually keratinise as the hair grows up the hair follicle. The hair bulb also contains melanocytes which will determine the pigment of the hair. Each hair consists of three distinct layers (Figure 2.6). The medulla running through the centre of the hair shaft consists of cells in which air is incorporated. The cortex is similar to the prickle cell layer of the skin, although keratinisation is further advanced. This is where the colour of the hair lies. The outer layer, or cuticle, is made up of overlapping keratinised plates, like tiles on a roof. The cuticle helps individual strands of hair to stay separate and not to matt together. Where the hair is subject to the greatest abrasion (at the tip), the cuticle may wear away allowing the keratin fibrils of the cortex and medulla to frizz out leading to split ends. Conditioners smooth the roughened surface of the cuticle helping the hair to look shinier. The structure of the hair is very strong and can stretch to up to 30% of its length.

Sebaceous glands

Each hair follicle has a sebaceous gland part way along its length. Sebaceous glands are simple branched alveolar glands which are found all over the body, except on the palms and soles. They are larger on the face, neck and upper chest and smaller on the limbs and trunk. The gland releases sebum onto the hair surface, thus lubricating it and the skin surface. The central cells of the alveoli accumulate oily lipids until they become so engorged that they burst, the gland is thus made up of cells that must 'die' as they release their secretory product. The cells are replaced by underlying cells.

Sebaceous glands are stimulated by hormones, particularly androgens, and therefore are key to the development of acne (see Chapter 10).

Attached to the hair follicle is a bundle of muscle called the arrector pili muscle. These contract when an individual is cold and pull the hair into an upright position. This causes goosebumps and is one of the body's ways of conserving heat. The erect hair traps warm air next to the skin surface. This biological phenomenon was much more effective when humans were hairier, now body hair is sparse and fine, this mechanism for keeping warm is relatively ineffective.

Nails

Nails provide protection for the delicate digital ends and make fine motor operations of the fingers more effective. Although humans do not rely on the use of their nails for scratching and grooming (as other primates do), they remain a useful tool for scratching when the skin is itchy!

Like the hair follicle, the nail bed and nail fold are formed from an invagination of the epidermis. Cell division (mitosis) occurs in the nail matrix and at the proximal end of the nail; new cells are then added to the nail plate. The process of growth is complex ensuring that the nail grows flat rather than as a claw (primates being the only other mammal with nails rather than claws) (Figure 2.7). Nails allow humans and primates to make much more delicate manoeuvres with their fingers. In humans, fingernails and toenails grow through the same mechanism; however, fingernails grow at the rate of 1 mm per week and toenails more slowly. The nail bed is highly vascularised and thus pink in colour. The 'half moon' white area that occurs just above the cuticle (the lunule) appears paler because a thicker basal layer obscures the dermal blood vessels from view. The shape and colour of the nail can be adversely affected by

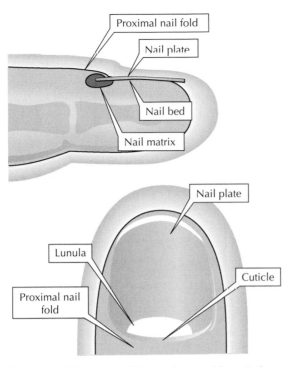

Figure 2.7 Nail structure. (Source: Reprinted from Graham Brown and Burns, 2006.)

Table 2.2 Nail anatomy.

Nail part	Definition
Nail bed	The skin on which the nail plate rests
Nail plate	The clear keratinised part of the nail
Root	Proximal end of the nail, underlying the nail fold
Body	Portion of the nail plate overlying the nail bed
Free edge	Portion of the nail plate that extends beyond the end of the finger
Hyponychium	The space beneath the free edge of the nail plate
Nail fold	The fold of skin around the margins of the nail plate
Eponychium	Dead epidermis that covers the proximal end of the nail: cuticle
Nail matrix	The growth zone of the proximal end of the nail. This corresponds to the stratum basale of the epidermis
Lunule	White crescent at the base of the nail

Source: Adapted from Saladin (2001).

trauma or inflammation. Table 2.2 gives further details on nail anatomy.

Sweat glands

It is estimated that there are around 2.6 million sweat glands in the skin, women have more than men but those in men are more active. There are two different types of sweat glands, eccrine and apocrine.

Eccrine sweat glands

Eccrine sweat glands are widely distributed across the skin surface, although concentrated in palms, soles, forehead and axillae. This type of sweat gland excretes a mildly salty fluid (99% water with small amounts of salts, ammonia, urea and uric acid) directly onto the surface of the skin when the skin surface temperature rises above 35°C (Hinchcliffe *et al.*, 1999). The main purpose of this is to encourage heat loss. The evaporation of 1 L of sweat requires 580 kcal (2,400 KJ) of energy. Heat provides this energy, thus using it up and cooling the skin. Sweat will not evaporate in a very humid climate as the atmosphere is already laden with water.

About 400–500 mL of fluid is lost per day mostly through sweat, although a small amount directly through the surface of the skin, lungs and bucal mucosa, known as insensible water loss. If the ambient temperature is particularly hot or the person is exercising, fluid loss may rise to as much as 12 L. Sweating from eccrine glands is also stimulated by fear particularly on the palms and soles; this phenomenon forms the basis of lie detector tests. Hot, spicy foods may also induce sweating, known as gustatory sweating.

Apocrine sweat glands

Apocrine sweat glands open into the hair follicle and are found mainly around the nipples, scalp in the groin and axillae. They are inactive in childhood, being activated during puberty under the influence of androgens.

The glands are affected by the sympathetic nervous system, during times of stress, pain or sexual arousal. The secretion is basically the same as eccrine sweat with the addition of proteins and fatty substances which make a thicker, stickier substance. Although this is odourless, it is vulnerable to the activities of bacteria found on the skin, and it is this action that makes the musty smell commonly known as body odour. It is thought that apocrine sweat is the human equivalent of a scent gland which, whilst vital for other animals, seems to have become less so for humans.

Mammary glands that produce breast milk and ceruminous glands that produce ear wax in the ear canal are modified apocrine glands.

Functions of the skin

The skin is a multifunction organ. Its structure is uniquely designed to enable it to undertake each of these functions and cope with a range of environments.

Barrier function

The skin is an incredibly effective barrier to the outside world – at its simplest, it keeps the outside world out and the inside in – quite literally it holds the human body together. However, the skin is not just a simple inert envelope; the barrier it provides is complex and offers physical, chemical and immunological protection.

Physical protection

The analogy that is most commonly used to describe the physical barrier properties of the skin is that of a brick wall. In this instance, the layer that really is of interest is the horny layer of the epidermis. Corneocytes form the top layer of skin, these heavily keratinised cells need to be well-hydrated to form a complete barrier – they are the bricks in the wall. These bricks are 'cemented' with lipids. As the skin is constantly shedding, it is physically difficult for pathogenic organisms to take hold.

When intact, this brick wall is very effective at keeping out allergens and pathogens. If the barrier function is compromised (and it only has to be relatively mildly damaged through an excoriation), pathogens or allergens can penetrate leading to an infection or an allergic reaction. Moving in the opposite direction, a break in the barrier also allows moisture and lipid to be lost. A more severe break in the skin barrier, for example following a burn, can be catastrophic, indeed life threatening, as the body struggles to cope with the challenge of extensive infection and imbalanced homeostasis.

Chemical protection

The surface of the skin is covered in commensal organisms. These 'friendly' bacteria and fungi live in harmony with humans and indeed offer a level of protection from pathogenic or disease-causing organisms. The commensals have evolved to be able to thrive in the slightly acidic environment of the skin surface (pH of 4.5–6).

Skin cells are provided with inbuilt protection from UV radiation by melanin. In the upper layers of the epidermis, melanin is scattered throughout the cells providing protection, whilst in the lower layers the protection is specifically targeted as the melanin granules form 'umbrellas' over the nuclei of the basal and spinous cells.

Physical and chemical barriers form part of the body's innate defence system.

Immunological surveillance

Understanding of the role that the skin plays within the immune system is ever increasing. The role of specialised cells such as Langerhans cells has already been discussed. However, other cells also have a role within immunological surveillance. For example, epidermal keratinocytes can, in certain circumstances, express immunological markers on their surface and produce cytokines which are known as signalling molecules (examples include immunomodulating agents such as interleukins) which in turn induce an inflammatory response.

Immunity is distinguished from innate non-specific resistance in two ways. Firstly, antigens are recognised and produce a specific response, which also involves distinguishing non-self molecules. Secondly, the body remembers previous encounters with antigens so that subsequent encounters prompt more rapid and vigorous responses. Generally the immune system works to protect the body from unwanted visitors (pathogens and allergens); however, if an individual is genetically predisposed to certain chronic skin conditions, the immune system can be triggered to produce responses that are not desired. For example, in psoriasis, T-cells are activated by the production of inflammatory mediators leading to hyperproliferation of skin cells and inflammation (see Chapter 9).

Storage

The skin acts as an organ of energy storage which can be drawn upon under physically challenging situations such as starvation and dehydration. The layer of fat acts as a reserve which can be metabolised to produce energy. This process involves fats being broken down into fatty acids which are in turn broken down into acetyl CoA which can feed directly into the Krebs cycle to produce energy.

Babies have a specialised type of fat known as brown fat which yields energy more easily than other types of fat. They also have a higher proportion of their body weight given over to fat than adults. This is important as babies have a large surface area relative to their weight and are unable to shiver; this makes them vulnerable to heat loss. Breakdown of this brown fat produces the energy required to stay warm. As a child develops muscular control and can use this muscular activity to generate warmth, the importance of the brown fat lessens. Generally adults do not have brown fat.

Temperature regulation

The skin is the organ of temperature regulation. Whilst thermoregulation (the maintenance of core body temperature at 37°C) is under the control of the hypothalamus, the receptors for temperature are found in the skin and likewise it is the structures within the skin that allow for heat conservation or heat loss. The mechanism involves stimulation of peripheral temperature receptors in the skin, which in turn affect the hypothalamus and the sympathetic nervous system which acts directly on the peripheral blood vessels in the skin. Vasoconstriction of the peripheral vasculature leads to heat conservation and vasodilation to heat loss.

Heat loss

There are four different mechanisms by which heat can be lost from the skin.

Radiation

Describes the movement of heat directly through the air and this can be a mechanism for heat loss if the skin is warmer than the surrounding air. However, on a sunny day the skin can be directly warmed by the sun's rays through radiation.

Convection

If there is movement in the air or of the body, hot air will rise and be replaced by cooler air. This mechanism is hampered by the presence of clothes (which will therefore keep a body warm) and facilitated by a fan.

Conduction

This simply describes the movement of heat through an object that the body comes into contact with.

Evaporation

When eccrine sweat is excreted onto the skin, the heat from the skin is used to evaporate it away into the atmosphere. The net effect is to cool the surface of the skin (see section on sweat glands for more details).

Sensation

Touch, a social phenomenon

The skin is the organ of physical sensation; it allows humans to experience the pleasure of sensual touch and the unpleasantness of pain. Heat, cold and pressure are all experienced through the skin. The skin is rich in sensory nerve endings, particularly the fingers, toes and lips. Touch is not only a physical experience but also a personal and social phenomenon; it is the way we connect physically to other humans and the way that we express a vast range of human experiences including power, love, abuse and caring. (Classen, 2005) describes touch as:

> ...a fundamental medium for the expression, experience and contestation of social value and hierarchy. The culture of touch involves all of culture. (Classen, 2005, p. 1)

Different cultures have unique ways of describing their experience of how the skin interacts with the world around it. The Cashinuahua tribe of Eastern Peru describes 'skin knowledge' as the knowledge of the world one acquires through the skin, through the feel of the sun, the wind, the rain and the forest. This allows them to find their way through the jungle and to locate the animals that they hunt for.

Western culture would advocate close contact between mother and baby as vital for bonding; however, this has not always been the case. In the late 19th and early 20th century, Dr L.E Holt wrote that babies should not be rocked and only kissed infrequently on the forehead. Dr Watson wrote in his 1928 book entitled *Psychological care of infant and child*:

> Mothers just don't know, when they kiss their children and pick them up and rock them, caress them and jiggle them upon their knee, that they are slowly building up a human being totally unable to cope with the world it must later live in (p. 42)

Thus, attitudes towards touch are not just related to cultural norms but also to time.

Sensation as a physical experience
The skin is part of the sensory nervous system and as such contains a number of mechanisms for sensation including touch, pressure, vibration, itch and tickle.

Touch
Touch sensation can either be crude or fine. Crude implies that there is knowledge that the skin has been touched but the exact location and size of stimulus may not be determined. Fine touch means that the exact part of the body, shape, size, texture and source of the stimuli can be distinguished.

Fine touch is experienced through the stimulation of Meissner's corpuscles which are found in hairless skin. They are an egg-shaped mass of dendrites enclosed in a capsule of connective tissue. These are rapid acting and generate nerve impulses at the beginning of a touch. They are abundant in fingertips, hands, eyelids, tip of the tongue, lips, nipples, soles, clitoris and the tip of the penis. Crude touch is experienced through the stimulation of hair-root plexuses. Again this produces a rapid response when movement on the surface of the skin which disturbs hairs stimulates free nerve endings wrapped around hair follicles.

Slowly adapting touch receptors are generally more sensitive to pressure, vibration and stretching. Type I receptors (Merkel discs) are saucer-shaped free nerve endings that contact Merkel cells in the epidermis. They are particularly prevalent in fingertips, hands, lips and external genitalia. Type II (Ruffini corpuscles) are elongated, encapsulated receptors found deep in the dermis (particularly in hands and soles) and in ligaments and tendons; they are sensitive to stretching.

Itch
Cutaneous itch is caused by the stimulation of free nerve endings of C fibres. These unmyelinated C fibres transmit impulses relatively slowly and although functionally they are the same as those that transmit pain, functionally they are distinct. There are a number of mediators which lead to the stimulation of these fibres and the consequent sensation of itch. These include histamine, cytokines, neuropeptides and prostaglandins.

Tickle is a curious sensation as it only occurs when an individual is touched by someone else. It is thought to be mediated by free nerve endings and lamellated corpuscles.

Pain

Whilst pain is generally considered an unpleasant experience, its biological functions are firstly to help protect us from noxious substances or dangerous situations and to help pinpoint an underlying cause of disease.

Nociceptors are free nerve endings which are found all over the body, except in the brain. Tissue irritation or injury releases chemicals such as potassium, prostaglandins and kinins, all of which can stimulate nociceptors. The pain may continue long after the stimulus is removed as the pain-stimulating chemicals may persist and the nociceptors exhibit very little adaptation.

Pain may be experienced as fast or slow pain, the sensation being determined by the type of fibres transmitting the pain impulses. Perception of fast pain occurs 0.1 seconds after the stimulus as impulses are sent along medium-diameter myelinated A fibres. This generates an acute, sharp, pricking pain. Generally fast pain is not felt in deeper tissues of the body. Slow pain begins a second or more after the stimuli has been applied and builds up in intensity over seconds or minutes. The impulses are transmitted by small-diameter unmyelinated A fibres and generate a more chronic, throbbing, burning or aching sensation. Pain can occur in skin, deeper tissues and internal organs.

Biochemical reactions in the skin

The most commonly reported biochemical function of the skin is the synthesis of vitamin D. This occurs mainly in the prickle and basal layers where UV light stimulates the conversion of 7-dehydrocholesterol to vitamin D3. Vitamin D is essential for the skeletal development as it controls the balance of calcium and phosphorous absorbed through the small intestine and mobilised from the bone. The amount of melanin in the skin affects the exposure time required to synthesise the vitamin; black skin requires 12 times the length of exposure to UVB than white skin. This is probably due to the fact that only 2–5% of UVB penetrates the epidermis in black skin whereas in white skin this is 20–30%.

Androgen metabolism also occurs in the skin; testosterone is converted to 5α-dihydrotestosterone by the enzyme 5α reductase.

Psychosocial

The skin is the organ of display, it is how humans present themselves to the world, and often judgements are made (rightly or wrongly) on appearance. The skin is often adorned in a multitude of ways in order to produce social signals of cultural significance. This may be through permanent marks such as tattooing, piercing and scarification or temporary decoration such as make-up and jewellery. The amount of skin that is displayed allows others to make judgements about lifestyle choices or religious convictions. Often one can determine racial groupings by the colour of the skin or hair, and age may be guessed by noting wrinkles, skin tone and hair colour. Of course, all judgements made on the basis of appearance may be wildly wrong, but this does not stop people making them!

In an appearance-based society, to appear 'abnormal' can have an enormous impact on an individual's psychological well-being. The feeling of being unwelcome or discriminated against because of the skin is a potentially devastating experience that means individuals have a range of negative responses including withdrawal from society, developing low self-esteem, having mental health problems or failing to achieve their full potential.

The profound almost instinctive distaste often engendered by skin disease, which more-often-than-not is totally out of proportion to its objective manifestation, may be related to a deeply held, almost primeval fear of contagious infection or infestation. It is clear through historic documents, including the Bible, that those with signs of disease through the skin were outcast, leprosy being the prime example of this. It is thought that many of those who were labelled as lepers actually had other skin diseases such as psoriasis. As communities who did not have the benefit of understanding of the modes of disease transmission, an outward sign such as a diseased skin was an obvious thing to 'blame'. These issues will be examined in more detail in Chapter 6.

In summary, our skin and hair can reflect both our physical and mental well-being. A 'bad hair day' can mean a day where everything seems to go wrong and where a person feels unprepossessing and incapable. Conversely, a new hair style can boost confidence and make an individual feel younger and more confident. General health will also affect the health of the skin, when someone is relaxed and healthy their skin is more likely to 'glow'. Good skin health not only means that the physical attributes of the skin are functioning well, but also that an individual feels psychologically comfortable in his/her own skin.

Skin and ageing

The skin structure and function changes throughout the human lifespan. The changes described in this section should be seen as inevitable biological processes, although it may be possible to slow down ageing, no one has yet worked out how to stop it happening altogether! Table 2.3 shows some terms which may be used to describe skin growth and skin death.

Table 2.3   Skin growth and skin death.

Skin death	Definition
Atrophy	Skin shrinking or reducing due to loss of cells either in size or number. This can be either through lack of use (disuse atrophy) or old age (senile atrophy)
Necrosis	Premature, pathological death of tissue caused by trauma, infections or toxins
Gangrene	Tissue necrosis resulting from insufficient blood supply
Skin growth	
Hyperplasia	Multiplication of cells
Hypertrophy	Enlargement of existing cells
Neoplasia	Tumour composed of abnormal non-functional tissue

Pre-birth

During embryogenesis, layers of cells known as germ cells are formed. Skin will eventually be formed by the cells in two of these layers; the ectoderm forming (amongst other structures) the epidermis and the mesoderm the dermis.

The baby is protected *in utero* by a thick layer of vernix caseosa, a very effective greasy substance which protects the infant's skin from the watery environment of the amniotic fluid. The words vernix caseosa come from a Latin derivation, *vernix*, meaning 'varnish' and caseosa 'cheesy'. The vernix is composed of sebum, which is secreted from the baby's sebaceous glands from around 20 weeks, and skin cells as they desquamate. Further protection is provided by the fine, downy hair known as lanugo. This falls out soon after birth to be replaced with vellus and terminal hairs.

At birth

If a baby is born after its due date, the vernix caseosa would have mostly gone which means the skin tends to be dry and peeling as it has not been effectively protected in the watery environment of the womb. If a baby is born prematurely, its skin will be more vulnerable as it would not have had chance to mature completely, making it more prone to infection and trauma. This being said, the skin of a newborn is generally quite vulnerable due to the immaturity of the skin barrier. It has not developed a complete flora and fauna, so does not have full protection of the commensal bacteria nor has it developed the acid mantle. For the first 6 weeks of life, it is recommended that water alone is used to cleanse the skin. Subsequently, any products that are used should have minimal levels of perfume and colourants in them. Bland emollients (see Chapter 5) may be helpful if a baby's skin gets dry.

Babies in neonatal units have particularly vulnerable skin. A survey carried out at the University of Southampton suggests that despite this fact, many neonates have their skin overly cleansed and frequently damaged with tape and dressings (Rapley, 2007).

Post-birth/early months

There are a number of skin changes in the early months which can be considered 'normal' that do not usually require any intervention except reassurance.

Milia

These are tiny white spots which appear over the nose and face of babies; they are common. Their formation is probably related to the stimulus of the sebaceous glands which become temporarily blocked. There is no need to squeeze them as they will resolve of their own accord. The sebaceous glands become small and inactive soon after birth and as they do the milia resolve. The sebaceous glands remain inactive until puberty.

Mongolian blue spot

These are also relatively common in babies of Indo-Asian or Afro-Caribbean origin and occur in over 90% of children of Mongolian extraction. They consist of a blue grey patch on the skin which often occurs on the sacrum but can occur anywhere on the body. The skin surface is normal. The cause is thought to be elongated melanocyte precursor cells in the dermis. They can be mistaken as trauma from non-accidental injury, so should be documented in the notes. For most children these patches will fade as they get older, some however will persist into adulthood.

Benign acquired melanocytic lesions

Both freckles and lentigo can be described as benign acquired melanocytic lesions. Freckles are areas of skin where melanocytes are seen to be more active than in neighbouring areas. As a result, small (less than 5 mm in diameter), flat areas of pigmentation appear, generally scattered over the face, neck and arms, appearing in a variety of shades depending on the individual and the time of the year (darker in summer). Lentigo (plural being lentigenes) are also flat and a similar variety of sizes as the freckles, but they do not vary with sun exposure. Unlike freckles where there is no increase in the number of melanocytes, in lentigo there are.

Congenital melanocytic naevi

These lesions may be small or giant and occur in approximately 1% of births. The surface of the lesion may be smooth or rough and warty; there may be one or more hair follicles in the lesion. Giant congenital melanocytic naevi (those that cover a large area of the body and may be accompanied by thousands of smaller lesions) are associated with malignant melanomas and parents will need careful counselling about what action to take. Sometimes, the lesions are too large to consider surgical excision and grafting.

Vascular naevi

Vascular naevi are caused by dilated and tortuous, but otherwise normal blood vessels. Where capillary vessels are involved, a superficial or deep type may be described.

The superficial capillary naevi are caused by abnormal dilated vessels in the superficial dermis leading to salmon-coloured patches often on the face that will fade quite quickly. They are relatively common, occurring in approximately 50% of all neonates. The deeper capillary naevi are known as 'port wine stains', and because the vascular abnormality extends deeper into the dermis, these do not resolve and may even extend throughout life. The colour of the patches varies from pale pinkish red to dark purple; the colours will deepen with age. These changes can be associated with intracranial vascular changes and neurological pathology, so any child with a facial port wine stain should be investigated.

Arterial naevi

Otherwise known as superficial angiomatous naevi or strawberry birth marks, these occur in around 10% of children by the age of 1. Commonly, they start growing within a few days to a few weeks of birth and are usually relatively soft and irregular in outline. Sometimes there is a deeper component to these naevi where the subcutis is involved, in these instances the changes may lead to a distortion of normal anatomy. Growth of the lesion usually stops at around 6 months and resolution is usually spontaneous and complete, although if the lesion was particularly large, lose skin or atrophy may be left. The following rule of thumb is usually quite accurate:

> Forty percent are gone by the age of 4 years; 50% by 5 years; 60% by 6 years; 70% by 7 years; 80% by 8 years and 90% by 9 years. (Graham-Brown and Bourke, 1998).

If the lesion interferes with feeding, breathing or sight, treatment may be recommended. For smaller areas, this is likely to be a steroid injection, but other options may be necessary including laser therapy. These types of naevi usually occur on the head, neck, buttocks or perineal areas. If they are associated with the lower back, sacrum or buttocks, a scan is usually recommended to exclude problems of tethering of the spinal cord.

Physiological jaundice (icterus neonatorum)

At about 2 days of age, parents may notice that their newborn is a yellowish colour. This is quite normal and results from the breakdown of the excess red blood cells that the child needed when they were *in utero*. As the child breaths following delivery, it no longer has any need of these red blood cells, so they break down leading to high serum bilirubin levels and the consequent yellow colour. This type of jaundice should not be confused with pathologic jaundice which occurs within 24 hours of birth and may be indicative of ABO or rhesus incompatibilities.

Puberty

Puberty is the time at which reproductive organs become functionally active. In both males and females, it is accompanied by the development of the secondary sexual characteristics including the growth of pubic hair and axillary hair and facial hair in boys. These changes are due to a large increase in the secretion of gonadal sex hormones. Androgens have a powerful effect on the hair follicle stimulating the sebaceous gland that has lain dormant since shortly after birth. This leads to an increased production of sebum causing teenage skin and hair to be greasier than prior to puberty. For some, this change in the sebaceous gland functioning will mean the appearance of acne. Most teenagers experience comedones, others will experience more extreme acne with pustule or even nodule formation. Chapter 10 discusses acne in greater depth. The apocrine glands are also stimulated leading to the experience of body odour for the first time.

Teenage years are also a time when young adults start to take a real interest in their appearance and is a good time to encourage healthy skin behaviour, including protection from UV radiation (see Chapter 4).

Pregnancy

Hormonal changes throughout the menstrual cycle can influence the skin and hair for some women. It is during the second half of the menstrual cycle, following ovulation when the progesterone levels peak, that women notice changes in their skin and those with a skin condition can experience an exacerbation.

During pregnancy some specific changes do occur, specifically a deepening of the normal pigmentation of the nipple, the areola, the genital area and the midline of the abdominal wall. Following delivery this pigmentation will fade, but seldom back to the usual colour. For a proportion of women (around 70%), the second half of pregnancy sees chloasmal pigmentation which is characterised by an irregular, sharply marginated area of pigmentation which develops in a symmetrical pattern over the cheeks and/or forehead. It is also common for women to see their moles darken whilst pregnant and it is also possible for new moles to appear. It is advisable for pregnant women to take additional precautions when going out into the sun; they should wear a hat and use a high factor sunscreen.

Vascular changes mean that women notice flushing of the palms of the hands and spider naevi appear on the face, upper trunk and arms. Oedema of the lower legs and increased appearance of varicose veins occur due to a rise in venous pressure caused by the increased pressure of the growing foetus impeding venous return. Dermal changes include stretch marks which occur due to weakened tensile strength of dermal fibres (caused by the increase corticosteroid output) and the stretching of the skin due to the growing foetus. A study carried out in Southern India showed that nearly 80% of women experienced stretch marks following pregnancy (Kumari *et al.*, 2007). Marks appear as raised reddish/purple lines during and just after pregnancy, which fade to more skin-coloured slightly depressed shiny lines. Avoiding stretch marks during pregnancy may be down to genetic good fortune; however, the following strategies may help decrease the likelihood of stretch marks or at least their severity:

- Gradual and moderate weight gain during pregnancy (a woman with a normal body mass index should aim to gain between 25 and 35 lbs during pregnancy.);
- Gentle exercise;
- A Cochrane review considered studies that looked at topical products which might alleviate stretch marks. The review highlights one product containing *Centella asiatica* extract, alpha tocopherol and collagen–elastin hydrolysates, which when compared to a placebo was associated with women developing fewer stretch marks. A second study suggested that a product containing tocopherol, panthenol, hyaluronic acid, elastin and menthol was associated with women developing fewer stretch marks. But this study did not include a control and the improvements may have been associated with the massage (Young and Jewell, 1996).

Old age

As humans get older, the skin becomes thinner, less elastic, drier and more finely wrinkled. The degree to which the skin becomes visibly aged is related largely to genetics and photo-ageing. In other words, wrinkle formation is determined by the traits inherited from parents and the extent to which someone has exposed themselves to sunshine over their lifetime. Intrinsic ageing describes the natural biological processes which it is not possible to control and extrinsic ageing the impact that the environment and exposure to it has on the skin. It is possible to get a sense of the impact of extrinsic factors by comparing the skin of a sun-exposed and non-sun-exposed site. In an elderly person, particularly, there is a marked difference between the texture and colouring, the former being much smoother and less wrinkled.

The changes highlighted in Table 2.4 mean that older skin is increasingly sensitive and less able to cope with external stressors on the skin. Thus the skin has less innate ability to cope with external agents such as perfumes in topical products, extremes of temperature, urine and faeces. These factors are discussed further in Chapter 4.

Overexposure to UV radiation is responsible not only for the effects of ageing but also more worryingly for skin cancers. Basal and squamous cell carcinomas are both closely associated with prolonged sun exposure and whilst they are rarely life threatening, they can be locally destructive and need to be properly diagnosed and treated. Malignant melanomas are also associated with sun exposure, although burning is generally thought to be a high risk factor. Skin malignancies are discussed later in Chapter 11.

Table 2.4 Skin changes caused by ageing.

Changes in the skin	Consequence
Epidermal turnover slows	Thinner skin
Less effective barrier function	More prone to infection/dryness
Less flexible and tough collagen	More prone to wrinkles and sheering
Less evenly distributed melanin	More prone to sun damage
Fewer sweat glands	Less effective temperature control
Less sebum production	Increased skin dryness

Conclusion

The skin provides humans with a flexible and dynamic outer layer. Its complex structure and function create a unique environment which protects the inner functionings of the body and provides an incredible interface with which to interact with the outside world. This chapter has formed the basis of a biological understanding of the skin; the rest of the book will look at what happens when skin fails, from a number of different perspectives.

References

Classen, C., Ed. (2005). *The Book of Touch*. Oxford: Berg Publishers.

Graham-Brown, R. and J.F. Bourke (1998). *Mosby's Color Atlas and Text of Dermatology*. London: Mosby.

Graham-Brown, R. and T. Burns (1996). *Lecture Notes in Dermatology* (7th edition). Oxford: Blackwell Science.

Graham-Brown, R. and T. Burns (2006). *Lecture Notes: Dermatology* (9th edition). Oxford: Blackwell Science.

Grimes, P., B. Edison, B.A. Green and R.H. Wildnauer *et al.* (2004). Evaluation of inherent differences between African American and white skin surface properties using subjective and objective measures. *Cutis*, 73(6): 392–396.

Hinchcliffe, S., S. Montague and R. Watson *et al.* (1999). *Physiology for Nursing Practice*. London: Bailiere Tindall.

Hoffjan, S. and S. Stemmler (2007). On the role of the epidermal differentiation complex in ichthyosis vulgaris, atopic dermatitis and psoriasis. *British Journal of Dermatology*, 157(3): 441–449.

Kingsley, P. (2003). *The Hair Bible: A Complete Guide to Health and Care*. London: Aurum Press Ltd.

Kumari, R., T. Jaisankar and D.M. Thappa *et al.* (2007). A clinical study of skin changes in pregnancy. *Indian Journal of Dermatology Venereology and Leprology*, 73(2): 141.

Lydyard, P., A. Whelan *et al.* (2000). *Instant Notes on Immunology*. Guildford: Bios.

Marieb, E. and K. Hoehn (2007). *Human Anatomy and Physiology* (7th edition). San Francisco: Pearson Benjamin Cummings.

Rapley, S. (2007). *A National Survey of Neonatal Skin Care Practices*. University of Southampton, School of Nursing and Midwifery. Unpublished report.

Roitt, E. and P. Delves (2001). *Roitt's Essential Immunology*. Oxford: Blackwell Science.

Saladin, K. (2001). *Anatomy and Physiology – The Unity of Form and Function*. New York: Magraw Hill.

Tortora, G. and B. Derrickson. (2006). *Principles of Anatomy and Physiology* (11th edition). New Jersey: John Wiley and Sons Inc.

Wesley, N. and H. Maibach (2003). Racial (ethnic) differences in skin properties: The objective data. *American Journal of Clinical Dermatology*, 4(12): 843–860.

Young, G. and D. Jewell (1996). Creams for preventing stretch marks in pregnancy. Cochrane Database of Systematic Reviews 1(Art No.CD000066).

Assessment and planning care

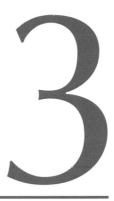

Steven J. Ersser

Introduction

This chapter will outline a systematic approach to assessment, introducing key concepts, their application and both physical and psychological assessment tools. Key principles and issues regarding the planning of care and relevant factors will be summarised. Details of the assessment process related to specific conditions in the relevant condition related chapters are provided. An overview will be given of common dermatological interventions and related psychological and educational interventions, although the detail will be discussed and signposted to the relevant chapters elsewhere. Finally, some issues of evaluation and the use of evaluative strategies are highlighted.

An effective plan of care requires careful assessment, the related planning of interventions and a systematic evaluation of its consequences. As the largest organ of the body, and the most visual, the skin is highly accessible to assessment, although the process is complex. The challenge of assessing abnormal changes in the skin is the sheer number of variation that may occur in site, colour, texture or surface features and the type of lesions that may be present. This chapter builds on the previous one on skin biology. Effective planning

of care requires an understanding of normal structure and function, its disruption by disease processes and the influence of psychosocial factors. The International Classification of Disease (ICD-10) index of dermatological diagnoses conveys the considerable and complex range of dermatological conditions, listing several hundred (www.who.int/classifications/icd/en/); however, the British Association of Dermatologists Diagnostic Index has over 4,000 preferred terms, with highly differentiated dermatological diagnoses. Many of these are rare in nature. The most common conditions fall into nine categories: skin cancer, atopic eczema, contact dermatitis and other eczemas, psoriasis, acne, blistering conditions, viral warts, other infective disorders, benign tumours and vascular lesions, leg ulceration (Williams, 1997). Indeed, a person may not have a skin disease *per se*, but a problem such as dryness (xerosis), which can be both uncomfortable and disruptive, leads to other problems with the skin barrier.

The purpose of assessment is to determine the nature of the clinical problem, its relative priority and the possible need for referral, given the nature and complexity of the person's condition. If the clinician does not have a diagnostic role then skill is required to accurately describe any changes observed that aid effective communication with clinical colleagues, and in particular to ensure appropriate referral. It is necessary to approach skin assessment in a systematic and holistic way, reviewing not only physical changes but also any psychological and social impact on the person and their family. This must also embrace a review of the impact on the quality of life of the person and their family. Assessment is not a one-off activity but rather an ongoing process, which involves monitoring changes in the patient's condition, their response to such changes and those related to treatment effects that are either therapeutic or adverse in nature.

Assessment

Normal skin

An assessment of a range of typical skin types is made by examining the person's tendency to burn and tan, using the following guide (Table 3.1). This is useful to assess and convey when appraising sun/ultraviolet (UV) damage, risk prior to phototherapy, or when providing a guide when engaging in health education related to UV exposure risk awareness. Key considerations in a person's skin typing include a person's pigmentation and erythema history and their genetic history (Leach *et al.*, 1996). Those with fair skin, which includes types 1 and 2, are more likely to develop skin cancer.

Table 3.1 Normal skin – skin typing.

Skin type	Characteristics
I	Always burns, never tans
II	Sometimes burn, rarely tan
III	Rarely burns, easily tans
IV	Never burns, always tans
V	Asian people
VI	Afro-Caribbean/Black African people

An assessment approach has been adopted that is suitable for use by a wide range of dermatology professionals and primary care staff based on the framework provided by Leach *et al.* (1996) and Ashton and Leppard (2005) to aid diagnosis, although it will also enable the clinician to describe and assess more precisely the condition of the skin, to aid effective team working, by enabling the referer to describe the lesion or rash in the absence of an established diagnosis.

Racial variations

Racial variations in skin are reflected in Table 3.1; these have implications for assessment, such as determining lesion colour and in the estimation of UV protection related to the presence of melanin (see Chapter 2). The most lightly pigmented (European, Chinese and Mexican) skin types have approximately half as much epidermal melanin as the most darkly pigmented (African and Indian) skin types. Research by Alaluf *et al.* (2002) highlights the analysis of melanosome size, which revealed a significant and progressive variation in size with ethnicity: African skin having the largest melanosomes followed in turn by Indian, Mexican, Chinese and European. Based on these findings, they propose that variation in skin pigmentation is strongly influenced by both the amount and the composition (or colour) of the melanin in the epidermis. Variation in melanosome size may also play a significant role. Further details of the relationship of skin typing to the person's genetic history and social heritage are given in Leach *et al.* (1996) and on racial influences on skin disease in Gawkrodger (1998).

Body surface area

As highlighted in the previous chapter, the skin covers an extensive surface area, covering approximately 2 m² of the body (Tortora and Derrickson, 2006). An important element of skin assessment is to determine the extent to which the body surface area (BSA) is affected by the disease and the nature and pattern of lesions. It is commonplace to use a simple body map *pro forma* in clinical practice to document the distribution of rashes and track their variations with

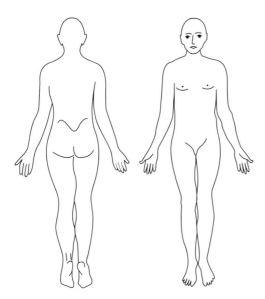

Figure 3.1 Body map.

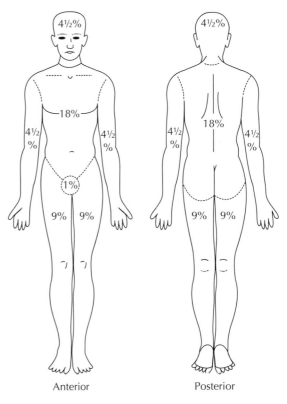

Anterior   Posterior

Figure 3.2 Rule of nines.

time. Figure 3.1 shows a body map depicting the front and back of the body, where the distribution of lesions (the affected area) may be crudely reflected by the degree of shading completed. It is possible to record on the body map the BSA affected, as a percentage.

The BSA can be estimated in various ways (Ashcroft *et al.*, 1999). The use of the flat hand palm provides an indicator of 1% of total BSA, whilst often accepted in clinical practice technical estimates put the area as up to 0.76% of the BSA. Another approach, the *rule of nines*, estimates different areas of the body comprising of 9% coverage for each of the following: head, anterior trunk (upper and lower each 9%), posterior trunk (upper and lower each 9%), each leg (anterior and posterior each 9%), each arm (4.5% each) and genitalia (1%) (see Figure 3.2). However, untrained observers tend to overestimate the extent of lesions, such as small psoriasis plaques. A challenge in dermatological assessment is securing sufficient consensus on the area of skin affected by disease, which is the variation between assessors or observers. High inter-observer variability is a problem of calculating BSA amongst clinicians (Ashcroft *et al.*, 1999).

Clinical monitoring of the course of disease over time may involve the documentation of the distribution of the affected area of skin; this is achieved by shading the affected area.

Increasingly, estimates of body surface are used in the assessment of disease severity measures, such as the PASI or Psoriasis Area Severity Index, which are discussed in more detail later in this chapter. Errors made in the estimation of BSA may well affect the severity score and, in turn, this may have implications for treatment decisions based on clinical protocols. For this reason, the estimation of BSA and the related calculation of severity measures require training and oversight within clinical teams, to ensure practitioner achieve a satisfactory standard of consistency and accuracy.

Understanding and describing lesions

With the very high number of dermatological diagnoses, it is particularly useful to be able to understand and systematically describe the different features and observable patterns of the underlying lesion or rash. This has the benefit of highlighting its observable features and enabling referral to other health professionals without a diagnosis. However, if undertaken effectively it should be an indication of a differential diagnosis for those with the appropriate training. Documenting the appearance of a lesion or rash can be challenging given their pattern of distribution and the sublety of their surface features. As such, it is necessary to gain familiarity with the typical types of lesions seen and rash patterns; these are introduced below. The process of describing lesions is therefore a precursor to making a full assessment and any subsequent differential diagnosis or the basis for referral. Guidance on how to describe skin lesions is summarised in Table 3.2.

Describing rashes

A rash is a change in the colour or texture of the skin and as such reflects the nature and pattern of a collection of individual lesions. A major consideration in dermatological assessment is to determine the specific patterns of such rashes and their specific characteristics as an aid to diagnosis. Some of the dimensions of

Table 3.2 Guidance on describing skin lesions.

1. Look first to identify:
   a. Sites involved: specify body area
   b. Number of lesions: single, multiple
   c. Distribution: includes symmetrical or not, localised or generalised
   d. Arrangement: includes discrete, coalescing, disseminated, linear, annular
2. Feel the lesions by:
   a. Surface palpation: with finger tips – smooth, uneven, rough
   b. Deep palpation: by squeezing between finger and thumb – soft, firm, hard
3. Describe a typical lesion using the following headings:
   a. Type of lesion (see Table 3.3)
   b. Surface features (see Table 3.3)
   c. Colour, including erythematous or non-erythematous
   d. Border of rash/lesion: well/poorly defined or an accentuated edge
   e. Size and shape of individual lesion: includes round, irregular, serpiginous

Source: Based on Ashton and Leppard (2005).

Table 3.3 A framework for skin assessment and lesion description.

1. Site

2. Erythematous, i.e. reddened skin (blanches on pressure) or **non-erythematous**

3. Acute (<2 weeks duration) or **chronic** (>2 weeks duration)

4. Surface features
   a. Normal/smooth (i.e. same as surrounding skin)
   b. Scaly
   c. Hyperkeratotic
   d. Warty
   e. Crust
   f. Exudate
   g. Excoriated

5. Type of lesion
   a. Flat: macules and patches
   b. Raised: papules, plaques and nodules
   c. Fluid-filled: vesicles, bullae and pustules
   d. Surface broken: erosions, ulcers and fissures

If non-erythematous describe the

6. Colour
   a. Due to blood: pink, purple, mauve
   b. Due to pigment: brown, black and blue
   c. Due to lack of blood/pigment: white
   d. Other colours: yellow, orange, grey

Source: Based on Ashton and Leppard (2005).

skin assessment are specified in Table 3.3. These include site, colour, acuity, surface features and type of lesion.

Owing to the wide-ranging nature of lesions, it is helpful to understand their different types. Therefore, specific definitions and clinical examples of particular surface features and lesions are now summarised in Table 3.4.

A useful distinction is also made of primary and secondary lesions. Primary lesions are caused directly by the disease process; this includes macules, papules, nodules, plaques, wheals, vesicles, bulla, pustules and cysts (Figures 3.3–3.8). Secondary lesions refer to the consequences of the disease process; these include scale, crust, fissures, lichenification, erosion, ulcers, excoriation, scar and atrophy (Johannsen, 1998). Further details of physical signs in dermatology, with excellent illustrative photographs, can be found in Lawrence and Cox (2002). Many skin

Table 3.4 Types and definitions: Surface features and lesions.

Types of lesion	
Normal	Smooth, the absence of other surface features
Scaly	Excess dead epidermal scales produced by shedding from the stratum corneum or abnormal keratinisation (e.g. erythrodermic psoriasis)
Hyperkeratotic	Increased keratinisation (cornification) of the epidermis, which appears clinically as thickened and rough skin or mucous membrane (e.g. foot psoriasis)
Warty	A wart-like lesion consisting of finger-like projections (e.g. filiform wart)
Crust	Dried exudate (comprised of dried serum, bacteria and possibly blood, mixed with epidermal debris – e.g. impetigo)
Excoriated	A superficial linear erosion caused by excessive scratching (e.g. atopic eczema)
Exudate	A leakage of fluid from blood vessels into nearby tissue (e.g. acute eczema)
Flat: macule	A flat lesion circumscribed area of altered skin colour <1 cm in diameter (e.g. vitiligo, solar lentigo)
Flat: patch	A flat lesion >1 cm in diameter (e.g. port wine stain)
Raised: papule	A raised lesion <1 cm in diameter (e.g. compound naevus)
Raised: plaque	A slightly raised flat-topped lesion >1 cm in diameter of surface skin (e.g. plaque psoriasis, pityriasis rosea)
Raised: nodule	A solid palpable mass that is larger than 1 cm whose greater part lies beneath the skin (e.g. erythema nodosum, basal cell carcinoma)
Fluid-filled: vesicle	A small lesion <5 mm in diameter, fluid-containing elevation (e.g. herpes simplex, eczema herpeticum)
Fluid-filled: bullae	A lesion >5 mm in diameter, fluid-containing elevation (e.g. bullous pemphigoid)
Fluid-filled: pustule	A lesion <1 cm filled with pus (e.g. acne vulgaris)
Due to broken surface: ulcer	Loss of epidermis and dermis (e.g. ducibitus [pressure] ulcer)
Due to broken surface: erosion	Loss of epidermis only (e.g. intertrigo – a rash in body folds)
Due to broken surface: fissure	Linear split in skin: foot psoriasis (e.g. a heel fissure)
Colour: due to blood	*Petechia* (pin head size) (e.g. Meningococcal disease – that do not disappear when pressure if applied) – they are purpuric lesions up to 2 mm across; *Purpura* (<2.5 mm): red, purple or orange/brown colour due to blood leaking from blood vessels (does not blanche under pressure) (e.g. drug eruption, allergic vasculitis); *Haematoma* (bruise); *Telangiectasia*: spider-like capillaries (e.g. due to chronic treatment with topical corticosteroids)
Colour: due to pigment	May be due to increase in melanin pigment following epidermal inflammation (e.g. lichen planus)
Colour: due to lack of blood/pigment	Depigmentation: complete loss of melanin (e.g. vitiligo) Hypopigmentation: partial melanin loss due to epidermal inflammation (e.g. eczema)
Colour: other	Yellow (e.g. xanthelasma)

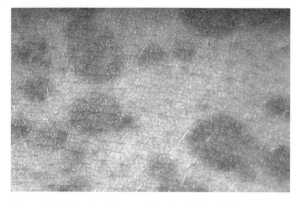

Figure 3.3   Macule. (Source: Reprinted from Graham-Brown and Burns, 2006.)

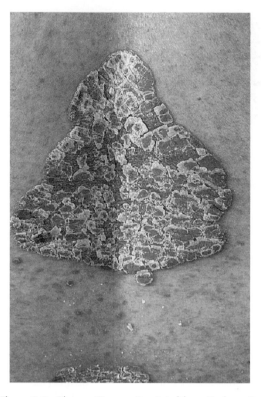

Figure 3.4   Plaque. (Source: Reprinted from Graham-Brown and Burns, 2006.)

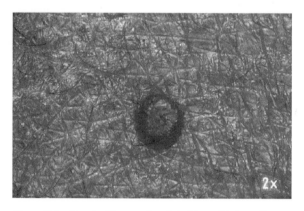

Figure 3.5   Papule. (Source: Reprinted from Graham-Brown and Burns, 2006.)

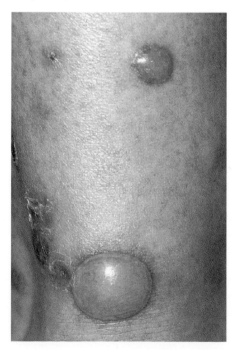

Figure 3.7   Bullae. (Source: Reprinted from Graham-Brown and Burns, 2006.)

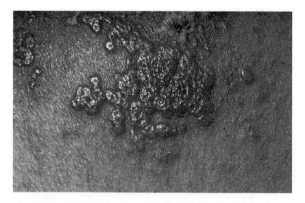

Figure 3.6   Vesicle. (Source: Reprinted from Graham-Brown and Burns, 2006.)

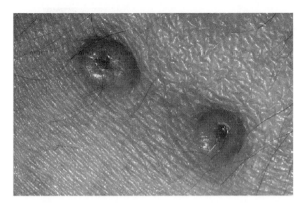

Figure 3.8 Nodule. (Source: Reprinted from Graham-Brown and Burns, 2006.)

diseases have a classic distribution which aids diagnosis; this is illustrated in Figure 3.9.

The process of skin assessment and history taking

Skin examination

The visual examination of the skin requires adequate light to ensure that the subtle changes in surface texture and colour are visible. Ideally natural sunlight is preferred, although additional artificial light may be used, such as a focused lamp with a magnification facility. Before examining for lesions, it is necessary to assess the general condition of the skin. One important general feature is skin turgor, which provides an indicator of hydration – by pulling the skin together in a gentle pinch-like movement and then examining the rapidity with which it returns to its original position – elasticity and moisture level. Good sites to test the skin turgor include the back of the hand and between the thumb and forefinger. A delayed period over which it returns to its normal shape may be an indication of dehydration. This is distinct but related to the elasticity of the skin, which is also dependant on its protein structure.

It is also necessary to assess the skin appendages such as nails and hair, which may provide an indication of generalised disease such as psoriasis or localised pathology. For example, nail infections (paronychia) can cause distortion and brittleness to finger and toenails and scalp psoriasis produces scalp scaling. Abnormalities in the appendages may also provide clues as to general health; for example clubbed nails may be an indication of poor nutritional status or disease such as pulmonary or inflammatory bowel disease (Fawcett *et al.*, 2004).

Palpation is important to distinguish some surface features such as warty, degree of scaling and the solidity of a lesion. Colour changes reflect the presence of factors such as the local microcirculation and inflammatory changes to the existence or absence of certain pigments, such as melanin (e.g. as in vitiligo). Other colour changes may be due to the presence of pigments such as haemosiderin, a brown-pigmented material found in skin affected by venous isease. To determine abnormal variations in colour change, it is often useful to examine the extremities such as the nails, lips and ear lobes, which can provide accessible indications of colour change. Technological aids may also enhance skin assessment; these are discussed later in this chapter.

History taking

History taking is more effective if undertaken systematically. Key areas to address are outlined in Table 3.5, with an illustration of two frameworks, which provide simple contrasting approaches to assessment and the use or not of a mnemonic reminder. These can be very useful when documenting a patient history, as say a nurse prescriber, as they prompt areas to explore and can aid clear reporting.

History taking is of course dependant on the ability of the patient to give an account of their medical history. A number of factors may limit this process, such as developmental stage, sensory impairment or mental health. Carers and parents can assist in the process. Patients may also be affected by their social confidence in disclosing information about their skin; for example they may be too embarrassed to discuss genital rashes or symptoms affecting sensitive areas or the effect of a skin condition on sexual activity. Aside to the use of empathy, receptiveness and sensitivity, continuity of contact with a health professional is desirable to

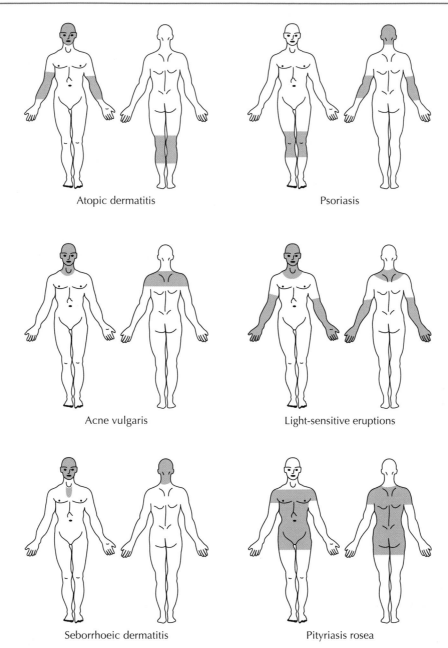

Atopic dermatitis

Psoriasis

Acne vulgaris

Light-sensitive eruptions

Seborrhoeic dermatitis

Pityriasis rosea

Figure 3.9 Classic lesion distribution in common skin disorders (Mackie, 2003).

develop a relationship and trust. This may lead to a greater willingness for patients to disclose sensitive information. The organisation of services may not permit such continuity, however, where possible it should be planned to ensure continuity of care; nurse-led clinics with agreed caseloads can assist this process. Consultation skills, within which history taking falls, are a neglected aspect of dermatology care and, indeed, they are an issue that has been given very limited attention in the speciality. Effective consultation skills provide a key

Table 3.5 History taking frameworks.

General	Oldcarts (mnemonic)
1. Presenting complaint	1. **O**nset
2. Previous history of presenting problem	2. **L**ocation
3. Previous medical history	3. **D**uration
4. Drug therapy	4. **C**haracter
5. Personal and social history	5. **A**ggravating factors
6. Systems review	6. **R**elieving factors
7. Overall appearance on examination	7. **T**iming
	8. **S**everity

basis upon which patients may be willing to disclose information relevant to their condition and how they are coping with it. Adequate attention needs to be given to the ability of the practitioner to create a helping or therapeutic relationship, including factors such as empathy, genuineness, self-awareness, ability to negotiate care with the patient, trust building and warmth (Ersser, 1997). This provides a key basis for effective support and education. Consultation skills are discussed further in Chapters 6 and 7.

Nursing diagnoses

Medical diagnoses are but one basis upon which health professionals may be guided to intervene in response to a health care need. Since 1973 work has been undertaken by the National Group for the Classification of Nursing Diagnosis in the USA to develop a system of nursing diagnoses. They refer to actual or potential health problems which nurses by virtue of their education and experience are capable and licensed to treat (Gordon, 1976). The benefit of this system is that it provides a method of framing patients' needs for nursing in ways other than by medical diagnosis alone, giving a partial

indication of the implications for nursing intervention to aid the process of care planning. It is also a reminder that nursing care of the skin is a fundamental consideration and transcends the scope of dermatological disease, by highlighting the range of causes of impaired skin integrity and skin at risk of impairment. The classification system has progressively developed taxonomy of nursing diagnoses since 1973. The development of nursing diagnoses is directed towards standardising nursing terminology; this process is now led by the North American Nursing Diagnosis Association (NANDA). This process aims to achieve the following outcomes (NANDA-International, 2007):

- name client responses to actual or potential health problems, life processes and wellness;
- documentation of nursing care;
- contribute to the development of informatics and information standards, ensuring the inclusion of nursing terminology in electronic health care records; and
- facilitates the study of the phenomena of concern to nurses to improve patient care.

Related developments have been led by the International Council of Nurses (ICN) to develop the International Classification for Nursing Practice (ICNP®).

The system used within the NANDA-I taxonomy utilises what are termed axes, which are defined as a dimension of the human response that is considered in the diagnostic process (NANDA-International, 2007). These include: (1) the diagnostic concept (fundamental root of the diagnostic statement), for example skin integrity, mucous membrane, bathing hygiene self-care; (2) the subject of diagnosis (individual, family and community); (3) judgement (impaired, ineffective); (4) location (e.g. skin); (5) age (infant, child, adult); (6) time (chronic, acute, intermittent); and (7) status of diagnosis (actual, risk, wellness, health promotion). Those nursing diagnoses directly related to skin care (NANDA-International, 2007) are summarised in Table 3.6.

Table 3.6   Nursing diagnoses directed related to skin health (NANDA-International, 2007).

Nursing diagnosis	Definition	Defining characteristics	Related or risk factors
Impaired skin integrity	Altered epidermis and/or dermis	Destruction of skin layers Disruption of skin surface Invasion of body structures	Related external factors: chemical substance, extremes of age, humidity, hyperthermia, hypothermia, mechanical factors (e.g. shearing forces, pressure, restraint), medications, moisture, physical immobilisation, radiation.
			Related internal factors: Change in fluid status, changes in pigmentation, changes in turgor, developmental factors, imbalanced nutritional status, immunological deficit, impaired circulation, impaired metabolic state, impaired sensation, skeletal prominence.
Risk for impaired skin integrity	At risk for skin being adversely altered		Related risk external factors: chemical substance, extremes of age, humidity, hyperthermia, hypothermia, mechanical factors, medications, moisture, physical immobilisation, radiation, secretions.
			Related risk internal factors: Change in fluid status, changes in pigmentation, changes in turgor, developmental factors, imbalanced nutritional status, immunological factors, impaired circulation, impaired metabolic state, impaired sensation, skeletal prominence, medication, psychogenic factors.

Of course, given the range of nursing diagnoses, generic needs for nursing may be manifested in a person with a skin health problem. For example, in supporting a child with severe atopic eczema, there may also be considerations regarding the following nursing diagnostic areas: for example, parenting, parental–child attachment, parental role conflict, caregiver role strain, infant feeding pattern, self-esteem, social isolation, anxiety and sleep deprivation – to name only some possible dimensions. Consideration of nursing diagnoses within a skin/dermatological nursing context may highlight a broader range of needs for nursing that may arise from a pathological problem (dermatological disease or other condition impacting on the skin) for which there may be a wide range of human responses and scope for nursing intervention through care planning.

Assessment tools

A variety of tools may be used to aid more effective assessment of the condition of the skin and patients responses to it; this includes physical assessment of lesions and clinical severity and psychological assessment. The former is discussed here and the latter (mainly disease-related quality of life measures) is examined in Chapter 6. Tools that examine the impact on the family, for example *The Dermatitis Family Impact Questionnaire* (Lawson *et al.*, 1998), reflect the wider psychosocial impact of chronic skin disease.

Severity tools

Tools to assess disease severity are important both in skin assessment and the evaluation of treatment effectiveness. Developed tools are now widely used for common chronic inflammatory skin conditions such as eczema and psoriasis. It is important to try to use valid and reliable standardised tools to ensure rigorous measurement. Valid tools measure what they are intended to measure and reliable tools ensure that the measure gained under the same conditions (such as degree of severity) is derived consistently. In addition, it is necessary to practise and develop skill in using some tools, for example the assessment of a *PASI* score to ensure reliability of assessment across observers and by the same clinician, under the similar clinical conditions. Details of commonly accepted valid tools are outlined in Table 3.7; copies of the PASI and SCORAD tools are reproduced in the Appendices 1 and 2 respectively. Acne severity is a core complex area for scoring; a recent review paper identified as many as 25 scales for the global assessment of acne, which indicates the lack of consensus on the issue and a gold standard (Lehmann *et al.*, 2002).

Table 3.7 Common chronic skin severity tools.

Tool	Disease parameters	Source material
PASI: Psoriasis Area Severity Index	This is the most widely used tool to assess psoriasis disease severity. The estimate is based on the percentage area affected of four body regions – head, trunk, upper and lower extremities – which is given a value of 0 (no psoriasis) to 6 (>90% present). The following clinical parameters are also used within a 0–4 scale – ranging from no symptoms to very marked symptoms, again for the different body areas. 1. Erythema (redness) 2. Induration (thickness) 3. Scaling (flaking or desquamation) 4. BSA affected A formula is used to calculate the PASI score. PASI scores: 1–10: mild to moderate; 11–20: moderate to severe and >20 severe; the theoretical maximum score being 72 (see Appendix 1).	Ashcroft *et al.* (1999); Ramsay and Lawrence (1991); Exum *et al.* (1996)
SCORAD Index	The European Task Force on Atopic Dermatitis has developed the SCORAD (SCORing AD) index to create a consensus on assessment methods for AD. 1. Objective items: a. Extent: Apply the rule of nines (see BSA given earlier) graded 0–100 on the front/back drawing. b. Intensity: consists of 6 items – erythema, oedema, excoriations, lichenification, oozing/crusts and dryness. Each item can be graded on a scale 0–3.	Kunz *et al.* (1997); Oranje *et al.* (2007); http://adserver.sante.univ-nantes.fr/Scorad.html

(continued)

Table 3.7   *(continued)*

Tool	Disease parameters	Source material

	2. Subjective items include:
	  a. Daily pruritus
	  b. Sleeplessness
	
	Both subjective items can be graded on a 10-cm visual analogue scale.
	
	SCORAD scores: The maximum SCORAD score is 103. The maximum subjective score is 20. The maximum objective SCORAD score is 83 (plus an additional 10 bonus points). Bonus points are given for severe disfiguring eczema (on face and hands). Mild <25, mild to moderate 25–50 and severe >50. There are criticisms of the tool including that it can be time consuming in clinical practice and that it has a bias for use with children (see Appendix 2).	

(Revised) Leeds Acne Score (1998)	Pictorial grading system – a photographic assessment system with severity criteria as: 1. Extent of inflammation 2. Range and size of inflamed lesions 3. Associated erythema Overall assessment is based predominantly on the number of *inflamed* lesions and their inflammatory intensity. The published photos demonstrate the extensive range of facial acne grades of increasing severity from 1 (least severe) to 12 (most severe). Different parts of the body are used, such as face, chest and back. The system is not suitable for those with non-inflamed acne or with highly localised acne or those with sporadic and asymmetrical large nodular lesions. Most patients have a combination of inflamed and non-inflamed lesions; the grading system focuses on inflamed lesions.	O'Brien *et al.* (1998) which builds on Burke and Cunliffe (1984)

Disease-related quality of life

The quality of life impact of skin conditions can be considerable. This factor needs to be taken into account when assessing patient's need and their response to treatment. The psychological and social impact of chronic skin conditions has been found to be of significance (Rapp *et al.*, 1999), especially when compared to other medical diseases. Irrespective of disease severity, the quality of life impact of many chronic skin diseases can be major. As such, it is necessary to assess disease-related quality of life effectively using valid tools (Chen, 2007). Due to the significance of this area, it is addressed in detail in Chapter 6, in an examination of the psychological and social impact of skin disease and treatment.

Technological aids

Λ range of technological and other diagnostic aids are available. Those listed below are typically used in clinical practice.

Dermatoscopy

It is also known as dermoscopy. This technique refers to the examination of the skin using skin surface microscopy. A dermatoscope (or dermoscope) is a device used for the examination of cutaneous lesions. It has a hand-held device with a magnifier with either cross-polarized or non-polarized light or a liquid medium of oil between the instrument and the skin to illuminate a lesion without glare from reflected light. The device is useful for examining pigmented lesions such as naevi and potential malignant lesions such as melanomas. There are specific dermoscopic patterns that aid in the diagnosis of the following pigmented skin lesions such as melanomas, moles (benign melanocytic naevi), freckles (lentigos), atypical naevi, seborrhoeic keratosis and pigmented basal cell carcinomas. Evidence suggests that while dermatoscopy improves the diagnostic accuracy for melanoma compared to the unaided eye, it requires sufficient training and is not recommended for untrained users (Kittler *et al.*, 2002).

Wood's light

Wood's light is a lamp emitting long-wave UVA used to examine pigmentary changes in the skin and fluorescent infections. This ultraviolet light source is used to screen for the fungal infection, tinea capitis; however, only certain species fluoresce (green) (*Microsporum canis* and *M. audouinii*). Other uses include highlighting patches of pityriasis versicolor caused by *Pityrosorum* yeast which fluoresces yellow; erythrasma, a bacterial infection affecting the skin folds, caused by *Corynebacterium* fluoresces green and vitiligo which delineates patches which can be otherwise missed.

Mycology

Mycology can be used to identify superficial fungal infections including yeasts (candidiasis and pityriasis versicolor), dermatophytes (ringworm/tinea – *tinea unguium*) or moulds (e.g. *Scopulariopsis)* using scales scraped from the edge of a scaly lesion, nails using a blunt instrument such as blunt scalpel blade or blunt edge of a stitch cutter. Scrapings of scale should be taken from the leading edge of the rash (as this is where active spores are most likely to be found) after the skin has been cleaned with alcohol, such as surgical spirit or 70% alcohol. This minimises contamination and is an aid to microscopy if greasy ointments or powders have been applied. Samples can be collected on kits providing black paper envelopes (e.g. Dermapak), which can be easily transferred to the lab. It is essential to have an adequate sample and provide full clinical details if the test is to be successful; whilst the precise quantity is difficult to quantify, as a general rule it is worth including as much material as possible so that full laboratory investigations can be carried out. It is always useful to have enough skin or nail to repeat the culture if necessary. Sample the discoloured, dystrophic or brittle parts of the nail only, gently digging as far back as possible from the distal part of the nail. For dermatophyte infections, samples should be taken from the distal nail and from debris under the nail (subungual debris). For superficial onychomycosis, the scraping should be from the nail surface and for Candida infections (e.g. a chronic paronychia) a swab should be taken from the proximal nail fold.

Hair can be plucked from the affected area with forceps; the infected hairs come out easily. The scalp may then be scraped with a blunt scalpel. Preferably, the sample should include hair stubs, the contents of plugged follicles and skin scales. Hair cut with a scissors is unsatisfactory as the focus of infection is usually below or near the surface of the scalp.

Biopsy

Where diagnosis is unclear but there is a differential diagnosis, an ellipse of skin can be taken through the edge of a lesion. There is a need to ensure that normal and abnormal skin (epidermis, dermis and fat) are included in the sample. Incisional, excisional and punch biopsies may be taken. Punch biopsies provide only limited sample, which may be inadequate for histological examination. Typically, the punch biopsy includes the full thickness skin and subcutaneous fat in the diagnosis of skin diseases. A round-shaped knife ranging in size from 1–8 mm is taken. The smaller size punch (1 mm) helps to minimise bleeding and assists in the vhealing of the wound without stitching. To diagnose many inflammatory skin conditions, the common punch size used is the 3.5- or 4-mm punch.

Bacteriology

The source of bacteria can be determined by swabbing a fluid sample pustules, vesicles, erosions and ulcers.

Patch testing

It is a technique used to diagnose contact allergic dermatitis based on the principle of delayed hypersensitivity (an immune response). Evidence of contact allergy is derived from a patient history (such as occupation), clinical examination and patch testing. The aim of the patch test is to ascertain allergic contact dermatitis by aiming to reproduce a rash on a small controlled area of skin using standardised batches or trays of allergens (termed batteries) or those commonly used at work or home. Standard batteries of substances (now often pre-prepared) are comprised of patches made up of Finn chambers and hypoallergenic tape that are applied to the patient's upper back; they should incorporate probable (standard battery) and possible substances (e.g. occupational specific) based on their history. The results are read at two stages, 48 hours and 72 hours; this timing sequence is related to the type IV hypersensitivity reaction, which is a delayed immune response. Care is needed to avoid misleading results from contact irritants that are distinct from hypersensitivity reactions. Differentiation is not always easy, however, the use of standard allergens and rigorous technique are required. A key reference source is a book on contact and occupational dermatology by Marks *et al.* (2002). Further details and sources are given in Chapter 9.

Planning care

A considerable amount of data is collected through the process of history taking and examination; however, the key outcome needs to be an informed clinical decision regarding the patient's need for nursing, medical support and a plan for intervention. Clinical judgements are made not only on information gathering, both clinical and about the person and their social context, but also account needs to be taken of other factors, such as the patient's own beliefs and priorities and the resources available to intervene effectively. Chapter 7 provides details of how to help patients to participate in decision regarding their treatment regimen and how to use this optimally. Here brief reference is made to the knowledge that informs clinical judgements and a brief outline of the key theories that describe and explain how clinical decisions are made. These are intended to raise awareness of the complexity of the decision-making process and what elements need to be considered when trying to formulate effective clinical judgements. Finally, the section briefly highlights issues of prioritisation in dermatology care and which 'red flag' skin conditions require a rapid response to minimise patient risk.

Knowledge sources informing clinical judgement

Clinical judgements underpinning care planning will draw on the different types of knowledge available. This includes empirical, aesthetic, ethical, personal and practical (Titchen and Ersser, 2001).

Empirical knowledge refers to scientific, technical or factual knowledge. This embraces research evidence including that from a systematic review to inform treatment choices or the selection of more effective methods to provide patient education. It also includes theoretical knowledge, such as those regarding the pharmacological action of drugs, which may influence judgements about the effective drug administration and, for example, ways to improve the absorption of a topical medication. Empirical knowledge is fundamental to the assessment process in which formalised knowledge has been categorised to aid systematic clinical assessment of the skin. Such knowledge provides the rational basis for explaining disease and its progression through, say, genetic, immunological or wider biological or pathological principles. Similarly, the behavioural sciences may explain social withdrawal due to poor self-esteem, how stress and anxiety may provoke a flare of a chronic skin condition or explain the inability of a person to cope with their self-management regime.

Personal knowledge or knowledge of self has been highlighted earlier in the discussion of effective consultation skills. Awareness is required of one's own individual perceptions, prejudices and bias shaped by own professional and personal history. These factors can lead to precipitant judgements on assessment and patient care.

Aesthetic knowledge refers to that knowledge that relies on an individualised appraisal of a unique situation – searching for patterns in the situation. This is based on how experienced clinicians formulate intuitive hunches on clinical situations and know how to mediate between empirical, practical and personal knowledge in the complex world of professional practice, using all the senses (Eisner, 1985; Titchen and Ersser, 2001). Experience can of course provide a template to aid recognition of similar assessment or treatment situations (such as the early recognition of infected atopic eczema) but this can also close off options for consideration. In the dermatological field, with the considerable number of dermatological diagnoses, it is probable that clinicians will typically gravitate to the common diagnostic groupings discussed earlier in this chapter. Intuitive impressions can be verified against empirical knowledge to better inform and explain clinical judgements.

Practical knowledge or 'know how' embraces skills such as those of a consultation, providing effective dressing or bandaging techniques. Here it is important to assess patient and carer or parental skills to manage their condition or that of their family member. One example would involve assessing if the patient is correctly utilising the appropriate topical medications and finding useful ways of supporting the person with a skin condition. Specifically, it is often necessary to assess both one's own and the patient's insight into their self-management and which knowledge and skills need to be developed.

Concepts and theories of clinical decision-making

A key concept in decision-making is that of heuristics; these are rules of thumb or strategies that assist in reasoning (Fonteyn and Ritter, 2008) and assist the processing of large amounts of data. These devices are important to clinicians, but are often taken for granted by those with experience. Familiarity with heuristics can enable health professionals to gain awareness of how these factors may influence their clinical judgements. Short cuts are developed with the processing of irrelevant data when formulating clinical judgements. Much of the time clinicians employ those heuristics most readily available in their mind, although these can introduce bias; for example, based on case examples from clinical experience which may or may not be relevant, with the individual being either representative or not of the cases typically seen. This may apply to initial clinical assessments or the evaluation of dermatological treatments. Anchoring heuristics are cognitive reference points or anchors, which can guide decisions. In dermatology, such devices are important in formulating assessment or diagnostic judgements about lesions. The classification systems described earlier in this chapter provide such heuristic aids to the pattern recognition of lesions and rashes.

One theory of reasoning, which gives an insight into the explanation of how clinical judgements are formed, is the Hypothetico-deductive theory. This is based on the work of Elstein *et al.* (1978), with the key processes being cue acquisition (such as a raised erythematous scaly plaque), hypothesis generation and cue interpretation (chronic plaque psoriasis) and hypothesis evaluation – that is, reviewing how well this fits with the clinical examination of the individual (Carnevali and Thomas, 1993). Such work is recognised to have relevance to nursing (Tanner *et al.*, 1987).

Dermatological 'red flag' conditions

Nurses working in any clinical setting require the skills to identify which skin conditions require immediate emergency referral or a response by other practitioners with appropriate advance practice skills and the relevant scope of practice. Some of the key 'red flag' conditions, which require prompt medical referral, are listed below:

■ Viral rashes if systemically unwell
■ Any rash that is purpuric in nature
■ Any rash associated with either temperature, multi-lymphadenitis headaches or stiffness of neck
■ Insect bites or stings that have a significant area of cellulitis or signs of vascular tracking
■ If the swelling from insect bites or stings compromises the patient's airway (to the face or neck)
■ Any sign of pharyngeal/facial swelling, difficulty in breathing or anaphylactic reaction
■ Shingles: herpes zoster
■ Raised skin lesions that show signs of infection

Acute dermatological situations which require a rapid treatment response include adverse drug reactions (e.g. toxic epidermal necrosis), herpes simplex affecting the eye, erythrodermic psoriasis – which is a very severe skin condition where there is a risk of shock and death and blistering disorders (e.g. epidermolysis bullosa) and where there is a significant disruption to the skin barrier (see Chapter 13).

Intervention

A key element of the care planning process is to formulate decisions regarding the appropriateness of treatment. As well as working within multi-professional teams and contributing to such decisions, nurses will be making some treatment choices in a growing number of countries with the appropriate nurse prescribing qualification or professional preparation. Each chapter, within the specific clinical area or condition discussed, will address issues of treatment, but as an overview, a summary is given here in Table 3.8 categorising the main treatment regimens commonly used within the dermatological field.

Treatment protocols and guidelines tend to stage therapy in accordance with the severity of disease and the patients response over time; assessment of the patient's response at each stage is required. For example, in the case of psoriasis, patients are likely to commence with topical therapy and be supported in self-management wherever possible. This may proceed to phototherapy or a combination of light therapy. For those with more severe disease, they may progress to systemic/oral therapy and thereafter possibly onto biological therapy.

Table 3.8 Categories of common dermatological treatments.

1. Pharmacological
a. Topicals: emollient (focus Chapter 5), tars, dithranol, topical immune-modulators, steroids, vitamin D analogues, retinoids, keratolytic agents, antibiotics, antifungal and antiviral drugs.
b. Systemic: immunosuppressive agents/ biological therapies, antibiotics and antifungals, retinoids, steroids, antiviral agents and antihistamines.

2. Phototherapy: UV, including narrow band (A and B), photodynamic therapy

3. Surgical, cryotherapy, laser: Skin biopsy (punch, shave, incisional biopsy and excision), curettage and cautery, skin grafting, Mohs microscopically controlled excision and cryotherapy (liquid nitrogen). Laser therapy: quasi-continuous wave and pulsed.

4. Psychological and educational: (details given in Chapter 7)

5. Iontophoresis (for hyperhidrosis, excessive sweating)

6. Bandages and dressings

Such progression would require assessment not only in changes in disease severity but also perhaps in disease-related quality of life and the patent's self-management ability, in relation to topical therapy.

Phototherapy assessment requires a systematic assessment of the patient's skin type and previous history of UV exposure and response to inform the assessment of a suitable dose regimen. The response to phototherapy needs to be assessed, both in terms of the disease severity and adverse effects, such as erythema and dryness of skin. The individual's skin response to UVB depends on their skin phototype, prior exposure to sunlight or other source of UV and the presence of photosensitivity. Typically for UVB therapy, the minimal erythema dose (MED) is measured; these vary widely within each skin type. A template is applied to a non-exposed area, such as the volar surface of the arm; test sites are outlined with a skin marker so that they can be identified. The response is measured 24 h later. The MED is the lowest dose that produces pink erythema with distinct borders.

The use of systemic therapy requires a complex monitoring regimen not only to determine suitability for treatment (to meet guideline requirements and patient protection, e.g. pregnancy) to monitor therapeutic effect, but also to assess for adverse effects in order to manage risk from cytotoxic agents. An increasing number of nurses are involved in monitoring patients on such therapy. For example, methotrexate use requires liver and renal monitoring, pulmonary review and a full blood count (Wakelin, 2002). Biologic monitoring is complex. A growing number of nurses are playing a key role in the monitoring of both treatments, shorter- and longer-term response, especially to pick up any adverse effects. Short-term monitoring will involve monitoring for infusion reactions with TNF inhibitors (e.g. Infliximab) such as hypotension, dyspnoea and urticaria (anaphylaxis). Adverse effects include headaches, gastrointestinal upsets and chills. Longer-term monitoring will involve the use of PASI and a review of risk such as infection (hepatitis B reactivation,

tuberculosis, hepatotoxicity and malignancy). For further details see Chapter 8.

Evaluation

Structured assessment tools may be used within clinical practice as well as in research evaluation. Specifically they are helpful as treatment or nursing care evaluation tools to monitor the progress of therapy or intervention. One such example of evaluation is the use of the PASI score. A 75% improvement (PASI75) is well established as a clinically meaningful endpoint for trials but PASI50 (50% improvement) is also considered by some to be a clinically valid endpoint. Common clinical guidelines, such as those for biological therapy for psoriasis, now incorporate PASI parameters to specify the level of disease severity required to permit treatment (Smith *et al.*, 2005; National Institute for Health and Clinical Excellence [NICE], 2008).

Consideration is required of the timing of the evaluation measurement; for example, if applying tar, there will be a slow response to treatment over a period of weeks. Both health professionals and patients need to give recognition of the duration over which interventions are typically effective, since patients may abandon treatments, which they believe are not working. Research evidence suggests patients may use timing of the treatment effect as a criterion for judging the effectiveness of their therapy in psoriasis care (Ersser *et al.*, 2002). Clinicians need to take account of the criteria that patients use in evaluating treatment regimens. Premature evaluative measurements may provide a misleading picture of the effectiveness of a particular therapy; therefore, there is a need to consider the evidence underlying the duration of treatments. Practitioners also need to be mindful of the role standardised tools play (see e.g. Table 3.7) as measures at key endpoints in the research evaluation of existing or new therapies; this will be useful when interpreting research results within clinical papers and understanding the way in which evidence may inform the clinical guidelines used by nurses.

Conclusion

This chapter has highlighted the significance of the assessment and planning process within dermatological care. Emphasis has been placed not on medical diagnosis, albeit important, but rather on the conceptualisation, description and categorisation of normal skin and then by contrast diseased skin through reference to the lesions and rashes commonly seen, to aid communication between health professionals and the patient. The process of assessment has been outlined and an illustration of the range of questionnaire and technological tools use to collect data. Then we have outlined the importance of effectively using data collected to inform clinical decisions and the planning and evaluation process. Finally, an outline has been given of common dermatological interventions used to manage and treating skin conditions and their sequelae. This chapter has set out the nature of dermatological and health-related needs and how these are assessed and subsequent care planned; these issues are then illustrated and discussed throughout the book, mainly focusing on common dermatological problems and their effective management.

References

Alaluf, S., D. Atkins *et al.* (2002). Ethnic variation in melanin content and composition in photoexposed and photoprotected human skin. *Pigment Cell Research*, **15**(2): 112–118.

Ashcroft, D.M., A. Li Wan Po *et al.* (1999). Clinical measures of disease severity and outcome in psoriasis: A critical appraisal of their quality. *British Journal of Dermatology*, **141**: 185–191.

Ashton, R. and B. Leppard (2005). *Differential Diagnosis in Dermatology*. Abingdon, Oxon: Radcliffe Publishing Ltd.

Burke, B.M. and W.J. Cunliffe (1984). The assessment of acne vulgaris – the Leeds technique. *British Journal of Dermatology*, **111**(1): 83–92.

Carnevali, D.L. and M.D. Thomas (1993). *Diagnostic Reasoning and Treatment Decision Making in Nursing*. Hagerstown, Maryland: Lippincott Williams & Wilkins.

Chen, S.C. (2007). Dermatology quality of life instruments: Sorting out the quagmire. *Journal of Investigative Dermatology*, **127**: 2695–2696.

Eisner, E. (1985). *The Art of Educational Evaluation: A Personal View*. London: Flamer Press.

Elstein, A.S., L.S. Shulman *et al.* (1978). *Medical Problem Solving: An Analysis of Clinical Reasoning*. Cambridge, MA: Harvard University Press.

Ersser, S. (1997). *Nursing as a Therapeutic Activity: An Ethnography*. Aldershot: Avebury Press.

Ersser, S.J., H. Surridge *et al.* (2002). What criteria do patients use when judging the effectiveness of psoriasis management? *Journal of Evaluation in Clinical Practice*, **8**(4): 367–376.

Exum, M.L., S.R. Rapp *et al.* (1996). Measuring severity of psoriasis. *Journal of Dermatological Treatments*, **7**: 119–124.

Fawcett, R.S., S. Linford *et al.* (2004). Nail abnormalities: clues to systemic disease. *American Family Physician*, **69**(6): 1417–1424.

Fonteyn, M.E. and B.J. Ritter (2008). Clinical reasoning. In: Higgs, J., Jones, M.A., Loftus, S., Christensen, N. (Eds), Nursing *Clinical Reasoning in the Health Professions*. Amsterdam: Elsevier Butterworth Heinemann.

Gawkrodger, D. (1998). Racial influences on skin disease. In: Burns, D.A., Breathnach, S., Cox, N., Griffiths, C. (Eds), *Rook's Textbook of Dermatology*. Oxford: Blackwell Science Ltd.

Gordon, M. (1976). Nursing diagnoses and the diagnostic process. *The American Journal of Nursing*, **76**(8): 1298–1300.

Graham-Brown, R. and T. Burns (2006). *Lecture Notes: Dermatology* (9th edition). Oxford: Blackwell Science.

Johannsen, L.L. (1998). Skin assessment and diagnostic techniques. In: Hill. M.J. (Ed.), *Dermatologic Nursing Essentials: A Core*

Curriculum, pp. 17–31. Pitman, New Jersey: Anthony J. Jannetti, Inc.

Kittler, H., H. Pehamberger *et al.* (2002). Diagnostic accuracy of dermoscopy. *The Lancet Oncology*, 3(3): 159–165.

Kunz, B., A.P. Oranje *et al.* (1997). Clinical validation and guidelines for the SCORAD index: Consensus report of the European Task Force on Atopic Dermatitis. *Dermatology*, **195**(1): 10–19.

Lawrence, C.M. and N.H. Cox (2002). *Physical Signs in Dermatology*. London: Mosby.

Lawson, V., M.S. Lewis-Jones *et al.* (1998). The family impact of childhood atopic dermatitis: The Dermatitis Family Impact Questionnaire. *British Journal of Dermatology*, **138**(1): 107–113.

Leach, E.E., P.B. McClelland *et al.* (1996). Basic principles of photobiology and photochemistry for nurse phototherapists and phototechnicians. *Dermatology Nursing*, 8(4): 235–241.

Lehmann, H., K. Robinson *et al.* (2002). Acne therapy: A methodologic review. *Journal of the American Academy of Dermatology*, **47**: 231–240.

Mackie, R.M. (2003). *Clinical Dermatology* (5th edition). Oxford: Oxford University Press.

Marks, J.G., V.A. DeLeo *et al.* (2002). *Contact and Occupational Dermatology* (3rd edition). London: Mosby.

NANDA-International (2007). *Nursing Diagnoses: Definitions and Classification 2007–2008*. Philadelphia: NANDA International.

National Institute for Health and Clinical Excellence (NICE) (2008). *Infliximab for the Treatment of Adults with Psoriasis*. London: NICE.

O'Brien, S.C., J.B. Lewis *et al.* (1998). The Leeds revised acne grading system. *Journal of Dermatological Treatments*, 9(4): 215–220.

Oranje, A., E. Glazenburg *et al.* (2007). Practical issues on interpretation of scoring atopic dermatitis: The SCORAD index, objective SCORAD and the three-item severity score. *British Journal of Dermatology*, **157**(4): 645–648.

Ramsay, B. and C.M. Lawrence (1991). Measurement of involved surface area in patients with psoriasis. *British Journal of Dermatology*, **128**: 69–74.

Rapp, S.R., S.R. Feldman, M.L. Exum, A.B. Fleischer Jr, D.M. Reboussin (1999). Psoriasis causes as much disability as other major medical diseases. *Journal of the American Academy of Dermatology*, **41**: 401–407.

Smith, C.H., A.V. Anstey *et al.* (2005). British Association of Dermatologists guidelines for use of biological interventions in psoriasis 2005. *British Journal of Dermatology*, **153**(3): 486–497.

Tanner, C.A., K.P. Padrick *et al.* (1987). Diagnostic reasoning strategies of nurses and nursing students. *Nursing Research* 36(6): 358–363.

Titchen, A. and S.J. Ersser (2001). The nature of professional craft knowledge. In: Higgs, J. Titchen, A. (Eds), *Practice Knowledge and Expertise in the Health Professions*. Oxford: Butterworth-Heinemann.

Tortora, G. and B. Derrickson (2006). *Principles of Anatomy and Physiology* (11th edition). New Jersey: John Wiley and Sons Inc.

Wakelin, S.H. (2002). *Systemic Drug Treatment in Dermatology*. London: Manson Publishing Ltd.

Williams, H.C. (1997). *Dermatology: Health Care Needs Assessment*. Oxford: Radcliffe Medical Press.

Protecting the skin and preventing breakdown

4

Steven J. Ersser

Introduction

Nurses spend considerable time protecting the skin and preventing its deterioration.

The intricately designed structure and function of the skin protects the body from a range of external physical and biological threats. Although barrier function is localised to the stratum corneum, protection is one of the primary functions of the skin as an organ. This includes defence against exposure to chemicals, irradiation, traumatic insult and microbiological threats such as bacteria, viruses and fungi. Chapter 2 has outlined the details of the skin's protective structural features and protective biological features. This chapter considers the processes involved in vulnerable skin and outlines the key factors associated with disruption of the skin barrier due to disease, biology and the impact of external physical factors, including treatment effects. It also highlights specific interventions for promoting skin barrier function, maintaining its integrity and preventing barrier disruption and breakdown.

The concept of skin vulnerability

The vulnerability of the skin reflects the susceptibility of the skin barrier's integrity and health due to the effects of a wide range of influencing factors, not only biological but also psychological and social. It therefore reflects a broader concept of health needs assessment rather than simply dermatological disease; this provides a wider basis for understanding the wide range of skin care needs met by health professionals. Skin vulnerability may result from difficulties such as the lack of self-care management skills, the influence of developmental factors (age and immaturity), stress and anxiety and the impact of socio-economic factors such as poverty and environmental factors, including climatic impact. The interplay of these factors can disrupt barrier functions of the skin, leading to breakdown, disease and further physical, psychological and social effects. The concept of skin vulnerability directly relates to that of nursing diagnosis (Chapter 3) that highlights the scope for nursing intervention.

What causes skin breakdown?

In this section, we examine some of the key pathological and physical factors that may directly lead to skin breakdown. These include the inflammatory response, pressure effects, poor perfusion, the effects of washing practices on the skin and those arising from urinary incontinence.

Inflammation

Inflammation is the body's response to injury, which may be acute or chronic. Acute inflammation is the immediate defensive reaction of tissue to any injury, which may be caused by infection, chemicals or physical agents and involves pain, heat, redness and swelling (Martin and McFerran, 2008). It has also been defined as a set of local cellular and vascular responses to tissue damage or infection, which accelerates the destruction and phagocytic removal of invading organisms and debris (McGeown, 2002). The fundamental inflammatory process occurs in many dermatological conditions, where there is the key indicator of redness or erythema over the area due to blood flow.

Inflammation has a protective function by helping to eliminate the cause of tissue damage, removing dead cells and maintaining stability within the internal physiological environment. In the case of a wound there may be also swelling; heat, pain and loss of function, with injury leading to vasoconstriction of vessels at the margins of the wound. Hyperaemia then occurs in which the blood vessels within the area dilate, increasing local blood flow and redness. The damaged cells release chemical mediators such as bradykinin, histamine and serotonin, which increase capillary permeability, allowing the leakage of fluid into the tissues, causing oedema and possibly pain. The loss of plasma proteins exerts an osmotic effect in the tissues slowing down the flow of blood in the dilated vessels. As part of the protective response, white blood cells, particularly neutrophils, migrate from the vessels to the inflamed area attracted by the chemicals released by injured tissue cells and microorganisms.

Antibodies within the exudate trigger neutrophils and macrophages phagocytosing these cells. Eventually fibrin builds up, with the inflamed area becoming sealed by the network of fibrin threads, localising the damaged tissues (McGeown, 2002; Hinchliff *et al.*, 2005).

Inflammation is a common pathological process within dermatological disease. This is evident in many of the lesions and rashes, as outlined in Chapter 3. The inflammatory dermatoses include common skin disease such as psoriasis and eczema; these are illustrated within Chapters 8 and 9.

Dry skin

Dry skin or xerosis is a common feature of skin disease, which reflects disruption to the skin barrier and the undue loss of moisture from the skin tissue. A list of common disease- or treatment-related causes of dry skin is given below:

- Atopic eczema
- Ichthyoses (inherited)
- Psoriasis
- Leprosy
- Drug induced (e.g. clofazimine given for leprosy)
- Phototherapy induced (e.g. PUVA therapy)

Disease processes lead to water loss because pathological or pharmacological effects will often disrupt the structure and processes that maintain the skin barrier integrity and retaining water within the dermis leading to transepidermal water loss (TEWL) and dehydration of the skin. Skin dryness may greatly vary in severity. It may occur without disease through factors such as over-washing of the skin or exposure to harsh climatic conditions. Because of severe environmental conditions or the presence of dermatological disease such as eczema or ichthyosis, the skin barrier will be impaired which will lead to dehydration of the skin by evaporation, develops cracking and fissuring of the skin, which will in turn further impair the integrity and effectiveness of the skin barrier.

Other external and intrinsic factors that cause dry skin and affect the skin barrier includes the following:

- Unsuitable skin hygiene, such as excessive washing, use of soap, water saturation due to undue soaking of the skin, rough skin drying technique, excessive routine skin washing and lack of moisturisation;
- Environmental factors both at home and externally including excessive UV exposure, centrally heated low humidity environments and use of air conditioning;
- Poor nutrition and inadequate hydration;
- Changes related to the maturity of the skin, with the risk of water loss from an immature infant's skin – with its high surface area to volume ratio and water loss from aged skin due to age-related changes in skin structure, such as the loss of sebum (see Chapter 2).

Poor perfusion and disrupted microcirculation of the skin

Poor perfusion of blood to the skin may result from a range of pathological factors such as cardiovascular disease due to arteriosclerosis and heart failure, the effects of oedema and trauma and the occlusion of blood vessels due to pressure. For critically ill patients, the circulatory failure associated with hypovolemia and low cardiac output is associated with redistribution of blood flow caused by increased vasoconstriction, which leads to a decrease in skin perfusion. Therefore, the degree of skin perfusion may reflect the adequacy of global blood flow. The clinical signs of poor skin perfusion include evidence of cold, pale, clammy and mottled skin.

Oedema and lymphoedema

Oedema and lymphoedema may disrupt the microcirculation thereby impairing the skin barrier. Oedema may be caused by heart failure, nephrosis, inflammation, venous hypertension, lymphatic impairment due to cancer and related therapy, filariasis, immobility and congenital and traumatic factors (Ryan, 2008) Chronic

oedema is a common problem with at least 100,000 patients affected in the UK alone; it is also poorly identified by health professionals (Moffatt *et al.*, 2003). Chronic oedema is tissue swelling that remains over 3 months, which is not relieved by elevation or diuretics. A useful indicator is a positive Stemmer's sign – the inability to pinch fold of skin at the base of second toe due to thickening. As a consequence this may impair the skin barrier leading to associated skin changes: these may include the following: dry flaky skin; hyperkeratosis – hard, scaly skin, development of skin creases around the toes and ankles; increased subcutaneous tissue; fibrosis of the tissue and lymphangioma, where there are blister-like bulging of dilated lymphatic vessels papillomatosis, with a cobblestone effect on the skin due to lymphangioma and fibrosis. The skin may be further impaired due to the greater subsequent risk of infection.

Lymphoedema is an accumulation of lymph in the tissues, producing swelling; the legs are most often affected, but arms and genitalia may also be involved. It may be due to a congenital abnormality of the lymphatic vessels, as in Milroy's disease, congenital lymphoedema of the legs or result from obstruction (Martin and McFerran, 2008).

Lymphoedema for clinical problems other than cancer treatment is much more prevalent than generally perceived, although the resources are mainly cancer service based.

Skin problems seen in lymphoedema include the following: (1) hyperkeratosis (an over proliferation of the keratin layer, (2) folliculitis, (3) fungal infections, (4) ulceration, (5) venous eczema, (6) contact dermatitis, (7) lymphangiectasia (soft fluid-filled projections caused by the dilatation of lymphatic vessels), (8) papillomatosis (firm raised projections of skin due to raised lymphatic vessels and fibrosis), (9) lymphorrhoea (the leakage of lymph from the skin surface) and (10) cellulitis/erysipelas.

Pressure

An efficient skin barrier is dependent on an adequate perfusion of blood. The primary effect of pressure on the skin is to occlude capillaries and thereby disrupt blood flow and the carriage of nutrients to the tissues. Pressure effects may arise due to immobility, commonly bed rest or spending prolonged periods in a chair. Pressure effects on the skin have been the subject of extensive research.

The European Pressure Ulcer Advisory Panel (EPUAP) website defines a pressure ulcer as an area of localised damage to the skin and underlying tissue caused by pressure or shear and/or a combination of these (EPUAP, 2008). Nixon (2001) outlines the distinction between the aetiology and pathology of pressure ulcers. Autoregulatory systems that affect blood flow during and following pressure effects are highly relevant to pressure ulcer aetiology. These include the raising of capillary pressure to maintain flow, intermittent flow at subcritical pressures and response to repetitive loading and the reactive hyperaemic response following partial or full occlusion. Such occlusion leads to anoxia and a related accumulation of metabolites. Following pressure release, the large and rapid increase in blood flow through the deprived tissues is termed reactive hyperaemia. Key mechanisms include those that are myogenic and metabolic, related to the metabolite release from either anoxic tissues or the lack of oxygen. The degree and duration of the hyperaemic response is related to the duration of occlusion (Walmsley and Wiles, 1990) and factors such as age (with the elderly being very vulnerable), smoking, vascular or related disease (e.g. diabetes) and conditions such as end-stage renal failure and spinal cord injury. Another important factor is the repetitive loading of pressure, which operates via an active vasomotor response mechanism (Bader, 1990).

The different types of pressure ulcer include those related to epidermal or dermal necrosis, deep pressure ulcers with necrosis occurring within the subcutaneous tissues and full thickness wounds of dry black eschar. The key pathological mechanisms include injury caused by abrupt reperfusion of the capillary bed following occlusion of blood flow, damage to the vasculature due to forces such as shear and cell death arising from prolonged direct occlusion of blood vessels (Nixon, 2001).

The effects of washing (skin hygiene) practices on the skin

Despite the significant amount of time nurses spend washing patients, the effects of washing activities on skin barrier function have received limited scientific appraisal. The evidence we have is largely based on the literature reviews, drawn from clinical observation, supported by limited experimental (quasi) study evidence and expert panel sources (Ersser *et al.*, 2005).

The use of very hot water may cause unnecessary drying of the skin by removing skin oils and accelerating water loss by evaporation (Gooch, 1989). As an emulsifying agent, soap acts by dispersing one liquid into another immiscible liquid and so it suspends the oil or debris in water, aiding rinsing. Sodium lauryl sulphate is one of the most common synthetic surfactants found in soaps and detergents (Kirsner and Froelich, 1998). It is also a potent skin irritant, especially after prolonged exposure (e.g. Held *et al.*, 2001), which may bind to keratin and cause denaturation of cell membranes, leading to an irritant response. Surfactants can also cause allergic contact dermatitis, but due to the high intensity effect of many, it can be difficult to differentiate an allergic reaction from contact irritation during patch testing (Flyvholm, 1993). Non-ionic surfactant, such as propylene glycol, is the least irritating group of surfactants. Products such as baby shampoo contain low-irritant, amphoteric surfactants, such as cocoamido-propyl betaine (Kirsner and Froelich, 1998).

Other physico-chemical effects of soap may disrupt the delicate skin barrier. Washing with soap may remove the natural protective emollient sebum oil from the skin (Baillie and Arrowsmith, 2001). Soaps and some cleansers may also raise the alkalinity of the skin (Korting *et al.*, 1987) and thereby negating the influence of the protective acid mantle (see Chapter 2). They may also change the balance of resident flora on the skin, leading to the proliferation or reduction of counts of common bacteria such as *Propionibacterium acnes* or *Staphylococcus aureus*, respectively (Korting and Braun-Falco, 1996); this may enhance the risk of skin colonisation and possible infection by pathogenic microorganisms.

Skin that is not dried carefully after washing can cause maceration and undue cooling. The mechanical and chemical drying of the skin can adversely affect barrier function, although the literature on this subject is limited.

The effects of urine and incontinence on the skin

The effects of urinary incontinence on skin vulnerability are another neglected area of nursing investigation (Ersser *et al.*, 2005). Despite the scale of the problem, the effects and prevention of urine exposure on skin barrier disruption has received limited research attention. The prevalence of urinary incontinence provides an indication of the potential significance of the problem (Getliffe and Dolman, 2003). It is estimated that 200 million people worldwide have significant urinary incontinence and many more with mild bladder problems (Abrams *et al.*, 2002), with a high occurrence among people living in institutional settings. Obesity affects 20% of the population in UK (National Audit Office, 2001). It is a major health problem in most affluent countries and is likely to lead to skin vulnerability due to the formation of skin folds. Children are another vulnerable group; it is estimated that in the UK 500,000 experience nocturnal enuresis (persistent bedwetting) (Department of Health, 2000). Although incontinence may not of course accompany older age, an increased incidence of multiple disabilities in this group may contribute to reduced ability to maintain continence, making this group vulnerable to skin damage.

The skin of an incontinent person will be exposed to regular contact with urine, sweat and possibly faeces. As such, the skin is vulnerable to chemical irritation by urine and physical effects caused by wetness of the skin that encourages maceration; these can disrupt the skin barrier and lead to breakdown. The decomposition of urinary urea by microorganisms release ammonia to form the alkali, ammonium hydroxide, thereby disrupting the acid mantle. Chemical irritation of the skin may arise from both the rise in alkalinity and bacterial proliferation. Perineal dermatitis may arise from urine exposure, which is characterised by inflammation of the skin, and may include redness, tissue breakdown, oozing, crusting, itching and pain (Brown and Sears, 1993; Gray, 2004) within the perineal area.

Faecal incontinence may present even more risk to skin integrity (Allman, 1986; Shannon and Skorga, 1989). It is more common in the general population than is often realised and the survey cited above suggests 5.7% of women and 6.2% of men over 40 years living in their own homes report some degree of faecal incontinence (Perry *et al.*, 2002). Overall, 1.4% of adults reported major faecal incontinence (at least several times a month) and 0.7% had disabling incontinence with a major impact on their quality of life.

Excess moisture can increase the friction coefficient, making the skin more vulnerable to breakdown due to friction forces (Nach *et al.*, 1981). This, coupled with frequent washing of the incontinent patient's skin, can disrupt skin barrier function by removal of skin lipids and the acceleration of epidermal water loss (further examination is given later). A number of studies reveal a general association between urinary incontinence and pressure sores, but few demonstrate a causal link. For example, a study of nursing home residents by Schnelle *et al.* (1997) demonstrated that skin problems tend to occur in areas where there has been consistent excessive skin wetness (hydration) through urine exposure. These findings are consistent with supporting experimental evidence that skin exposed to urine due to infrequent pad change can increase the wetness of the skin; the increase in friction and abrasion predisposing it to breakdown (Fader *et al.*, 2003). Prolonged exposure to water alone may cause hydration dermatitis (Kligman, 1994; Tsai and Maibach, 1999) and prolonged occlusion of the skin (as within a continence product) may reduce skin barrier function (Fluhr *et al.*, 1999) and significantly raise microbial counts and pH (Aly *et al.*, 1978; Faergemann *et al.*, 1983).

Consideration also needs to be given to the effects of drying practices related to washing practices. An excessively dry stratum corneum can develop cracks and fissures and can be as ineffective a barrier as an over-hydrated one (Tsai and Maibach, 1999). Dry and scaling skin contributes to the risk of pressure ulcer development, although only limited evidence has been found. Those with dry or scaling skin have been found to be at least 2.5 times more likely to develop wounds from skin breakdown compared to a matched control group (Gulralnik *et al.*, 1988), based on one of the largest studies ($n = 5, 193$) examining predictors of pressure sores in the community (55–75 years). As a risk factor, dry skin is not reflected in pressure risk scales, which focus on the key role of moisture. Aside to dry and over-hydrated skin, some patients also develop sore skin in which there is erythema due to inflammatory effects and a damaged skin barrier. Again, the issue of sore skin is another area given scant attention in the literature.

Other factors affecting skin breakdown

Malignancy can affect the skin barrier when the pathological process leads to a breakdown in skin integrity, such as a malignant fungating wound, which may include mycosis fungoides, a type of cutaneous T-cell lymphoma. Whilst such problems will require wound care, the effects of cancer treatments can have implications for skin care. Iatrogenic effects or the effects of medical treatment on the skin such as radiotherapy effects and adverse drug reactions (ADRs) are now examined.

Radiotherapy

Radiotherapy may cause acute radiation dermatitis, with the reaction intensity depending on the dose, the treated area and individual variation (Tucker *et al.*, 1984). Common effects on the skin include erythema, which resembles severe sunburn, and peeling or desquamation; rarely it can lead to necrosis (Porock and KristJanson, 1999). Skin reactions tend to be short lived; they are also uncomfortable for patients, with accompanying itch and pain at times (Campbell and Illingworth, 1992).

Adverse drug reactions

Adverse drug reactions (ADRs) or side effects can have a significant cutaneous effect, which may lead to a significant breakdown of skin integrity. They can account for 5% of all hospital admissions in the UK and between 10% and 20% of hospital inpatients (The National Prescribing Centre, 1998) and hence can be a common reason for dermatological contact with other hospital areas. Whilst a rash is a common skin reaction, drug eruptions can be severe and lead to skin barrier breakdown (see Chapter 13 for more details on drug reactions).

The mechanisms of ADRs include anaphylactic reactions (type I), cytotoxic reactions (type II) and immune complex–mediated reactions (type III), in which combinations of some of these mechanisms may occur (Mackie, 2003). Typical cutaneous reaction patterns due to ADRs are summarised in Table 4.1.

In countries such as South Africa, which have high HIV-AIDS prevalence and so a highly immuno-compromised population, some

Table 4.1 Cutaneous reaction patterns due to ADRs.

Reaction pattern	Likely drugs
Toxic erythema	Antibiotics, sulphonamides, barbiturates, anti-rheumatics
Erythema multiforme and Stevens–Johnson syndrome	Antibiotics, sulphonamides and anti-rheumatics
Erythema nodosum	Contraceptive pill, sulphonamides
Erythroderma	Antibiotics and anti-rheumatics
Vasculitis and purpuric eruptions or aggravation of psoriasis	Phenytoin, indomethacin
Very severe blistering eruption (toxic epidermal necrolysis)	Sulphonamides, allopurinol and phenylbutazone
Photosensitivity	Tetracyclines, phenothiazines
Acne	Phenytoin
SLE-like syndrome	Hydralazine, penicillin and sulphonamides
Exfoliative dermatitis	Gold, isoniazid and phenylbutazone

Source: Based on Mackie (2003).

conditions such as severe blistering condition toxic epidermal necrolysis are much more common, which has a significant effect on skin breakdown and perhaps a major challenge for nursing and medical care. Strong (1998) gives further details on dermatological emergencies from a nursing perspective.

Preventative practices

Skin washing and drying practices

The earlier section on washing the skin highlights the importance of several factors in maintaining the skin barrier; avoiding excessive use of soap and where possible using soap substitutes or cleansers, not using water that is too hot and minimising rough drying technique.

For those with chronic skin conditions such as psoriasis and eczema, emollients may be used as soap substitutes (see Chapter 5). For routine skin care for those requiring regular washing, such as the incontinent patients, skin cleansers may provide an alternative means to maintain skin hygiene. They may reduce some of the adverse effects of soap, due to their chemical composition, and help to maintain a pH level that minimises barrier disruption. Several studies have compared the use and effect of skin cleansers with soap and water use, but design weaknesses are common, such as small sample size, and hence conclusions are often unclear. For example, Whittingham (1998) compared the relative effectiveness of one of two cleansers (*Triple Care, Smith & Nephew* and *Clinisan, Vernacare*) with that of using soap and water on skin condition among a sample of highly dependent elderly patients with some degree of incontinence. Other studies have compared the combined use of cleansers with a barrier cream with the effectiveness of soap and water, although again design weaknesses are common (e.g. Byers *et al.*, 1995; Dealey, 1995) compared to skin washing and cleansing regimens and their effect on skin integrity using a 'multi-baseline cross-over design', with soap and water as the baseline control. Although a small study, repeated

observations revealed statistically significant differences between the regimens, and there was no clinically observable evidence of skin breakdown. Based on the transepidermal water loss (TEWL) and erythema measurements, the soap and water regimen was the least efficient in promoting skin health. There were statistically significant differences on TEWL measures between the soap and water control and the use of cleanser alone ($p = 0.02$), soap and barrier cream ($p = 0.01$) and cleanser plus barrier cream ($p = 0.03$). Soap also produced a more alkaline skin (pH 7.5), but barrier function improved with the use of a barrier cream and was even greater with the cleanser and cream regimen. As such, for use with vulnerable skin, the use of carefully selected cleansers and emollients should be considered (see Chapter 5).

The capillary action of the towel wicks water away from the surface and various authors have suggested drying the skin gently, patting it rather than rubbing to reduce frictional damage (Fiers, 1996). Unpublished preliminary observations from the authors' group would support the fact that a minimal rubbing drying technique, such as patting, may reduce frictional damage. Measurements of skin barrier function (including TEWL) were significantly increased following a single wash with towel drying by rubbing, the mean pre-wash TEWL ($\pm$SEM) being 8 ± 0.12 g/hm^2 increasing to 12.6 ± 0.52 g/hm^2 after a single wash, representing a significant disruption to skin barrier function (p < 0.01) (Ersser *et al.*, 2005).

Promoting skin hydration

The principles of improving skin hydration are twofold: firstly the need to promote the retention of moisture (and prevent dehydration) and secondly to support the process of adding water to the skin structure. Emollient therapy is a key technique for achieving both approaches by reducing water loss by moisturisation (occlusive effect), promoting water retention and helping water to penetrate directly into the skin, as in the application of creams. Emollient therapy is examined in detail in Chapter 5 and in a best practice review document (Ersser *et al.*,

2007). Even in situations and countries where pharmaceutical emollients are scarce, the effect of safe oils on the skin barrier can be effective (Darmstadt *et al.*, 2002).

Details have been given on washing and drying practices to prevent or minimise water loss from the skin. In summary this includes minimising soap use and considering the use of soap substitutes, avoiding very hot water which enhances evaporation and removes natural skin oils such as sebum, sealing the skin with emollients after soaking, drying to minimise trauma to the skin barrier. Occlusive techniques are the other main techniques that enhance the hydration of the skin and minimise trauma to the skin barrier related to scratching.

Wrapping or bandaging techniques involve a process of occluding the skin to promote skin hydration and skin protection. These techniques may be wet or dry, depending on the relative need for hydration and skin protection, respectively. Hydration is achieved by the application of liberal quantities of emollients under the wrapping, which may be a bandage or cotton clothing. Occlusion increases emollient absorption. Wraps can be very helpful for parents of children with eczema who can be resistant to treatment in order to improve the quality of life and sleep (Goodyear and Harper, 2002). This requires nursing support to ensure parents and the child are need to be taught to prepare them apply the wraps suitably, maintain effectiveness and to minimise any adverse effects. Box 4.1 outlines the principles of wrapping techniques; these apply to both adults and children requiring wrapping.

There are various elements of the basic wet wrapping technique; the following describes some of the core elements which may be adapted according to the need. Two layers of wrapping are used – tubular bandages, ordinary soft cotton clothing or designed commercial garments such as Tubifast. A warm damp inner wrapping layer (produced using comfortably hot water) is placed over skin onto which an emollient and possibly a topical treatment (e.g. steroid) has been applied. Keep tight fitting to prevent fast cooling. The outer dry layer is placed over the wet layer. The frequency of application will

> ### Box 4.1   Principles of wrapping techniques
>
> - Helps to interrupt the scratch – itch cycle
> - May reduce topical steroid use – wet garments can help aid penetration of topical treatment
> - Acts as a mechanical barrier preventing further damage to the skin
> - Cools and soothes the skin as water evaporates
> - Prevents emollients being wiped off and protects clothing
> - Maintains hydration
> - Reduces inflammation and allergen load

depend if the condition is severe or not, if so the parents can wrap each day and night, then once under control apply approximately thrice per week. Overnight use is particularly useful with the utilisation of existing night clothing and the opportunity to ameliorate night-time scratching. Wet wraps can be used for children from 3 months of age.

Dry wraps – A single dry layer is applied over an emollient to aid the occlusive and protective effect. As with wet wrapping, this can be applied to the badly affected areas with either the tubular bandage or the Tubifast garments (e.g. vest, leggings or socks). The garments stretch easily and are more comfortable to wear; they are washable/reusable.

Wraps can normally be used for children from 3 months of age. These principles equally apply to adults requiring wrapping, due to either the need for hydration or to alleviate the effects of damaging scratching behaviour. This process helps to disrupt the scratch–itch cycle, in which scratching aggravates the pruritic experience and thereby may lead to further damage in a cyclic manner.

Medicated paste bandages may also be used under medical supervision. These are used to treat conditions such as eczema that affect the limbs and vary according to their constituent medication, including substances such as zinc oxide, ichthammol and coal tar (both of which alleviate pruritus). As well as acting as a barrier to prevent damage from scratching they can have a cooling and soothing effect on pruritic skin, as well aiding the penetration and effectiveness of topical medications, as with other forms of occlusion. Guidance on how to apply paste bandages has been developed by the BDNG (British Dermatological Nursing Group, 2008). Application should be preceded by bathing and use of a soap substitute and the application of the topical agent. The bandages are applied from the base of the limb, i.e. starting from the wrist or the ankle upwards. There are two methods illustrated in the BDNG 'how to article'. (1) Cut and overlap method: The limb is then bandaged around the limb through one and half turns creating an overlap by half the width of the bandage each time – it is then cut; this process is repeated as the limb is ascended. (2) The second 'pleating method' involves wrapping the bandage around the limb and then folding back or pleating upon itself and then applying in the reverse direction, also overlapping by half the width of the bandage, avoiding pleats near bony prominences. Bandages are covered with a further outer cotton tubular or self-adhesive bandage which prevents staining of clothes and slippage. The final process involves checking that the bandage is not too tight and so the fingers and toes are moveable and perfused normally.

Caution is needed when using wraps, which must be intimated to the patients or their carers. Careful parental teaching is therefore needed, which can be initially time consuming. Occlusion can intensify the activity of active topical treatments such as steroids – always use the lowest strength required to bring condition under control. It is important not to use wet wraps if the skin is infected; as such there is a need to monitor the skin – pulling back the bandages to ensure skin has not got worse. Avoiding the use of occlusion is necessary since – the warmth and moisture favour the build up of microorganisms. Application should also be avoided if the child is unwell. It is advised not to cut holes for fingers or toes too small, as this can lead to swelling in these areas if tight.

Useful guidance on wet wrapping is provided by Goodyear *et al.* (1991), whilst evidence for the efficacy and safety is usefully summarised by Devillers and Oranje (2006), although further research evaluation of these techniques and their optimal usage is still required.

Maintaining skin integrity

Alleviating pressure

The focus of pressure ulcer prevention remains the mitigation of the effects of immobility despite some uncertainty regarding the precise nature of pressure sore aetiology (Clark, 2001). Specifically, this requires reducing the time of weight bearing of the body's bony prominences, through repositioning or using support devices, such as air pressure alleviating mattresses. The latter may also reduce the magnitude of the forces applied during tissue loading. Guidelines from EPUAP (2008) highlight the importance of the following key preventative strategies (see Box 4.2). The new guidelines from EPUAP and the National Pressure Ulcer Advisory Panel (NPUAP) are due to be published soon (www. epuap.org and www.npuap.org, respectively).

The Panel for the Prediction and prevention of Pressure Ulcers in Adults published by the Agency for Health Care Policy and Research (AHCPR) (1992) reflects guidance of US national importance. They recommend that patient repositioning be performed 'at least every 2 hours'. Discussions on the issues related to prevention through patient turning are examined effectively (Clark, 2001). The EPUAP website in 2008 indicated that their own and the AHCPR guidelines remain the current internationally recognised ones available, although they acknowledge these need updating.

Support surfaces such as pressure-relieving beds, mattresses and seat cushions may be used as aids to prevent pressure ulcers both at home and in institutions. The evaluation of pressure-relieving support surfaces has investigated such support systems through a rigorous trial ('PRESSURE') (Nixon *et al.*, 2006) and a Cochrane review (McInnes *et al.*, 2008). The PRESSURE trial undertaken for the Health Technology Assessment

---

Box 4.2 Key pressure ulcer prevention strategies based on EPUAP guidance (1998)

(1) Systematic risk assessment, using tools combined with clinical judgement,

(2) Maintaining and improving tissue tolerance to pressure to prevent injury by conducting skin assessment of the bony prominences and skin condition (dryness, cracking, erythema, maceration, fragility, heat and induration) and optimising the skin's condition (e.g. reducing excessive moisture),

(3) Minimise friction and shear forces through correct positioning and transferring techniques,

(4) Identify nutritionally compromised individuals through assessment and plan for nutritional support to meet individual needs,

(5) Improve the patient's activity level where possible,

(6) Protect against the adverse effects of external mechanical forces: pressure, friction and shear through frequent and correct repositioning and the use of suitable support surfaces, and

(7) Education directed at health professionals, patients, family and caregivers (e.g. teach able patients to redistribute weight every 15 minutes).

---

programme was a multicentre, randomised controlled parallel group trial. They found no difference between alternating pressure mattress replacements and overlays in terms of the patients developing new pressure ulcers (Nixon *et al.*, 2006). However, alternating pressure mattress replacements were found more likely to be cost saving. It is suggested that patient preference can be supported without risk, if they prefer an overlay to a replacement mattress. The review by McInnes *et al.* (2008) aimed to assess the effectiveness of support surfaces in the prevention and treatment of pressure ulcers. They concluded that higher specification foam mattresses should be considered rather than standard hospital foam mattresses. They propose that organisations consider the use of pressure relief for high-risk patients in the operating theatre, as this is associated with a reduction in the post-operative incidence of pressure ulcers. The review also suggests that the evaluation of seat cushions is limited.

Assessing and limiting the effects of incontinence on the skin

Incontinence is identified as a risk factor in many published pressure ulcer assessment tools (Norton *et al.*, 1962; Gosnell, 1973; Waterlow, 1988). Tools such as the Braden Scale (Bergstrom *et al.*, 1987a, b) specify the moisture factor, considering sweat and or incontinence as possible sources. The literature includes analyses of the rigour by which risk can be predicted (e.g. Haalboom *et al.*, 1999). The review by Cullum *et al.* (1995) indicated that such tools have been developed in an *ad hoc* fashion without the use of statistical regression models to choose and weigh the factors that may predict development. As such, their validity remains problematic. Morison (2001) argues that incontinence or moisture may not be a primary factor but rather an indicator of poor physical condition, stating that it has not been identified by prospective cohort studies, which identify key diagnostic factors using multivariate statistics. However, there are indications of the importance of moisture in pressure ulcer risk from some studies (Haalboom *et al.*, 1999). This study revealed that the incontinence factor increased the incidence of pressure ulcers by a factor of 6.2 (Odds Ratio), although the wide 95% confidence interval (2.3–17) revealed the low precision of the point estimate.

The EPUAP (1998) identified incontinence and 'moistness' as key pressure ulcer risk factor and therefore as clinical issues to be managed. Halfens *et al.* (2000) examined the evidence to support the established Braden scale (Bergstrom *et al.*, 1987a, b); analysis revealed that only age and incontinence of urine and/or faeces were related to the external criteria for risk of pressure sore (including non-blanchable oedema and skin loss).

Preventing and minimising iatrogenic effects

Health professionals may adversely disrupt the skin barrier in a range of ways; these may include through poor washing practices, the impact of ADRs on the skin and a lack of adequate pressure-relieving interventions. As washing practice and pressure ulcer prevention are discussed elsewhere, here we will focus on the adverse effects of drugs on the skin and their prevention.

Preventing ADRs

The nature and effects of ADRs have been described earlier. Central to prevention is familiarity with the drugs commonly causing drug eruptions and risk factors such as medication history or medical conditions such as an allergy history and renal or liver impairment that may affect elimination. Other risk factors include new drugs and first doses and contraindicated drugs, which are by definition those drugs where risk of patient harm is high. Assessment is therefore essential with a review of medical and medication history, allergy and the nature of any prior ADRs.

Managing lymphoedema

Evidence suggests that a combination of physical treatments are effective for managing lymphoedema (Ko *et al.*, 1998), although there is limited evidence to identify which components are most important. The key elements include compression using bandaging or garments, massage, exercise and skin care. The international consensus document on lymphoedema management provides an evidence-based guideline on effective service models (Lymphoedema Framework, 2006). The skin care component highlights the importance of maintaining skin integrity and the care management of skin problems to minimise the risk of infection. Whilst the principles are summarised in Box 4.3, the guidelines specify the details.

Vaqas and Ryan (2003) examined the management of lymphoedema in resource-poor settings. Those affected may include people with lymphatic filariasis, which affects up to 40 million people (Global Alliance to Eliminate Lymphatic Filariasis [GAELF]). Vaqas and Ryan highlighted the importance of ankle movement to improve lymph flow, limb elevation to reduce venous pressure in the lower limb and breathing exercises to support clearance of the central lymphatics. The role of skin care has been highlighted – especially maintaining epidermal integrity through careful washing of the skin and use of emollients to help maintain skin barrier integrity which in turn will help to prevent bacterial penetration. This is important given that recurrent inflammatory episodes are a common complication of lymphoedema and correlate with its grade of severity (Pani and Srividya, 1995).

Protecting the skin during radiotherapy

The consensus in the literature is that the severity of skin reactions can be reduced by washing the skin with mild soap or a cleansing agent and moisturising with a light moisturising cream or emollient (e.g. National Breast and Ovarian Cancer Centre, 2008). Mild soaps are typically considered those that are less irritant to the skin

---

Box 4.3   General principles of skin care for lymphoedema management.

- Wash daily using pH neutral soap or a soap substitute and dry thoroughly.
- Ensure skin folds, if present, are clean and dry.
- Monitor for affected and unaffected skin for cuts, abrasions or insect bites, paying specific attention to any areas affected by sensory neuropathy.
- Apply emollients.
- Avoid scented products.

Source: Lymphoedema Framework (2006).

and have reduced levels of irritating additives such as perfumes. Furthermore, patients should also use sunscreen or wear protective clothing, avoid irritants (such as deodorant, perfume, hair dye) and keep the skin folds dry. Trial evidence in the breast cancer context suggests that washing irradiated skin during radiotherapy can be undertaken as it is not associated with increased skin toxicity (Roy *et al.*, 2001). In a key study, Campbell and Illingworth (1992) found no statistically significant difference in the severity reaction between those washing with water alone and those using soap, although skin reactions were worse in patients who were not allowed to wash at all.

A review indicates that two preparations reduce the severity of skin reactions experienced by patients, i.e. sucralfate cream and hyaluronic acid cream (Naylor and Mallett, 2001), however, these may are not now available through the standard formulary (BNF). Furthermore, it is suggested that some cream (non-steroidal water in oil preparations) can limit the effects of radiation. A paper by Leonardi *et al.* (2008) evaluated a cream containing hyaluronic acid (which is a major component of the extracellular matrix of the skin) and shea butter. They found a statistically significant difference with the control vehicle on the severity of skin toxicity, burning and desquamation in favour of the cream, although the small number of patients may limit the study. Hyaluronic acid is the most powerful moisturising agent known because of its significant hygroscopic properties that enable it to attract 1,000 times its weight in water. Shea butter resembles sebum in its fatty acid composition and as such can help to restore skin barrier function, by supporting the skin elasticity and turgidity (Abramovits and Boguniewicz, 2006).

Well and MacBride (2003) gave an excellent summary of radiation skin reactions and their management. They highlight that there is limited data depicting patients' experiences of skin reactions and much conflicting evidence on their prevention and management. The importance of patient information targeting at risk patients is also emphasised on the risks of breakdown and self-care strategies to minimise problems. Those at high risk include people with greater UV

sensitivity, smokers, those with heavier breasts or larger tumours.

Nursing intervention to support behavioural change (prevention) in relation to sun exposure

Despite the significance of skin cancer as a growing health issue, evidence indicates limited knowledge and unsafe sun practices in the UK (Office of National Statistics, 1999). Further research is required to promote and evaluate behavioural change to prevent cancer and promote early detection (National Cancer Research Institute, 2005). The Cancer Research UK *Sunsmart* campaign aims to achieve this by 'action ... to inform and empower patients so that they can play an active role in decisions', but there is limited discussion about delivery models, other than UV awareness campaigns (Department of Health, 2007). Review evidence of primary care prevention proposes caution when drawing from US and Australian strategies (Melia *et al.*, 2000). The Royal College of Physicians' (2007) guidelines on the prevention of skin melanoma highlight the need for sun avoidance and effective sunscreen and clothing use.

The International Cancer Research Portfolio (International Cancer Research Funding Organisations, 2008) highlights US research using an educational preventive intervention with young people. Although sun exposure in children is an important preventable factor since risk develops in childhood (Armstrong and Kricker, 2001) through genetic mutation and learnt risk behaviour, educational intervention with this group remains problematic since adolescents continue to report intentional sun exposure to get a tan (e.g. Melia *et al.*, 2000; Cokkinides *et al.*, 2002). The key risk factors for skin cancer are well established (Gandini *et al.*, 2005; South West Public Health Observatory, 2008); this includes young adults' frequent use of sun beds (Armstrong and Kricker, 2001). A review paper argues prevention is also valuable later in life, especially in people who have heavy exposure to solar radiation in childhood (Armstrong and

Kricker, 2001). Also, achieving attitude and UV protective behavioural change in adults, many of whom will be parents, may result in good practice being passed to children (e.g. parental UV risk behaviour is a predictor of that by young people; Cokkinides *et al.*, 2002). However, adults have received little focused attention in preventive studies.

Using evidence of theory related to effective behaviour change is likely to maximise the effectiveness and efficiency of lifestyle interventions (Berwick *et al.*, 2000; National Institute for Health and Clinical Excellence, 2007). Relevant theories include *Bandura's Construct of Self-efficacy* (Bandura, 1977, 1996) and *Theory of Planned Behaviour* (Ajzen, 1991, 2001). Self-efficacy is derived from Bandura's (1977, 1996) social learning theory, highlighting a person's belief and their capacity to undertake a health behaviour, such as to prevent skin cancer and engage in effective self-examination. A body of research highlights self-efficacy as an important predictor of engagement in healthy behaviours (Havas *et al.*, 1998; Rosal *et al.*, 1998; Clark and Dodge, 1999). The theory of planned behaviour is the most widely applied model of beliefs, attitudes and intentions that precede action (Ajzen 2001; Connor and Sparks, 2005). Both theories are likely to bolster intentions and sustain action.

Nurses are a substantial resource with a potential to deliver effective health education (Latter, 2000; Runciman *et al.*, 2006). Evidence suggests primary care nurses could play an effective role in reducing the risks of cancer by promoting early detection and fast referral (Austoker, 1994; Oliveria *et al.*, 2002). Studies of nurse-led interventions to increase awareness or change behaviour related to cancer have been successful (Koinberg *et al.*, 2004; Sharp and Tischelman, 2005). However, most previous initiatives have been applied in cancer contexts other than skin cancer prevention, with many involving self-examination only (e.g. Oliveria *et al.*, 2002) and limited theoretical underpinning. A nurse-led teaching intervention, using images, can enhance patient skin self-examination (Oliveria *et al.*, 2004); however, this study did not incorporate the evaluation of

education to reduce risk behaviours. A good example of a self-examination guide is that provided by the Wessex Cancer Trust (Hancock, 2007).

A key challenge for nurse-led prevention is to establish how best to raise awareness about skin cancer but in particular change behaviour. A systematic review by Saraiya *et al.* (2004) argues for research focused on health outcome, patient behaviour and examination of the 'role of the non-physician provider to help identify if counselling skills to change behaviour might be better suited to providers with the time and skills, such as a nurse' (p. 444); however, there is little evidence of such studies. Also, resource-efficient models of service delivery are required for primary care–based health promotion. One possibility for consideration is telephone consultation. Nurses have been found to increase patient self-efficacy in targeted telephone interventions with patients (Wong *et al.*, 2005) with systematic review evidence finding them to be safe and acceptable to patients (Bunn *et al.*, 2004).

Details of key health education messages related to skin cancer prevention are given in Chapter 11.

Nutrition to support skin integrity

Requirements of the skin barrier/ nutrients for a healthy skin

The effective structure and functioning of healthy skin is dependent on an adequate level of nutrition. It is evident from the deficiency of certain essential nutrients that certain diseases may arise. This includes, for example, vitamin deficiency such as scurvy due to vitamin C deficiency, which can lead to bleeding gums, easy bruising and sometimes purpura, and pellagra (including dermatitis) due to nicotinic acid (niacin or vitamin B_3) deficiency, which include signs such as dermatitis to sun exposed sites, scaly erythema and hyperpigmentation (Mackie, 2003). Another condition is kwashiorkor that is due to protein malnutrition and leads to dry skin, erythematatous eruption and dry brittle hair. Table 4.2 summarises the key nutrients related to skin health, based on Allen (2000), Dealey (2005) and Patel (2005).

Malnutrition remains a significant problem among outpatients (Neelemaat *et al.*, 2008) and indeed may occur when patients are hospitalised (O'Flynn *et al.*, 2005). Other common forms of malnutrition, such as obesity, are responsible for changes in skin barrier function, sebaceous glands and sebum production, sweat glands, collagen structure and function, wound healing and the microcirculation and are implicated in a wide spectrum of dermatological diseases (Yosipovitch *et al.*, 2007).

When the skin is under stress the demand for nutrients will alter and specific items play an important role in countering disease, such as essential fatty acids (EFA) in eczema and psoriasis and zinc in wound healing (Allen, 2000). Extensive skin inflammation increases its requirements for energy and fluid and for specific nutrients such as folic acid and protein.

Nutritional support is required for the healing of wounds (Dealey, 2005) and may help protect against pressure ulcer development and improve

Table 4.2 Key nutrients related to skin health.

Nutrient	Relevant function	Good sources
Carbohydrate	Energy for fibroblast, macrophage, leucocyte function and collagen synthesis	Wholegrain cereals, potatoes, wholemeal bread
Essential fatty acids (EFAs)	Formation of new cells (cell wall phospholipids), energy formation, skin barrier function	Dairy products, vegetable oil, oily fish, nuts
Minerals		
Zinc	Enzymatic activity – intermediary in metabolism, cell proliferation and epithelisation, collagen synthesis	Meat, wholegrain cereals, cheese
Iron	Collagen synthesis	Meat, eggs, dried fruit
Copper	Collagen synthesis	Shellfish, liver, meat, bread
Protein	Collagen synthesis (about a third of the body's protein), fibroblast proliferation, angiogenesis, immunity	Meat, fish, eggs, cheese, pulses, wholegrain cereals
Vitamin A	Membrane stability, normal growth and differentiation of the epidermis	Leafy vegetables (broccoli, spinach), carrots, apricots, liver
Vitamin B complex including		
B_3 (niacin)	Collagen cross-linking, Enzymatic activity – intermediary in metabolism	Cereal grains, meat, nuts and some fruit and vegetables
B_2 (riboflavin)	Deficiency can cause fissuring and inflammation around the lips/mouth and tongue	
B_6 (pyridoxine)	Amino acid metabolism	
Vitamin C	Enzymatic activity, collagen synthesis, blood vessel maintenance, immunity	Citrus fruit and fresh vegetables
Vitamin D	Cell signalling, keratinocyte proliferation	Solar irradiation of Vitamin D_3 (cholecalciferol) in the skin and some fish (mackerel, tuna and salmon); Cheese, eggs, beef, liver

the rate of healing (Houwing *et al.*, 2003). However, a systematic review suggests that more evidence is required to identify effective dietary interventions (Langer *et al.*, 2003). Nutrition guidelines for pressure ulcers have been developed (Schols and de Jager-v d Ende, 2004).

Preventing skin damage by scratching

Breaking the scratch–itch cycle and behavioural management

A fundamental management problem with eczema is the disruption of the skin barrier due to scratching in response to itch. Itching evokes scratching that further damages the skin leading to more itching, a vicious itch–scratch cycle is established (see Figure 4.1) and therefore breaking this cycle is a primary clinical aim (Hagermark and Wahlgren, 1995).

Behavioural management is a strategy that may help manage damaging habit of the itch–scratch cycle. The key principle of classical conditioning views learning as a behavioural response to itch may take place if it is paired with a positive or aversive stimulus. Cognitive behavioural approaches focus on the ability and intention to change behaviour to the benefit of the individual and others. Habit reversal is a well-established method of eliminating nervous habits and tics, whereby an alternative or competing behaviour was adopted in place of the undesirable behaviour (Azrin and Nunn, 1973). The empirical base emerged from the early studies of Azrin. Classic studies include work on nervous habits in adolescents (Allen, 1998; Rapp *et al.*, 1998); these include small numbers of cases and the use of direct observation techniques.

One the clearest accounts of habit reversal remains that by Bridgett *et al.* (1996) in London, based on the work of Melin, Noren and colleagues in Uppsala Sweden, as cited previously (Noren, 1995). They advise that this does not require a trained behavioural therapist – and as such this technique can be used by those that are delivering dermatology care and could be applied for all ages.

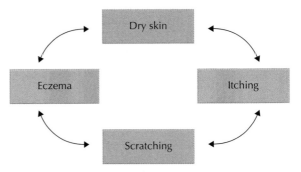

Figure 4.1 The itch–scratch cycle.

Miltenberger *et al.* (1998) provide an overview of the elements of habit reversal and evidence regarding its effectiveness. This paper highlights the mechanisms responsible for its success and its effectiveness in reducing nervous habits, such as scratching, in a replicable way. Research over time has attempted to elucidate the key elements of effectiveness. Miltenberger *et al.* (1998) summarises these three components as follows, as relevant to the parent–child situation.

It comprises of three main elements: awareness raising, introducing a competing response and motivational training to maintain engagement. The book by Bridgett *et al.* (1996) is a useful and detailed practical guide to supporting adults and children with atopic skin disease through habit reversal. The following outline on the nature of training is focused more on supporting the parent and the child, although of course the same principles apply to adult patients.

Awareness training (registration) is concerned with demonstrating the occurrence of the habit and bringing it more closely to the child and parent's attention. This involves helping them to describe the topography of the behaviour, i.e. identifying when it is about to occur and what antecedent factors are most reliably predicting occurrence. One practical way to implement this is to ask parents to keep a scratch diary to record episodes of when their child scratches and any influencing factor that seems to be implicated. The nurse or dermatologists can review this with the parent and child to raise awareness of how their child is responding to the problem of itch.

The next stage (competing response training) involves replacing the damaging behaviour with a new individualised pattern which does not lead to damage to the skin, with the following features: the new behaviour was opposite to the old habit, could be maintained for several minutes and was socially acceptable. Alternative behaviours may include clenching the fists, gently pinching the skin or patting it. The substitute behavioural may be planned as a play activity for children, with a behavioural response linked to a story.

Motivational training involves reviewing all ways in which the habit is inconvenient or embarrassing to the child and parent prompting the child to use competing response and praising and encouraging them when successful.

They emphasise from clinical experience that habit reversal in this application is only successful when individualised and combined with an effective topical treatment. Key to the success of the approach is the person being enabled to manage their own condition. The approach can be delivered as a group approach to improve cost-effectiveness, as illustrated by Ehlers *et al.* (1995); this could be adapted to the setting of a nurse-led clinic. Increasingly, computer-based or multimedia educational programmes will promote behavioural treatment and aid in effective self-management through programmed instruction. This represents an area where there is further scope for development and evaluation research.

Conclusion

This chapter has focused on the topic of universal relevance to nurses and many other health professionals, the need to protect the skin and prevent breakdown. The significance of the skin barrier has been highlighted, including the need to support its structures and functions. The concept of skin vulnerability has been introduced – which conveys the need to understand both biological and behavioural basis of skin vulnerability as a platform for preventing and managing breakdown of the skin barrier;

this we would argue is a fundamental nursing role. The causes of skin breakdown have been outlined followed by the related approaches to its prevention, as the initial therapeutic priority. Attention has also been given to the role of the individual in preventing breakdown, with an examination of the strategies that can be used for the nurse to support appropriate behavioural change. Other therapeutic strategies have been outlined, such as the importance of nutritional support – all of which is within the scope of the nursing role – with opportunities for supporting contributions from other members of the multidisciplinary team.

References

Abramovits, W. and M. Boguniewicz (2006). A multicenter, randomized, vehicle-controlled clinical study to examine the efficacy and safety of MAS063DP (Atopiclair) in the management of mild to moderate atopic dermatitis in adults. *Journal of Drugs in Dermatology*, 5(3): 236–244.

Abrams, P., L. Cardozo, S. Khoury and A. Wein (Eds) (2002). Incontinence: Report of the Second International Consultation on Incontinence, 1–3 July 2002. Paris: Health Publications.

Agency for Health Care Policy and Research (1992). *Pressure Ulcers in Adults: Prediction and Prevention*. A.S.C.P. Guidelines.

Ajzen, I. (1991). The theory of planned behaviour. *Organizational Behavior and Human Decision Processes*, 50: 179–211.

Ajzen, I. (2001). Nature and operation of attitudes. *Annual Review of Psychology*, 52: 27–58.

Allen, B.R. (2000). *Skin, Hair and Nails. Human Nutrition*, pp. 731–746. Edinburgh: Churchill Livingstone.

Allen, K.D. (1998). The use of an enhanced simplified habit-reversal procedure to reduce disruptive outbursts during athletic performance. *Journal of Applied Behavioral Analysis*, 31(3): 489–492.

Allman, R.M. (1986). Pressure sores among hospitalized patients. *Annals of Internal Medicine*, **105**: 337–342.

Aly, R., C. Shirley *et al.* (1978). Effect of prolonged occlusion on the microbial flora, pH, carbon dioxide and transepidermal water loss on human skin. *Journal of Investigative Dermatology*, **71**(6): 378–381.

Armstrong, B.K. and A. Kricker (2001). The epidemiology of UV induced skin cancer. Journal of Photochemistry and Photobiology B, Biology, **63**(1–3): 8–18.

Austoker, J. (1994). Melanoma: Prevention and early diagnosis. *British Medical Journal*, **308**(3944): 1682–1686.

Azrin, K.D. and R.G. Nunn (1973). Habit-reversal: A method of eliminating nervous habits and tics. *Behaviour Research and Therapy*, **11**(4): 19–28.

Bader, D.L. (1990). The recovery characteristics of soft tissues following repeated loading. *Journal of Rehabilitation Research and Development*, **27**(2): 141–150.

Baillie, L. and V. Arrowsmith (2001). *Meeting Elimination Needs. Developing Practical Nursing Skills*. London: Hodder Arnold.

Bandura, A. (1977). *Social Learning Theory*. Englewood Cliffs, New Jersey: Prentice Hall.

Bandura, A. (1996). *Social Foundations of Thought and Action: A Social Cognitive Theory*. Englewood Cliffs, New Jersey: Prentice Hall.

BDNG (British Dermatological Nursing Group) (2008). How to apply a paste bandage, from www.bdng.org.uk/news/patients/How_to_Apply_Paste_BandagesBDNG.pdf.

Bergstrom, N., B.J. Baden *et al.* (1987a). The Braden scale for predicting pressure sore risk. *Nursing Research* **36**: 205–210.

Bergstrom, N., P.J. Demuth *et al.* (1987b). A clinical trial of the Braden scale for predicting pressure sore risk. *Nursing Clinics in North America* **22**(2): 417–428.

Berwick M, Oliveria S, Luo ST, Headley A, Bolognia JL.

Berwick, M., S. Oliveria, S.T. Luo, A. Headley and J.L. Bolognia (2000). A pilot study using nurse education as an intervention to increase skin self-examination for melanoma. *Journal of Cancer Education*, **15**(1): 38–40.

Bridgett, C., P. Noren *et al.* (1996). *Atopic Skin Disease: A Manual for Practitioners*. Petersfiled: Wrightson Biomedical Publishing Limited.

Brown, D.S. and M. Sears (1993). Perineal dermatitis a conceptual framework. *Ostomy/Wound Management*, **39**(7): 20–22, 24–25.

Bunn, F., G. Byrne *et al.* (2004). Telephone consultation and triage: Effects on health care use and patient satisfaction. *Cochrane Database of Systematic Reviews*, **18**(4): CD004180.

Byers, P.H., P.A. Ryan *et al.* (1995). Effects of incontinence care cleansing regimens on skin integrity. *Journal of Wound Ostomy Continence Nursing*, **4**: 187–192.

Campbell, I.R. and M.H. Illingworth (1992). Can patients wash during radiotherapy to the breast or chest wall? A randomised controlled trial. *Clinical Oncology (Royal College of Radiologists)*, **4**: 78–82.

Clark, M. (2001). *Pressure Ulcer Prevention. The Prevention and Treatment of Pressure Ulcers*. Edinburgh, Mosby: M. J. Morison.

Clark, J. and N. Dodge (1999). Exploring self-efficacy as a predictor of disease management. *Health Education and Behavior*, **26**: 72–89.

Cokkinides, V.E., M.A. Weinstock, M.C. O'Connell and M.J. Thun (2002). Use of indoor tanning sunlamps by US youth, ages 11–18 years, and by their parent or guardian caregivers: Prevalence and correlates. *Pediatrics*, **109**(6): 1124–1130.

Connor, M. and P. Sparks (2005). Theory of planned behaviour and health behaviour. In: Connor, M., Sparks, P. (Eds), *Predicting Health Behaviour: Health and Practice with Social Cognition Models*. Maidenhead: Open University.

Cullum, N., J.J. Deeks *et al.* (1995). Preventing and treating pressure sores. *Quality in Health Care*, **4**(4): 289–297.

Darmstadt, G.L., M. Mao-Qiang *et al.* (2002). Impact of tropical oils on the skin barrier: Possible implications for neonatal health in developing countries. *Acta Paediatrica*, **91**(5): 546–554.

Dealey, C. (1995). Pressure sores and incontinence a study evaluating the use of topical agents in skin care. *Journal of Wound Care*, **3**: 103–105.

Dealey, C. (2005). *The Care of Wounds: A Guide for Nurses*. Oxford: Blackwell Publishing.

Department of Health (2000). *Good Practice in Continence Services*. London: Department of Health.

Department of Health (2007). *What the Cancer Reform Strategy means to Patients*. London: Crown.

Devillers, A.C. and A.P. Oranje (2006). Efficacy & safety of wet wrap dressings as an intervention treatment in children with severe and /or refractory atopic dermatitis: A critical review of the literature. *British Journal of Dermatology*, **154**: 579–585.

Ehlers, A., U. Gieler *et al.* (1995). Treatment of atopic dermatitis: A comparison of psychological and dermatological approaches to relapse prevention. *Journal of Consulting and Clinical Psychology*, **63**(4): 624–635.

Ersser, S.J., K. Getliffe *et al.* (2005). A critical review of the inter-relationship between skin vulnerability and urinary incontinence and related nursing intervention. *International Journal of Nursing Studies*, **42**(7): 823–835.

Ersser, S., S. Macguire *et al.* (2007). *Best Practice in Emollient therapy: A Statement for Health Care Professionals*. Aberdeen: A supplement of Dermatological Nursing.

European Pressure Ulcer Advisory Panel (EPUAP) (1998). Pressure Ulcer Prevention Guidelines. Retrieved 23 April 2009 from http://www.epuap.org/glprevention.html.

European Pressure Ulcer Advisory Panel (EPUAP) (2008). Pressure Ulcer Classification. Retrieved 2008 from http://www.puclas.ugent.be/puclas/e/page3480.html.

Fader, M., S. Clarke-O'Neill *et al.* (2003). Management of night-time urinary incontinence in residential settings for older people an investigation into the effects of different pad changing regimes on skin health. *Journal of Clinical Nursing*, **12**: 374–386.

Faergemann, J., R. Aly *et al.* (1983). Skin occlusion effect on *Pityrosporum orbiculare*, skin PCO2, pH, transepidermal water loss, and water content. *Archives of Dermatological Research*, **6**: 383–387.

Fiers, S.A. (1996). Breaking the cycle: The etiology of incontinence dermatitis and evaluating and using skin care products. *Ostomy/Wound Management*, **42**(3): 32–34, 36, 38–40.

Fluhr, J. W., S. Lazzerini *et al.* (1999). Effects of prolonged occlusion on stratum corneum barrier function and water holding capacity. *Skin Pharmacology and Applied Skin Physiology*, **4**: 193–198.

Flyvholm, M.A. (1993). Contact allergens in registered agents for industrial and household use. *British Journal of Industrial Medicine*, **50**: 1043–1050.

Gandini, S., F. Sera *et al.* (2005). Meta-analysis of risk factors for cutaneous melanoma: III. Family history, actinic damage and phenotypic factors. *European Journal of Cancer*, **41**(14): 2040–2059.

Getliffe, K. and M. Dolman (2003). *Promoting Continence: A Clinical and Research Resource*. Edinburgh: Elsevier Science.

Global Alliance to Eliminate Lymphatic Filariasis (GAELF). Retrieved 7 May 2009 from http://www.filariasis.org/.

Gooch, J. (1989). Skin hygiene. *The Professional Nurse*, **5**(1): 13–18.

Goodyear, H.M. and J.I. Harper (2002). Wet wrap dressings for eczema: An effective treatment but not to be misused. *British Journal of Dermatology*, **146**(1): 159.

Goodyear, H.M., K. Spowart *et al.* (1991). 'Wet-wrap' dressings for the treatment of atopic eczema in children. *British Journal of Dermatology*, **125**(6): 604.

Gosnell, P.J. (1973). Assessment tool to identify pressure sores. *Nursing Research* **22**: 55–59.

Gray, M. (2004). Preventing and managing perineal dermatitis: A shared goal for wound and continence care. *Journal of Wound, Ostomy and Continence Nursing*, **3**(1): S2–S11.

Gulralnik, J.M., T.B. Harris *et al.* (1988). Occurrence and predictors of pressure sores in the national health and nutrition examination survey follow-up. *Journal of American Geriatrics Society*, **36**: 807–812.

Haalboom, J.R., J. den Boer *et al.* (1999). Risk-assessment tools in the prevention of pressure ulcers. *Ostomy/Wound Management*, **45**(2): 20–26, 28, 30–34.

Hagermark, O. and C.F. Wahlgren (1995). Treatment of itch. *Seminars in Dermatology*, **14**(4): 320–325.

Halfens, R.J.G., R.M. Achterberg *et al.* (2000). Validity and reliability of the Braden scale and the influence of other risk factors: A multi-centre prospective study. *International Journal of Nursing Studies*, **37**: 313–319.

Hancock, D. (2007). *How to Check Your Skin for Skin Cancer: Skin Examination*. Southampton: Wessex Cancer Trust.

Havas, S., K. Treimen *et al.* (1998). Factors associated with fruit and vegetable consumption among women participating in WIC. *Journal of American Dietetic Association*, **98**: 1141–1148.

Held, E., H. Lund *et al.* (2001). Effects of different moisturizers on SLS-irritated human skin. *Contact Dermatitis*, **44**: 229–234.

Hinchliff, S.M., S.E. Montague *et al.* (2005). *Physiology for Nursing Practice*. Oxford: Bailliere Tindall.

Houwing, R., M. Rozendaal *et al.* (2003). A randomised, double-blind assessment of the effect of nutritional supplementation on the prevention of pressure ulcers in hip-fracture patients. *Clinical Nutrition*, **22**(4): 401–405.

International Cancer Research Funding Organisations (2008). International Cancer Research Portfolio. From http://www.cancerportfolio.org/index.jsp.

Kirsner, R.S. and C.W. Froelich (1998). Soap and detergents understanding their composition and effect. *Ostomy/Wound Management*, **44**(3A Suppl.): 62s–70s.

Kligman, A. (1994). Hydration injury to human skin. In: Elsner, P., Berardesca, E., Mailbach, H. (Eds), *Bioengineering of the Skin: Water and the Stratum Corneum*. Boca Raton: CRC Press.

Ko, D.S.C., R. Lerner *et al.* (1998). Effective treatment of lymphoedema of the extremities. *Archives of Surgery*, **133**: 452–458.

Koinberg, I.L., B. Fridlund *et al.* (2004). Nurse-led follow-up on demand or by a physician after breast cancer surgery: A randomised study. *European Journal of Oncology Nursing*, **8**: 109–117.

Korting, H., M. Kober *et al.* (1987). Influence of repeated washings with soap and synthetic detergents on pH and resident flora of the skin of forehead and forearm. *Acta Dermato-Venerologica*, **67**: 41–47.

Korting, H.C. and O. Braun-Falco (1996). The effect of detergents on skin pH and its consequences. *Clinics in Dermatology*, **14**: 23–27.

Langer, G., G. Schloemer *et al.* (2003) Nutritional interventions for preventing and treating pressure ulcers. *Cochrane Database of Systematic Reviews*, **4**: CD003216 (DOI: 10.1002/14651858).

Latter, S., P. Yerrell, J. Rycroft-Malone and D. Shaw (2000). Nursing, medication education and the new policy agenda: The evidence base. *International Journal of Nursing Studies*, **37**(6): 469–479.

Leonardi, M.C., S. Gariboldi *et al.* (2008). A double-blind, randomised, vehicle-controlled clinical study to evaluate the efficacy of MAS065D in limiting the effects of radiation on the skin: Interim analysis. *European Journal of Dermatology*, **18**(3): 317.

Lymphoedema Framework (2006). *Best Practice for the Management of Lymphoedema. International Consensus*. London: MEP Ltd.

Mackie, R.M. (2003). *Clinical Dermatology* (5th edition). Oxford: Oxford University Press.

Martin, E. and T. McFerran (2008). *A Dictionary of Nursing*. Aylesbury, England: Aylesbury Market House Books Ltd.

McGeown, J.G. (2002). *Physiology*. Edinburgh: Churchill Livingstone.

McInnes, E., S.E.M. Bell-Syer *et al.* (2008) Support surfaces for pressure ulcer prevention. *Cochrane Database of Systematic Reviews*, **4**: CD001735 (DOI: 10.1002/14651858).

Melia, J., L. Pendrey *et al.* (2000). Evaluation of primary prevention initiatives for skin cancer: A review from a UK perspective. *British Journal of Dermatology*, **143**: 701–708.

Miltenberger, R.G., R.W. Fuqua *et al.* (1998). Applying behaviour analysis to clinical problems: Review and analysis of habit reversal. *Journal of Applied Behaviour Analysis*, **31**(3): 447–469.

Moffatt, C.J., P.J. Franks *et al.* (2003). Lymphoedema: An underestimated health problem. QJM, **96**(10): 731–738.

Morison, M.J., Ed. (2001). *The Prevention and Treatment of Pressure Ulcers*. Edinburgh: Mosby.

Nach, S., J. Close *et al.* (1981). Skin friction coefficient changes induced by skin hydration and emollient application and correlation with perceived skin feel. *Journal of the Society of Cosmetic Chemists*, **32**: 5565.

National Audit Office (2001). *Tackling Obesity in England*. London: The Stationery Office.

National Breast and Ovarian Cancer Centre (2008). *Skin Care during Radiotherapy*. Australia: NBOCC.

National Cancer Research Institute (2005). *Strategic Plan 2005–2008*. London, NCRI.

National Institute for Health and Clinical Excellence (2007). *The Most Appropriate means of Generic and Specific Interventions to Support Attitude and Behaviour Change at Population and Community Levels*. London: NICE.

Naylor, W. and J. Mallett (2001). Management of acute radiotherapy induced skin reactions: A literature review. *European Journal of Oncology Nursing*, **5**: 221–233.

Neelemaat, F., H.M. Kruizenga *et al.* (2008). Screening malnutrition in hospital outpatients. Can the SNAQ malnutrition screening tool also be applied to this population? *Clinical Nutrition*, **27**(3): 439–446.

Nixon, J. (2001). The pathophysiology and aetiology of pressure ulcers. In: Morison, M.J. (Ed.), *The Prevention and Treatment of Pressure Ulcers*. Edinburgh: Mosby.

Nixon, J., E.A. Nelson *et al.* (2006). Pressure relieving support surfaces: A randomised evaluation. *Health Technology Assessment*, **10**(22): iii.

Noren, P. (1995). Habit reversal – a turning point in the treatment of atopic dermatitis. *Clinical and Experimental Dermatology*, **20**(1): 2–5.

Norton, D., R. McLaren *et al.* (1962). *An Investigation of Geriatric Nursing Problems in Hospital*. Edinburgh, Churchill Livingstone.

O'Flynn, J., H. Peake *et al.* (2005). The prevalence of malnutrition in hospitals can be reduced: The results from three consecutive cross-sectional studies. *Clinical Nutrition*, **24**(6): 1078–1088.

Office of National Statistics (1999). Attitudes to protecting self from sun exposure: By gender. Social Trends 32. From http://www.statistics.gov.uk/StatBase/ssdataset.asp?vlnk=5238&Pos=3&ColRank=2&Rank=272.

Oliveria, S.A., J.F. Altman *et al.* (2002). Use of nonphysician health care providers for skin cancer screening in the primary care setting. *Preventive Medicine* **34**(3): 374–379.

Oliveria, S.A., S.W. Dusza *et al.* (2004). Patient adherence to skin self-examination – Effect of nurse intervention with photographs. *American Journal of Preventive Medicine*, **26**(2): 152–155.

Pani, S.P. and A. Srividya (1995). Clinical manifestations of bancroftian filariasis with special reference to lymphoedema grading. *Indian Journal of Medical Research*, **102**: 114–118.

Patel, G.K. (2005). The role of nutrition in the management of lower extremity wounds. *The Journal of Lower Extremity Wounds*, **4**(1): 12–22.

Perry, S., C. Shaw *et al.* (2002). The prevalence of faecal incontinence in adults aged 40 years or more living in the community. *Gut*, **50**(4): 480–484.

Porock, S. and L. KristJanson (1999). Skin reactions during radiotherapy for breast cancer: The use and impact of topical agents and dressings. *European Journal of Cancer Care*, **8**(3): 143–153.

Rapp, J., R.G. Miltenberger *et al.* (1998). Simplified habit reversal treatment for chronic hair pulling in three adolescents: A clinical application with direct observation. *Journal of Applied Behavior Analysis*, **31**: 299–302.

Rosal, M.C., J.K. Ockene *et al.* (1998). Coronary Artery Smoking Intervention Study (CASIS): 5 year follow up. *Health Psychology*, **1**(7): 476–478.

Roy, I., A. Fortin *et al.* (2001). The impact of skin washing with water and soap during breast irradiation: A randomized study. *Radiotherapy and Oncology*, **58**(3): 333–339.

Royal College of Physicians (2007). *The Prevention, Diagnosis, Referral and Management of Melanoma of the Skin: Concise Guidance to Good Practice. Number 7 Clinical Standards: Royal College of Physicians and British Association of Dermatologists*. London: Royal College of Physicians.

Runciman, P., H. Watson *et al.* (2006). Community nurses' health promotion work with older people. *Journal of Advanced Nursing*, **55**(1): 46–57.

Ryan, T.J. (2008). *Healthy Skin for All: A Multi-faceted Approach*. Oxford: Parchment Press.

Saraiya, M., K. Glanz *et al.* (2004). Interventions to prevent skin cancer by reducing exposure to ultraviolet radiation: A systematic review. *American Journal of Preventive Medicine*, **27**(5): 422–466.

Schnelle, J.F., G.M. Adamson *et al.* (1997). Skin disorders and moisture in incontinent nursing home residents intervention implications. *Journal of American Geriatrics Society*, **45**: 1182–1188.

Schols, J.M.G.A. and M.A. de Jager-v d Ende (2004). Nutritional intervention in pressure ulcer guidelines: An inventory. *Nutrition*, **20**(6): 548–553.

Shannon, M.L. and P. Skorga (1989). Pressure ulcer prevalence in two general hospitals. *Decubitus*, **2**(4): 38–43.

Sharp, L. and C. Tischelman (2005). Smoking cessation for patients with head and neck cancer. *Cancer Nursing*, **28**(3): 226–235.

South West Public Health Observatory (2008). Factsheet No 2: Malignant Melanoma in the South West. ICD-10: C43, 15 September 2005 (date created) from http://www.swpho.nhs.uk/.

Strong, D. (1998). Dermatologic Emergencies. Dermatologic Nursing Essentials: A Core Curriculum. New Jersey: Anthony J. Jannetti.

The National Prescribing Centre (1998). MeReC bulletin. Prescribing new drugs in general practice. *Liverpool*, **9**: 21–24.

Tsai, T.F. and H.I. Maibach (1999). How irritant is water? An overview. *Contact Dermatitis*, **41**: 311–314.

Tucker, S., I. Turesson *et al.* (1984). Evidence of individual differences in the radiosensitivity of human skin. *International Journal of Radiation Oncology Biology Physics*, **10**: 607–618.

Vaqas, B. and T.J. Ryan (2003). Lymphoedema: Pathophysiology and management in resource-poor settings – relevance for lymphatic filariasis control programmes. *Filiaria Journal*, **2**: 4.

Walmsley, D. and P.G. Wiles (1990). Reactive hyperemia in the skin of the human foot measured by laser doppler flowmetry – effects of duration of ischemia and local heating. *International Journal of Microcirculation – Clinical and Experimental*, **9**(4): 345–355.

Waterlow, J. (1988). The Waterlow card for the prevention and management of pressure sores: Towards a patient policy. *Care Science and Practice*, **6**(1): 8–12.

Well, M. and S. MacBride (2003). Radiation skin reactions. In: Faithfull, S., Wells, M. (Eds), *Supportive Care in Radiotherapy*, pp. 135–159. Edinburgh: Churchill Livingstone.

Whittingham, K. (1998). Cleansing regimens for continence care. *Professional Nurse*, **3**: 167–172.

Wong, K., F.K. Wong *et al.* (2005). Effects of nurse-initiated telephone follow-up on self-efficacy among patients with chronic obstructive pulmonary disease. *Journal of Advanced Nursing*, **49**(2): 210–222.

Yosipovitch, G., A. DeVore *et al.* (2007). Obesity and the skin: Skin physiology and skin manifestations of obesity. *Journal of the American Academy of Dermatology*, **56**(6): 901–916.

Emollients 5

Rebecca Penzer

Introduction

Throughout human history it is possible to find references to the use of emollients. Ancient Egyptians used sesame, almond and olive oils to anoint their skin and to care for the wigs that were fashionable at the time. Natural oils were also used to perfume these. Cleopatra famously bathed in asses' milk believing that it would be good for her skin. Lanolin, extracted from sheep wool, was widely used as an emollient in medieval Europe. In 1872 a patent was filed for 'Vaseline', a product which 140 years later is still immensely successful. Today there are a myriad of cosmetic emollients available, all making various claims towards creating or maintaining youthful looks in the user. The choice of medicinal emollients is also extensive. The British National Formulary lists at least 34 topical emollient products (this does not include the bath oils), which can make selecting a suitable product something of a challenge (British Medical Association and Royal Pharmaceutical Society of Great Britain, 2007) (see Appendix 3 for list of emollients). This chapter will explore what emollients are and how they work, it will also provide some practical guidance for

selecting and using emollients to ensure that they are being used to best therapeutic effect.

Definition

A standard definition for emollients is not widely available, although they are commonly referred to as substances that '...reduce the signs and symptoms of dry, scaly skin, making the rough surface soft and smooth' (Kligman, 2000). This definition does not, perhaps, do justice to the complex nature of emollients. Not only are modern day formulations complex, but their effects are numerous and generally not entirely understood (Marks, 2001). Their usefulness is well recognised by those who work in the field of dermatology; however, there is little good science to back up how they should be used, although increasingly scientific attention is being given to how they work.

Often the words moisturiser and emollient are used synonymously. The British National Formulary makes no distinction between the two. However, some sources do differentiate between an emollient and a moisturiser; these differences are discussed here.

The New Zealand online dermatology resource, Dermnet NZ, refers to an emollient as a substance that softens the skin and a moisturiser as one which adds moisture (www.dermnet.nz). Voegeli (2007) suggests that the following distinctions should be made:

■ Emollients are lipids that occlude the skin surface thus preventing water loss from the stratum corneum.
■ Moisturisers are lipid emulsions that actively hydrate the skin by the application of a humectant to the skin surface (often glycol or urea). Humectants are water loving and draw water from the dermis into the epidermis thus hydrating it.

It is worth noting that some products have emollient properties only and some have both emollient and moisturising properties. In this book, the word emollient will be used to refer to products that soften the skin by increasing the level of moisture in the stratum corneum, i.e. an emollient moisturises the skin. The mechanisms for this are discussed later in this chapter.

Constituents of emollients

Emollient products are composed of a variety of constituent substances. Broadly speaking these can be divided into active ingredients and excipients. Active ingredients are those ingredients that exert a therapeutic benefit. Excipients can be described as the ingredients that allow the product to be effective but have no direct therapeutic benefit themselves. They will include preservatives and emulsifiers. Manufacturers are obliged to list the active ingredients and excipients of their products. It is worth noting that this listing does not always highlight the potential sensitisers within a product. For example, emulsifying wax contains cetostearyl alcohol which is a potential sensitiser. On products, only emulsifying wax will be listed. In general the British National Formulary will highlight when a product has a potential sensitiser in it. Other common constituents and their purpose are listed in Table 5.1.

Emollients will always have some level of lipid in them. Lipid is a broad term used to describe different types of waxes, oils and fats (Marks, 2001). Oils are the most common lipids found in emollient products; these include vegetable oils such as sunflower oil, mineral oils such as petrolatum or synthetic man-made oils such as polysiloxane. The only animal fat that is regularly used is lanolin.

Lanolin (also known as a wool alcohol or a wool wax) is extracted from sheep's wool. It is excreted by the sheep's sebaceous glands and keeps the fleece soft whilst also protecting it from the elements. Historically, it has a reputation for being highly allergenic. Whilst this may have been of some concern in the past, modern extraction and purification methods mean that lanolin has a very low incidence of sensitisation and should not be considered a common allergen (Stone, 2000; British Medical Association and Royal Pharmaceutical Society of Great Britain, 2007).

There is evidence to show that lanolin is an effective emollient. This is summarised by Harris and Hoppe (2000) who report a number of studies. These suggested that lanolin:

■ Reduces transepidermal water loss in xerotic skin and has long-term effects (up to 14 days after 21 days of application);
■ Restores barrier function in normal skin that has been perturbed by acetone;
■ Can act as a barrier to virus particles and irritants;
■ Increases the rate of re-epithelisation;
■ Decreases levels of skin roughness for up to 8 hours after application (Harris and Hoppe, 2000).

Lipids may be mixed with differing amounts of water to produce the various consistencies of emollient. The absolute quantity of water and the amount relative to the level of lipid present will affect the consistency and efficacy of the product. Therefore, products with high lipid content (and no water) will tend to be greasy and heavy whilst those with low lipid content (and high levels of water) will be less greasy and lighter. Most cosmetic emollients (usually

Table 5.1 Potential sensitisers as listed in BNF and found as excipients in emollients.

Excipient	Property
Benzyl alcohol	Preservative
Butylated hydroxyanisole	Preservative
Butylated hydroxytoluene	
Cetostearyl alcohol (including cetyl and stearyl alcohol)	Has moisturising properties (and emulsifying properties)
Chlorocresol	Preservative
Edetic acid (EDTA)	Improves product stability towards the air
Fragrances	To make a product smell pleasant or to mask unpleasant odours
Hydroxybenzoates (parabens)	Preservative
Imidurea	Preservative
Isopropyl palmitate	Thickening agent
N-(3-Chloroallyl)hexaminium chloride (quaternium 15)	Preservative
Polysorbates	Emulsifier
Sodium metabisulphite	Preservative
Propylene glycol	Humectant, preservative and stabiliser
Wool fat and related substances including lanolin (*not generally thought of as excipient, but rather an active ingredient*)	Emollient
Sorbic acid	Preservative

lotions) have a high water content, which ensures that they sink into the skin quickly without leaving greasy traces. However they are less effective at retaining water in the skin than their greasier counterparts, creams and ointments.

Potential side effects

Emollients are commonly thought to have few side effects and it is true that generally patients can use these products without fear of unwanted outcomes. However, there are some factors that it is important to be aware of.

Contact dermatitis

Contact dermatitis is the term given to adverse inflammatory changes that occur in the skin when it comes into contact with certain products. Patients will sometimes complain of transient stinging or discomfort when a product is applied. This is not unusual and may be caused by the application of a substance to inflamed and broken skin rather than by any true sensitivity. This cannot be described as a true contact dermatitis. However, if the discomfort is more than just transient it may represent a true contact dermatitis; in other words, the patient is experiencing an irritant or allergic reaction to some ingredient within the product.

An allergic contact dermatitis is an immune-mediated response to a product; once the patient has been sensitised they will react to the product even if they come into contact with only a small amount of it. The severity of the reaction may increase if exposure to the allergen is increased. The reaction may be immediate or can be delayed for 48–96 hours after the contact (Nicol *et al.*, 1995). An immediate response is known as a Type 1 or an IgE-mediated response. It can be mild or in severe cases the individual may go into anaphylactic shock. A delayed response is known as a Type 4 or T-cell-mediated response.

In contrast an irritant contact dermatitis is a non-immune-mediated reaction where the skin reacts immediately or within hours. The adverse response can occur after a period of cumulative use, e.g. after frequent hand washing. In this instance no response is seen initially, but repeated use of a product causes inflammation. Alternatively, an irritant contact response can occur immediately after contact with a substance.

If a contact dermatitis is suspected, patch testing may be an appropriate way to investigate the precise cause of the inflammation (see Chapter 9 for further details on patch testing). Whilst this process may be able to determine the nature of the allergen or irritant, it may then be almost impossible to determine whether it is present in commercial preparations.

It is most common for the excipients to act as sensitisers rather than the active ingredients themselves. Common irritants/allergens include perfumes and preservatives (de Groot, 2000). It is thought that for around 1% of the population, fragrances act as sensitisers and that for those with eczema this percentage increases to around 14% (de Groot, 2000). It is good practice, therefore, to recommend that people with sensitive skin use products that are truly fragrance free. It can be difficult to find absolutely fragrance-free products as many contain masking fragrances. Most prescribable products in the UK are fragrance free.

In order to reduce the impact of any potential adverse reactions when applying emollients, patients should be advised to apply a small 'test patch' to an area of their body (the inner arm is a good place to use). This should be left for 48 hours; if no adverse reaction is seen, the product is most likely to be safe to use extensively.

Another issue when considering potential adverse effects of emollients is the importance of using the product correctly, both the correct amount and in the correct way. For example a product that is used extensively in a way that it was not designed for, is aqueous cream. Originally designed as a wash product (i.e. to be applied to the skin as a soap substitute and then washed off), it has become a commonly used leave-on emollient. For many people this does not create any problems, although it is not a particularly effective emollient for those with dry skin. However, Cork *et al.* carried out an audit which showed that when aqueous cream was used as a leave-on product for children with eczema, it caused a significantly higher level of stinging and discomfort than other emollient products (Cork *et al.*, 2003). Interestingly, the same audit showed that when aqueous cream was used as a wash product, it did not cause the same level of adverse reactions, and was an acceptable product. This audit emphasises the importance of using products in the way that they were designed for; this will help reduce adverse reactions.

Adverse effects caused by the occlusive nature of emollients

Greasy topical emollients can result in painful pustules caused by the blockage and consequent infection of the hair follicle; this is known as folliculitis. This can usually be avoided by correct application of emollients, i.e. in the direction of the lie of the hair. Changing the emollient to a lighter, less greasy one may be enough to resolve the problem; if not it may be necessary to stop emollient application for a time until the folliculitis resolves. Occasionally, topical or even oral antibiotics may be needed. If there is a high bacterial load on the skin caused by poor hygiene, folliculitis may be more likely if an occlusive emollient is applied. This will be aggravated further by hot, humid climatic conditions.

In dry, hot environments occlusive emollients may reduce heat loss through the skin. The lipids act as an insulator decreasing evaporation from the skin and thus affecting thermoregulation. This may be particularly important in small children who have a high surface area to volume ratio. In an adult or older child, thick occlusive emollients may feel very uncomfortable in hot weather. So choosing a lighter, less greasy emollient is preferable.

Other safety concerns

Emollients of all types, but particularly bath oils and soap substitutes, can make the skin and the bath or shower feel slippery. Caution needs to be taken especially with vulnerable groups like babies and older people to prevent accidents.

Another potential safety concern involves the flammability of paraffin-based emollients when they are soaked into a fabric. Thus dressings or clothing that have absorbed quantities of emollients that are primarily paraffin based (which includes most ointments) are at risk of catching fire if they come into contact with a naked flame. Patients should be advised not to smoke or come into contact with any type of flame if they are wearing paraffin-soaked garments or bandages (British Medical Association and Royal Pharmaceutical Society of Great Britain, 2007).

Emollient formulations

In order to ensure the maximum impact of emollients, it has become common practice to use them at every stage of the skin-care process. This means that there are emollient cleansers, emollient bath additives and topical emollients which are left on the skin (Holden *et al.*, 2002). These three elements are often collectively referred to as 'total emollient therapy'. This section will give an overview of the available emollient formulations.

Bath additives

These are liquid, lipid products usually based on liquid paraffin but may be formulated using vegetable oils such as soya. When added to water, they are dispersible and therefore appropriate for use within washing water. Their primary aim is to form a thin layer of oil over the surface of the skin thus helping to rehydrate it. Most will also cleanse the skin thus removing the need for further skin cleansing products.

Method of application

A quantity, as identified by the manufacturer, should be added to the wash water and the water then agitated to ensure the product is dispersed properly. Some bath additives can be used directly onto the skin in the shower, although clearly it is much harder to measure the amount used. This may be important in the case of an antibacterial bath product as it may be irritant if overused. There is little independent research evidence that proves the therapeutic benefit of bath emollients (Drugs and Therapeutics Bulletin, 2007); however, patients may find them helpful and some company-funded research does suggest they are beneficial (Bettzuege-Pfaff and Melzer, 2005).

Many of the greasier ointment emollients (e.g. emulsifying ointment) can also be added to bath water. They must first be dissolved in hot water and then added to a bath of normal temperature water. It may not disperse as well as a trade name bath additive but there is no evidence to suggest it is any more or less effective.

Most bath additive products will make the bath and the person who has been immersed in them, slippery.

Skin cleansers

For most people with dry skin conditions and certainly for those who have eczema, using soap is not recommended. Soap works by removing natural oils from the skin and with those oils go the debris that builds up on the skin over a day. This will cause those with a dry skin to become even drier. Therefore, skin cleansers should be used instead of soap. Rather than stripping the skin off their natural oils, skin cleansers (also known as soap substitutes) help to trap moisture in the skin, whilst removing the surface dirt.

Box 5.1   Amounts of emollient measured in spoonfuls

A formal topical regime of emollient would be, for example, 10 g to each of the following areas:

Each arm
The chest
The abdomen
Each thigh
Each shin
Upper back
Lower back
2 g to the face
10 g is the equivalent of a desert spoonful. If someone is less dry, the same ratios should be used by 5 g (a teaspoon) per area or 20 g (a tablespoon) per area if more dry.

---

who gives three possible regimes as guidance (Britton, 2003) (see Box 5.1). This is particularly helpful when explaining to patients as it may be easier for them to understand measures such as spoonfuls rather than grams or millilitres. Custom and practice has become that an adult with a dry skin condition should use around 500 g of topical emollient a week and a child should get through 250 g per week. This is only guidance and really only serves to ensure that patients with dry skin conditions are not prescribed quantities less than 500 g (unless it is for the convenience of having a smaller quantity to carry around.)

How frequently to apply emollients?

The usual advice for patients with a dry skin condition is to apply a topical emollient at least twice daily. Better advice is to apply emollients to the skin whenever it gets dry, which in reality may be every 2 hours. This is likely to be impractical for most people, so the patient needs to be able to experiment with emollients to find the one that suits them best and hydrates the skin most effectively without too many

compromises in terms of impact on quality of life. It is generally thought that greasier emollients are effective for a longer period of time than creams and gels, but this will depend to some extent on the individual.

When to apply emollients?

It is generally agreed that an optimal time to apply emollients is after a bath. This helps to trap water into the stratum corneum and the warmth of the skin makes applying emollients easier. The trapping of moisture in the skin can be enhanced if the skin is left slightly damp after washing. Whilst it is important that flexures are well dried, to prevent intertrigo, the rest of the skin can be left slightly moist and emollients then applied. This process of 'soaking and sealing' moisture into the skin is key in helping rehydrate the skin (Nicol and Boguniewicz, 2008). To reduce the likelihood of the skin becoming very dry overnight, it is always advisable to apply emollient just before going to bed.

There is considerable debate about when to apply emollients in relation to other topical products, particularly topical steroids which are used for patients who have eczema. It is agreed that emollients are of key importance in the treatment of eczema (Akdis *et al.*, 2006); the debate centres around when they should be applied. A number of authors have shown that use of emollients appears to reduce the amount of topical steroid needed to control eczema (Watsky *et al.*, 1992; Lucky *et al.*, 1997; Hanifin *et al.*, 1998; Grimalt *et al.*, 2007). However, these are in no way universally accepted findings. Using biological principles, some would argue that applying an emollient prior to a steroid may reduce its efficacy. The argument used is that the emollient saturates the layers of the stratum corneum preventing effective penetration of the topical steroid to the deeper layers and therefore reducing its efficacy. Currently no robust clinical data exists to support or disprove this point.

Where does this leave the practitioner who is caring for someone with eczema who is using emollients and topical steroids? If an emollient is applied prior to a steroid, consideration should be given to how long it is given to 'soak' into the skin before a steroid is applied. The timing will vary, but it is generally accepted that the skin should be tacky but not slippery. Around 30 minutes is usually long enough for this to have happened, but may need to be up to an hour. Similar thoughts should be given to the circumstances around applying a steroid before an emollient. If a steroid is not allowed to sink in properly concerns around diluting the effect of the steroid or smearing onto parts of the body where it is not required may be valid, although Smoker could not find any evidence to back up these concerns (Smoker, 2007). If occlusion is to be applied over topical treatments allowing a time period to elapse may be less important. In the case of wet wrapping for example, applying topical steroid to the areas that need it and then applying emollient elsewhere is a sensible approach (see Chapter 9 for further detail).

In other disease areas like psoriasis, the evidence is even weaker as to the order in which to apply treatments. One unpublished experiment reported by Finlay suggested that the use of emollient improved outcomes for patients treated with dithranol (Finlay, 1997). Whilst it is generally accepted that emollients are helpful adjuvants for the treatment of psoriasis (National Institute for Clinical Excellence, 2001; Hall, 2003), their exact use is hardly explored at all in the literature (Penzer, 2005).

In conclusion, all it is possible to say categorically is that the lack of evidence in this field makes definitive recommendations for practice in this area difficult. The general principles that should guide practice include:

(a) Applying active topical medications (e.g. steroids) to well-moisturized skin, is generally preferable than applying them to dry skin;

(b) Around 30 minutes should elapse between applying an emollient and an active topical medication. The exact time period will depend upon how dry the skin is and how greasy the emollient;

(c) If both emollient and topical steroid have to go on at the same time, applying the steroid to the inflamed areas and the emollient everywhere else is acceptable;

(d) If products are being applied under occlusive bandages or dressings, it is probably less important for there to be a gap between the active topical medication and the emollient.

How to apply emollients?

The literature in general agrees that emollients should be applied using a gentle stroking motion following the lie of the hair on the body. This said, no specific scientific evidence could be found to back this up. The rationale for this is based on a biological principle that rubbing the skin with a greasy emollient could lead to an irritated or blocked hair follicle and the resulting folliculitis (see the section on potential side effects). The only possible exception to this is when an emollient is being used as part of another therapeutic process, e.g. lymphatic drainage massage. In these instances, going against the lie of the hair may be necessary; it is generally recommended to use a lighter, less greasy emollient in this case as these are less likely to adversely affect the hair follicle.

Most cream emollients now come in pump dispensers, which makes their use much more straightforward. It also prevents potential contamination caused by the introduction of debris (especially skin scales) when a hand is put into a pot. If a pump dispenser is not available, emollient should be taken out of a pot using a clean spoon or a spatula. Individuals should be encouraged not to share pots to maintain infection control.

Where to apply the emollient?

Whilst the answer to this may seem obvious, it is always worth clarifying with patients that emollient can be applied all over the skin without any adverse side effects. If the dry skin is very localized, then application to just those areas may be acceptable, but often dry skin is diffuse and a general all over application is recommended.

There is a lot to remember to tell a patient about using emollients. Box 5.2 is a checklist to act as an aide memoir to make sure that everything is covered. The order the list is written in here may not suit you or your patient; as

> ### Box 5.2   Aide memoir for discussing emollient use with patients
>
> (1) Why emollients are important and how they work?
> (2) How much to use (described in a way that the patient can understand, but spoonfuls may be helpful)?
> (3) When to apply an emollient and in particular emphasise the importance of applying after bathing?
> (4) Where to apply the emollient?
> (5) How to apply the emollient?
> (6) When to apply emollients in relation to the other topical treatments that they are using?
> (7) Health and safety issues;
> (8) Which emollient they will use and whether they need more than one for different times of the day?

long as everything is covered (and makes sense to the patient) the order is not that important. Appendix 3 might be helpful as it lists available emollients in Britain.

How emollients work?

The science of emollient therapy is constantly developing. This reflects an increased understanding of what happens at a cellular level when an individual experiences dry skin or a dry skin condition. For an in-depth look at emollients, their chemistry and function, Loden and Maibach's book provides an excellent, detailed overview (Loden and Maibach, 2000).

Skin becomes dry for two main reasons:

(a) Natural moisture from within the stratum corneum is lost due to barrier dysfunction.
(b) The natural moisturising lipids that are normally found within the skin are for some reason deficient.

The level of water in the epidermis is greater at the interface with the dermis and is least in the stratum corneum. The natural lipids (mainly ceramides) which are found in the intercellular spaces of the epidermis impede the movement of the water from the deeper layers to the stratum corneum. When there is a deficiency of these natural lipids, the movement of water is less effectively impeded and therefore more readily lost from the surface of the skin.

Because the outer layer of the stratum corneum contains only approximately 10% water, any reduction in this quantity causes the skin to loose its flexibility (Marks, 2001). When water is lost from the stratum corneum, the corneocytes become shrivelled, shrink and gaps in between them develop. These gaps allow further moisture and natural lipid to 'escape' leading to even drier skin. The analogy that is often used is a brick wall. The corneocytes are the 'bricks' which in normal skin are held together with 'cement', i.e. the natural lipids. As soon as either the 'bricks' or 'cement' are compromised, the impermeable, smooth structure of the skin is affected and it becomes dry. It feels rough, often sore and itchy. More detail is given about how dry skin manifests itself in specific dry skin conditions in Chapters 8 (psoriasis) and 9 (eczema).

Desquamation, the loss of skin cells from the surface of the skin, is also thought to be an important factor in skin dryness. Normally corneocytes are shed from the skin surface singly. At the correct point in time (i.e. at the skin surface), they lose the binding forces that hold them together and shed in such a manner that is not visible to the naked eye. However, in dry scaly conditions, the corneocytes 'stick' together and shed in a way that is visible to the naked eye. Emollients seem to correct this problem. One suggested mechanism is that water trapped in the skin by emollients activates an enzyme which breaks the desmosomal contacts that keep corneocytes stuck to one another (Marks, 2001). In doing this, corneocytes are shed normally again.

In order to increase the level of water in the skin, emollients exert an occlusive or humectant effect, or both depending on their constituents.

Occlusive effect of emollients

Lipids have an occlusive effect, trapping natural moisture into the skin by mimicking the role played by sebum. Transepidermal water loss is reduced particularly when greasy emollients with a high level of lipid, for example liquid paraffin, are used (Rawlings *et al.*, 2004).

Humectant effects of emollients

Humectants are substances which attract water. The dermis has a high level of water in it (70% of the dermis is water). Thus when humectant substances such as urea and glycerine are added to emollients and then applied to the skin, they attract water from the dermis into the epidermis thus helping to rehydrate it. In this way, they mimic the role of natural moisturising factor (NMF). NMF is comprised of a group of humectant substances (e.g. pyrrolidone carboxylic acid) which occur naturally within the upper epidermis. Because of its water-loving properties, NMF is responsible for maintaining water in this part of the epidermis (Marks, 2001). An emollient containing humectants can only be effective if it also contains an occlusive substance such as soft paraffin. Without this the water drawn into the epidermis would not be trapped there and would be lost transepidermally.

Although not particularly well understood, it does appear to be the case that emollients have an antimitotic, anti-inflammatory and antipruritic properties.

Antimitotic effects of emollients

An experimental study on mice whose skin had been stimulated through tape stripping showed that application of emollient decreased the mitotic activity in the epidermis (Tree and Marks, 1975). The authors suggested this may have been due to either repair of the barrier function of the skin or a reduction in prostaglandin synthesis which is caused by use of emollients high in petrolatum.

Anti-inflammatory effects of emollients

Studies in the field of eczema have shown that even minor damage to the skin (through scratching) can cause the release of powerful inflammatory agents such as IL-1α. Wood *et al.* showed that by occluding tape stripped skin with polythene, release of IL-1α could be prevented (Wood *et al.*, 1996) and Cork speculated that this action is replicated when a layer of occlusive emollient is applied to the skin (Cork, 1997).

On a practical note, it is worth noting that the physical motion of applying the emollient can make the skin look more inflamed. Two mechanisms are possible. Firstly, whilst vigorous rubbing in of emollients is to be avoided, the very process of emollient application can increase blood flow to the skin surface which mimics the appearance of inflammation. Secondly, if the skin is scaly this will cover up the underlying inflammation and make the skin look a duskier colour. As an emollient will help to reduce the level of scale, it may, in turn, make the skin look more inflamed when it is applied to the skin. Patients should be reassured in both instances that the emollient is not causing further inflammation.

Antipruritic effects of emollients

Experience shows that applying emollients to dry, itchy skin usually provides some transient relief (even those without specific antipruritic agents in them). Emollients containing high levels of water may be more relieving as there is a cooling effect caused by water from the product evaporating from the skin.

Effects of added active ingredients to emollients

A number of different effects can be created by adding further substances to a basic emollient base.

Anti-infective agents: Whilst independent evidence for the impact of anti-infective agents is hard to come by, it would appear that these products do reduce the bacterial load on the skin which can be very helpful for people who suffer recurrent infective episodes of their skin, e.g. those with atopic eczema. Examples of the anti-infective ingredients are chlorhexidine hydrochloride and benzylkonium chloride.

Antipruritic agents: Lauromacrogols have an antipruritic effect which, whilst not entirely understood, probably work by inhibiting the transmission of itch sensations through the unmyelinated C fibres. They also act as an anaesthetic when applied to mucous membranes or bruised skin (Bettzuege-Pfaff and Melzer, 2005).

Descaling agents: An example of these is salicylic acid which is used to break down hyperkeratotic skin and thus remove the build up of scale.

Considerations that will effect how patients use emollients

Encouraging patients to concord with treatment is a key role for nurses; the concept of concordance is examined in some depth in Chapter 7. With regards to emollient use, one of the key considerations is the usability of the product. The Skin Care Campaign reminds us that patients have to 'wear' topical products and this is of course true for emollients. Products that suit one person will not suit another and so choice is key to successful selection and subsequent use. 'Psychorheology' is the name given to the study of the response an individual has to the application of a topical product (Marks, 2001).

In practical terms, the best way to get patients to use emollients is to provide them with a number of samples that they can go away and try before getting large quantities prescribed. To make this a reality, a team approach with the pharmacy department or advisor within the workplace is essential. Consideration needs to be given to workplace policies on getting free samples from the pharmaceutical industry and on giving non-prescribed items to patients. Having emollient formularies within a workplace helps

in the process of establishing the emollients which can be given out as samples.

Patient choice of emollient might be affected by something related to the product, the environment or themselves. Each of these are considered in turn.

The product

A common concern for patients is the consistency of the product, how greasy it is and how it smoothes onto the skin. This is not as simple as saying people do not like greasy products and do like creamy ones, because this is simply not the case. The product needs to be easy to apply to the skin and not to sting. Although most pharmaceutical products have no fragrance added to them, some do have a slight aroma. Indeed, it is probably because there is no fragrance to 'mask' the smells of the ingredients that people complain. Smell is a very personal issue. So, if someone does not like the smell of a product (even if it does not appear to have a smell) it is important that another product is tried. The physical presentation of a product may also have a bearing, e.g. a pump dispenser may be much easier than having to scoop a product out of a pot.

The environment

One of the major environmental factors that can impact on and individual's choice of emollient is the ambient temperature. Thick greasy emollients can also act as insulators and in hot weather may be too uncomfortable to use. It is also true that when the atmosphere is dry, the skin is more likely to become dry as there is less natural moisture in the air. Windy conditions can have a similar effect. Thus in hot conditions a lighter cream might be preferred whereas in cold, dry, windy conditions an ointment might be more suitable.

The person

The condition of an individual's skin will impact on the type of emollient that they may feel able to use. If the skin is very dry, a greasy ointment may feel most comfortable; if it is only moderately dry, a cream might be more appropriate. What a person does on a day-to-day basis will also make a difference; someone who is at work in smart clothing is unlikely to want to put on greasy emollients prior to getting dressed, but the same person may well be willing to use the greasier products under their pyjamas before going to bed. A greasy product may be fine on the feet where it can be covered up with socks and shoes, but totally unbearable on the face.

To get the most out of emollients, health care professionals need to engage in a conversation with their patients ascertaining as much information on the above as possible. It is not as straightforward as thinking 'very dry skin, needs very greasy emollients'. Therapeutically this may be the best decision to make, but in reality, if a patient does not like the product, it will stay in the pot where it has no therapeutic benefit at all!

Conclusion

Emollients are vital therapeutic products in the field of dermatology. They are not just simple inert products, but complicated mixtures of carefully formulated compounds with a range of impacts on the skin. Whilst the knowledge relating to how emollients work on the skin is increasing, and there is a significant body of scientific knowledge in relation to this, there is an enormous scarcity of experimental data to inform how emollients are physically used. This leaves practitioners to make decisions based on first principles and custom and practice. This is a field that would benefit from further research to ensure that emollients are used to maximum effect.

References

Akdis, C., M. Akdis *et al.* (2006). Diagnosis and treatment of atopic dermatitis in children and adults: European Academy of Allergy and Clinical Immunology/American Academy of Allergy, Asthma and Immunology/PRACTALL Consensus Report. *Allergy,* **61**(8): 969–987.

All Party Parliamentary Group on Skin (2006). Report on the enquiry into the adequacy and equity of dermatology services in the United Kingdom. London: APPGS.

Bettzuege-Pfaff, B. and A. Melzer (2005). Treating dry skin and pruritus with a bath oil containing soya oil and lauromacragols. *Current Medical Research and Opinion,* **21**(11): 173501739.

British Medical Association and Royal Pharmaceutical Society of Great Britain (2007). British National Formulary 54. Retrieved 7/01/08, 2007, from www.bnf.org.

Britton, J. (2003). The use of emollients and their correct application. *Journal of Community Nursing,* **17**(9): 22–25.

Cork, M.J. (1997). The importance of skin barrier function. *Journal of Dermatological Treatment,* **8**: s7–s13.

Cork, M.J., J. Timmins *et al.* (2003). An audit of adverse drug reactions to aqueous cream in children with atopic eczema. *The Pharmaceutical Journal,* **271**: 747–748.

de Groot, A. (2000). Sensitizing substances. In: Loden, M., Maibach, H. (Eds), *Dry Skin and Moisturizers.* Boca Raton: CRC Press.

Drugs and Therapeutics Bulletin (2007). Bath emollients for atopic eczema: Why use them? *Drugs and Therapeutics Bulletin,* **45**(10): 73–75.

Ersser, S., S. Maguire *et al.* (2007). A Best Practice Statement for Emollient Therapy. Retrieved 7 January 2008, from www.dermatology-uk.com/educational_projects.shtml.

Finlay, A.Y. (1997). Emollients as adjuvant therapy for psoriasis. *Journal of Dermatological Treatment,* **8**: s25–s27.

Grimalt, R., U. Mengeaud *et al.* (2007). The steroid sparing effect of emollient therapy in infants with atopic dermatitis: A randomised controlled study. *Dermatology,* **214**(1): 61–67.

Hall, M. (2003). Target skin. In: Kirkness, B. (Ed.). London: The Association of the British Pharmaceutical Industry.

Hanifin, J., A. Herbert *et al.* (1998). Effects of a low potency corticosteroid lotion plus a moisturizing regimen in the treatment of atopic dermatitis. *Current Therapeutic Research Clinical and Experimental*, **59**(4): 227–233.

Harris, I. and U. Hoppe (2000). Lanolins. In: Loden, M., Maibach, H. (Eds), *Dry Skin and Moisturizers – Chemistry and Function*. Boca Raton: CRC Press.

Holden, C., J. English *et al.* (2002). Advised best practice for the use of emollients in eczema and other dry skin conditions. *Journal of Dermatological Treatment*, **13**(3): 103–106.

Kligman, A.M. (2000). Introduction. In: Loden, M., Maibach, H. (Eds), *Dry Skin and Moisturizers: Chemistry and Function*. Boca Raton: CRC Press.

Loden, M. and H. Maibach, Eds (2000). Dry skin and moisturizers: Chemistry and function. Boca Raton, CRC Press.

Lucky, A.W., A.D. Leach *et al.* (1997). Use of an emollient as a steroid-sparing agent in the treatment of mild to moderate atopic dermatitis in children. *Paediatric Dermatology*, **14**(4): 321–324.

Marks, R. (2001). *Sophisticated Emollients*. Stuttgart: Thieme.

National Institute for Clinical Excellence (2001). *Referral Advice: A Guide to Appropriate Referral from General to Specialist Services*. London: NICE.

Nicol, N. and M. Boguniewicz (2008). Successful strategies in atopic dermatitis management. *Dermatology Nursing*, **Oct**(Suppl): 3–18.

Nicol, N., A. Ruszkowski *et al.* (1995). Contact dermatitis and the role of patch testing in its diagnosis and management. *Dermatology Nursing*, **Feb**(Suppl): 5–27.

Penzer, R. (2005). What advice do nurses working with adult patients with moderate plaque psoriasis give on the use of topical emollients? *Dermatological Nursing*, **4**(4): 21–22.

Rawlings, A.V., D.A. Canestrari *et al.* (2004). Moisturizer technology versus clinical performance. *Dermatologic Therapy*, **17**(Suppl 1): 49–56.

Smoker, A. (2007). Topical steroid or emollient – Which one do you apply first? An investigation into the sequencing of topical steroid and emollient application and the most clinically effective method of application. University of Southampton.

Stone, L. (2000). Medilan: A hypoallergenic lanolin for emollient therapy. *British Journal of Nursing*, **9**(1): 54–57.

Tree, S. and R. Marks (1975). An explanation for the 'placebo' effect of bland ointment bases. *British Journal of Dermatology*, **92**: 195–198.

Voegeli, D. (2007). Factors that exacerbate skin breakdown and ulceration. In: Pownell, M. (Ed.), *Skin Breakdown – The Silent Epidemic*, pp. 17–22. Hull: The Smith and Nephew Foundation.

Watsky, K.L., L. Freije *et al.* (1992). Water-in-oil emollients as steroid-sparing adjunctive therapy in the treatment of psoriasis. *Cutis*, **50**: 383–386.

Wood, L., P. Elias *et al.* (1996). Barrier disruption stimulate interleukin-1 alpha expression and release from a pre-formed pool in murine epidermis. *Journal of Investigative Dermatology*, **106**(3): 397–403.

Psychological and social aspects of skin care

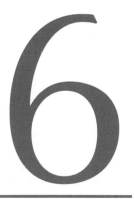

Rebecca Penzer

Introduction

This chapter seeks to explore the issues around the psychological and social impacts of skin disease. Often these two concepts get grouped together and psychosocial issues are discussed with no distinction being made. This is a tempting approach as there are many overlaps; however, here they will be considered as two sides of the same coin. The psychological aspect refers to issues related to the mind, about how the individual copes with their surroundings and experiences. The social aspect is about how the individual interacts with other people and how they feel to be part of human society.

The interplay between the skin and the mind and individuals and their communities, is not in any way a new concept. Indeed, the nursing literature has made mention of it years before more scientific work examined the nature of the relationship between the brain and the skin. In an attempt to understand this relationship, this chapter will look at the pathophysiological changes that affect both the brain and the skin in what has become known as the brain–skin axis. Once these are understood, it is then helpful to gain some insight into the coping mechanisms

that people employ to enable them to live with chronic skin conditions. At the same time, it is important to bear in mind that some people struggle to cope and as such, the chapter will look at some nursing interventions that can improve mental well-being and the ability to cope with adverse health experiences.

Mention will be made of mental illness, however, the focus of the chapter is on promoting mental health well-being and knowing when to refer on if a mental disorder is suspected.

The chapter starts with consideration of the social impacts of skin disease and particularly the social pressure that individuals with skin disorders experience on a day-to-day basis.

Social impacts

Historical context

Skin disease throughout history has been associated with contagion and dirt. This is at least partially due to the fact that many contagious diseases had skin manifestations (e.g. the plague) so that the relationship between some skin rashes and infectivity were indeed real. It is also thought that the natural human response of scratching has evolved to ensure that humans are made aware when something unpleasant is on their skin and the scratching is a way of getting rid of it. These two facts seem to be deeply buried within the human psyche. Thus it remains a common reaction to recoil from someone who has a visible skin condition and someone who scratches may be viewed as somehow dirty or unclean. Indeed this almost instinctive response to skin disease is very often totally out of proportion to the objective manifestation of the condition. The media and entertainment industry seem to play on this deeply held 'fear' making the 'bad guys' in films appear with facial defects such as acne scars or severe burns, thus reinforcing our instinct that 'bad' skin equals evil and thereby of course that 'beautiful' skin equals good.

Stigma

As a consequence, people with chronic skin diseases such as acne, eczema or psoriasis may suffer ridicule and rejection. Even if this response is anticipated rather than real, an individual may choose to avoid social interactions or avoid certain activities to ensure that they do not have to face unpleasantness from others (Hong *et al.*, 2008). Individuals may describe themselves as being stigmatised by their condition, where stigma can be described as a 'connotation of disgrace associated with certain thing'(Allen, 2000). As this definition highlights, people with skin disease often associate it to issues of morality, in other words, there is some level of (perceived) disgrace associated with it. This may in part be due to religious teachings emphasising the importance of cleanliness and because of skin diseases' association with dirt it becomes associated with Godlessness.

A study looking at feelings of stigmatisation in patients with psoriasis noted six different dimensions of stigma experience, many of which echo what has already been stated (Ginsburg & Link, 1989). Those dimensions were:

- anticipation of rejection
- feeling of being flawed

- sensitivity to others' attitudes
- guilt and shame
- secretiveness
- positive attitudes

In this study, different people had these experiences to different levels; however, the single factor that was most likely to predict for feelings of stigma and despair was bleeding skin. Whilst stigma may be thought of as a social construct, feelings of stigmatisation can have significant impact on psychological well-being. It was shown that a group of psoriasis patients who had felt stigmatised by people deliberately avoiding touching them, had significantly higher depression scores than a group with similar level of disease who did not feel stigmatised (Gupta *et al.*, 1998).

Disability and impairment

These words are sometimes used in relation to skin disease particularly to express a level of impact that the condition has on a person. Some of the outcome measures used to document the level of impact of the disease are expressed as a disability index, e.g. the Psoriasis Disability Index. The term 'disability' is an emotive word and different models view it in very different ways. For example, the medical model would define disability as a lack of ability as compared to a standard or norm. It may involve a physical, cognitive or intellectual impairment, mental disorder, or various types of chronic disease. This definition focuses on what the individual cannot do because of something that society might consider an impairment (Open University, 2006). A social model of disability takes a very different view labelling disability as a disadvantage or restriction on doing things that is the fault of society and the way that it is run. Thus the focus is on the way that society is set up and as such people become disabled because of the lack of preparedness of the society, rather than any personal intrinsic factor. (Open University, 2006) When considering the disability caused by skin disease, this definition is helpful as it is so often the responses from society at large that creates a disability for the individual sufferer. An impairment (that may have once been referred to as a handicap) is when a person has an injury or an illness for a long time that makes them different from other people. Impairment does not cause disability.

A piece of research carried out by Jowett and Ryan in 1985 looked at what they then labelled the handicapping impact of skin disease. This was early work looking at not only the physical, but also psychological and social burden of skin disease. Whilst the term handicap may no longer be used, this work clearly outlined how significant a range of skin conditions were on peoples' psychological and social well-being (Jowett & Ryan, 1985).

Body image

Body image can be described as a subjective concept of one's physical appearance based on self-observation and the reaction of others. Thus the image that individuals form of themselves has two parts to it, firstly how they see themselves and equally important how they perceive others reacting to them. When discussing body image, people are said to have a good or a poor body image, which in effect refers to the level of contentment that someone has with their body. Perception of body image is not necessarily related to the reality of what is before a person, for example someone with what outwardly would seem like a 'normal' body, may have a poor body image. Papadopoulus and Bor (1999) suggest a list of behaviours that those with poor body image might exhibit. Thus those with poor body image might:

- Edit social experiences to reinforce existing negative perceptions of themselves;
- View their bodies only as aesthetic objects;
- Minimise other positive aspects of their appearance;
- Have a heightened sense of body awareness;
- Comply with narrow social standards in terms of what is attractive.

(Papadopoulus & Bor, 1999)

What do these points mean with regard to someone with a skin condition? Editing social experiences means that an individual will choose to remember the unpleasant things that happen to them which in turn reinforce their beliefs about themselves. For example, someone with acne will remember how someone stared at them because this reinforces their belief that their acne is incredibly noticeable and ugly. They will not remember the pleasant instances where people smile and say hello. When someone has a skin disease they are likely to have a heightened sense of body awareness. Every day they are reminded of how their body is not 'working' for them because they have to treat it with creams, because it feels itchy or sore or because they have to display it to a health care professional. When parts of the skin are felt to be uncomfortable and unattractive, it is easy to forget or ignore the other parts of the body which are still normal, working well and attractive. All these factors can help to create a poor body image.

Social pressures

In a review article, Hong *et al.* (2008) outlines the many pressures that people with chronic diseases, such as eczema and psoriasis, experience. For many, family relationships are affected with families reporting that they too are negatively affected by the conditions. For adults, sexual functioning is affected with significant numbers reporting decreased sexual desire.

Economic pressures

Economic burden can be considered in a number of different ways. Firstly, there is a burden to the health service in terms of the amount that it costs to provide the direct care to patients. 1994 figures suggested that the costs were around 2% of the total NHS budget (Williams, 1997). New drugs (particularly the biologics) and increased levels of skin cancer are likely to mean that this figure has increased;

Table 6.1 Possible personal costs of a skin disease.

Modification	Personal costs
Environmental modifications particularly for patients with eczema	• Changing curtains for blinds • Changing carpets for hard flooring • Cotton clothing/special clothing • Water softener • Extra cleaning • Special mattress and bedding covers
Extra washing of clothes and bedding due to greasy treatments	• Increased water usage • Increased energy usage (electricity) • Increased washing detergent • Need to replace washing machine more frequently
Attempts to find 'magic cure'	• Money and emotion wasted on unproven and potentially dangerous treatments

however, they may have been offset by decreases in the amount of care provided on an in-patient basis. Secondly, there is an economic burden to society as a whole, as people with skin disease have to take time off work and are therefore unproductive. Williams sites that skin disease was one of the most common reasons for claiming injury and disablement benefit in the period 1977–1983. Finally, the personal economic burden has not been evaluated in terms of cost. However, a US study found that around 10% of people believed that their skin condition was a handicap to them while working or doing housework (Johnson & Jones, 1985). The economic impact of eczema is discussed in Chapter 9.

For some, the social stigma felt because of their skin disease prevents them from applying for jobs, and anecdotal reports from patients make it clear that it can be difficult to get jobs that involve face-to-face contact with members of the public. Whilst potential employers should not discriminate against employees because of their skin disease, there are still some instances where employment may be prevented because of the condition. For example, the British Armed Forces list chronic eczema, severe

psoriasis and severe acne as conditions that would make a person permanently unsuitable for entry into the services. There is also a very real direct cost to patients with skin disease in terms of what they need to do to manage their condition. Thus, unless the individual is eligible for free prescriptions, costs of these can be very high especially as often 2, 3 or even more items are required. It is sometimes cheaper for individuals to buy a season ticket, where they pay a lump sum up front and then receive free prescriptions regardless of the number they need. In England, details can be found at www.nhsbsa.nhs.uk/1127.aspx and in Scotland at www.psd.scot.nhs.uk/doctors/prepayment-certificates.html. However, the costs do not stop at prescriptions. Table 6.1 shows some of the other additional costs that someone with skin disease may incur.

Psychological impact

There are many issues to consider when looking at the psychological impact of skin disease. This section will begin by looking at some of the most recent thinking on the physical responses to stress that have an impact on the brain and the skin.

Brain–skin axis

There is varying degrees of evidence to support the relationship between stress and skin disease. For psoriasis and atopic eczema that evidence is well-established, it is less well so for urticaria, herpes simplex virus and vitiligo and only a weak association exists for lichen planus, pemphigus vulgaris and acne (Pavlovsky & Friedman, 2007). Whilst there is still much research needed to untangle the mechanisms that link the brain and skin with associated stress, current opinion suggests that there are three areas of interest: the hypothalamic–pituitary–adrenal axis (HPA), the peripheral nervous system (PNS) and biological barriers. The skin appears to have a dual role in relation to its response to stress. It is a target for key stress mediators (such as corticotrophin releasing hormone, adrenocorticotrophic hormone, cortisol, catecholamines, prolactin, substance P and nerve growth factor) but also a key *source* of these mediators of the stress response (Arck *et al.*, 2006).

Hypothalamus–pituitary–adrenal axis

The interplay between these three glands describes the classic stress response. Following experience of a stressor, the hypothalamus releases corticotrophin-releasing hormone, this acts on the pituitary gland to release adreno-corticotrophic hormone which finally induces the adrenal gland to produce cortisol. It is thought that cortisol protects the body under stress, although the mechanism is not clear, and it has a well-known anti-inflammatory effect. What appears to happen in some chronic inflammatory disorders (particularly psoriasis and eczema) is that there is a muted HPA response with cortisol levels that are lower than those seen in a general population. Richards *et al.* (2005) demonstrated that patients with psoriasis had lower levels of serum cortisol following an experimentally induced emotional stress, than controls. More significantly, those who rated their psoriasis as stress-responsive had even lower serum cortisol levels than those who did not rate so. Thus psoriasis patients do not seem to show an appropriate response of the HPA axis (Richards *et al.*, 2005). As a result of this reduced HPA reactivity, the body is not protected by the release of cortisol in response to stress.

Peripheral nervous system (PNS)

The PNS is all nervous tissue other than the brain and the spinal column (which are known as the central nervous system). Part of the PNS is not under voluntary control and as such is labelled the autonomic nervous system (ANS). The ANS can be divided further into the para-sympathetic and sympathetic nervous systems. The parasympathetic system maintains the body in a normal resting state. Stimulation of the sympathetic nervous system occurs during times of stress. At a gross physiological level there are a number of changes that happen to the body in order to deal with that stress. These responses are based upon an innate 'flight or fight' response that were useful when stressors were large dangerous animals, threatening life and limb. Whilst humans rarely run away literally, or fight the stressors in their lives, the biological responses still prepare us to be able to do so (see Table 6.2).

Table 6.2 Changes in the sympathetic nervous system in response to stress.

Target organ	Sympathetic effect
Brain	Becomes alert and focused in order to prepare for finding safety
Circulatory system	Heart beats faster
	Blood flow diverted to muscles ready for activity
	Blood flow away from skin leading to pallor (classic look of fear)
	Blood clotting ability increases, preparing for possible injury
Lungs	Airways open up allowing for increased oxygenation
	Rate of breathing increases
Gut	Less activity in digestion
	Vomiting may occur
	Constriction leads to feeling of butterflies or knot in the stomach
Liver	Releases more sugar and blood sugar levels go up in order to provide more energy
Bladder and bowel	Tend to be more irritable with decreased bladder capacity. May lead to involuntary emptying of either
Sexual organs	Erectile dysfunction in men
	Loss of lubrication in women

Besides the more familiar role of the sympathetic nervous system in relation to stress, it also has a crucial immune-related role to play through the release of catecholamines. These appear to stimulate stress-induced lymphocytosis and lead to particular changes in lymphocyte trafficking, circulation, proliferation and cytokine production. Another neurohormone which has a crucial role to play is nerve growth factor (NGF), which is a potent immunomodulator, aiding cell communications and facilitating monocyte/macrophage migration through vascular endothelium (Arck *et al.*, 2006). NGF modulates the synthesis of substance P which probably has a role in the activation of mast cells to secrete specific cytokines, chemokines and tumour necrosis factor α (Pavlovsky & Friedman, 2007).

Biological barriers

Studies in both human and animal models suggest that psychological stress has a direct impact on skin barrier and the ability for it to repair. A study looking at two groups of women who were put under psychological stress in a laboratory, one group through interview stress and another through sleep deprivation, both experienced a delay in barrier function recovery (Altemus *et al.*, 2001). Further work on mouse models suggest that this occurs because psychological stress leads to decreased epidermal proliferation, decreased epidermal differentiation and decreased the density and size of corneodesmosomes. Decreased production of lamellar bodies and decreased secretion from them leads to a lower level of natural lipid in the skin that affects barrier function (Choi *et al.*, 2005).

Coping

Internal factors

The internal factors related to coping with a chronic skin disease are those personal skills and abilities that an individual has to manage their condition. The intrinsic capability of somebody to cope with a stressful situation is complex and will be influenced by previous experience and inherited tendencies. The relative importance of nurture and nature is not going to be debated here, instead attention is drawn to the importance of self-efficacy. Self-efficacy is defined as: 'an individuals' belief in their capacity to successfully execute a health related behaviour' (Bandura, 1997). This concept is discussed in greater depth in Chapter 7 with a particular emphasis on improving self-efficacy in order to help people make the most of their treatments. However, in a more general capacity, if an individual has belief in their ability to manage their condition effectively, they are likely to feel more inclined to cope.

External factors

Typology of the disease
One of the factors that patients report as being hard to cope with about skin disease is its unpredictable nature. The typology of a disease relates to its nature, onset, course and appearance, thus a condition may be progressive, episodic or acute. A progressive disease follows a well-documented course and although the timings of the progression may not be entirely predictable, there are key indicators which allow an understanding of where the disease has progressed to. Mycosis fungoides is an example of a progressive condition. As explored in Chapter 13, a biopsy can determine the stage of the disease, which will then determine its subsequent progression.

An acute condition in this instance is used to describe a one off-event that occurs as a response to an external agent, e.g. a drug reaction. Although the response may be extremely unpleasant and may occur again if the individual is exposed to the offending drug, it is very clear what has caused the problem and how it may be avoided in the future.

Episodic conditions are, as their name implies, unpredictable, appearing for a time and then going away again. Most chronic skin conditions explored in this book belong in the episodic category. Psoriasis, eczema, urticaria and vitiligo are all examples of skin diseases that often seem to worsen for no apparent reason and may go into remission similarly for no apparent reason.

The seemingly random nature of these conditions can make it very difficult to cope with as it is impossible to plan for special events to take place in periods of remission, as these cannot be predicted. Clearly, treatments can improve the likelihood of remission occurring, but patients will report that treatments that have once worked are no longer doing so, adding to the stress incurred by an episodic condition.

It is helpful to turn to documented patient experience to really begin to understand, how this episodic nature can impact on the psychological well-being of an individual (Kennaway, 2008). Here, Guy Kennaway describes the appearance of psoriasis on his face.

'The stuff on my face was quick to establish itself in my life, providing a commentary on all my activities. Some things I did, like drink heavy red wine and party late into the night, it disapproved of, and it would be waiting in the morning to reprove me at its most blotchy. But it wasn't just a party-pooping bore. Another long night on the Scotch could result in a clear complexion the next day. Above all it wasn't predictable although I never gave up trying to second-guess it. It seemed to have a preference for some of my friends over others, appearing all over my face and neck, bright red almost pulsating with rage, in the pub with some and then calmly disappearing entirely with the departure – or arrival of others.' (p. 6)

Treatment

Whilst treatments may physically improve the skin condition, the process of using them can in itself make the condition difficult to cope with. Topical treatments may be greasy, smelly, may irritate the skin or change its colour. Systemic therapies bring their own stressors with them. For example, light therapy requires frequent trips to the hospital and methotrexate regular blood tests along with the life-style change of not consuming alcohol. Unlike many chronic conditions where the behaviour change may involve taking an oral drug regularly, skin diseases require a commitment to ongoing application of topical treatments for an indeterminate length of time. Many patients cite the time element as a major negative impact that influences

how they cope with their disease. Washing and getting dressed are not straight forward activities that take half an hour, applying of emollients and other topical products may take over an hour and may need to be done at least twice a day.

Discomfort

Skin that is affected by disease can be physically uncomfortable in a number of ways, but most commonly, patients will describe itch, soreness, tightness and pain.

Itch is associated with a number of skin conditions particularly eczema and urticaria and perhaps to a lesser extent psoriasis. It is thought to be the most common symptom of dermatologic disease (Gupta *et al.*, 1994). It causes extreme discomfort and patients will often say they would rather have pain than live with itch. Indeed some will scratch themselves raw in order to experience soreness rather than itch. It has been rated second only to disfigurement as a source of patient distress for those with pruritic dermatoses (Gilchrest, 1982). Skin disease often provides the sufferer with a constant reminder of its presence, as humans 'wear' their skin it is impossible to escape from it. Whilst techniques for managing pain have improved over time, there is still relatively little development of novel ways of treating itch.

Mental health well-being

Whilst it is important to acknowledge the role of stress and coping on the experience of a skin disease, perhaps the most important focus for nurses is on enhancing the mental health well-being of their patients in order to help them cope with the stress of life. It is clear from all that has gone before in this chapter that stress can lead to a flare up or deterioration of chronic skin conditions. Whilst the mechanisms for this are complex and only partly understood, it would seem that for many conditions it is an irrefutable truth. What is also the case is that experiencing a skin condition is stressful in itself. Thus, intervening to improve mental health may improve the physical state of the skin by reducing the physiological stress responses and also by improving an individual's ability to cope with stressful events in their lives. In this way a therapeutic objective is to break this vicious circle (see Figure 6.1).

Mental health can be viewed on a spectrum, which does not have any absolutes associated with it. For example, an individual may have a tendency towards being anxious, but not have an anxiety disorder. Helping that individual to cope better with their anxiety would, in all likelihood help to improve their mental health well-being and may in turn help them to cope better with their skin disease. An individual can be said to have a mental health disorder when their mental state interferes with their daily living. The World Health Organisation (WHO) describes it thus: 'Mental disorders comprise a broad range of problems, with different symptoms. However, they are generally characterised by some combination of abnormal thoughts, emotions, behaviour and relationships with others.' (WHO, 2009)

Thus, anxiety is a normal emotion that we feel when we are asked to do something that is outside our 'comfort zone'. But an anxiety disorder includes a range of responses which become problematic. For example, most people do not enjoy being sick, but for some it becomes a phobia known as emetophobia. Most people will go through rituals of checking keys and locking windows when they leave the house; however, someone with obsessive compulsive disorder will go through elaborate, repetitive behaviours that make leaving the house difficult and time consuming.

Skin manifestations of mental disorders

Along the spectrum of mental disorders, there are some conditions that manifest themselves through the skin, and are reflections of true mental health issues. It can be very difficult to help these patients as they are often adamant that their skin lesions are true dermatological conditions rather than self-induced.

Trichotillomania describes hair pulling, which results in fractured hair and bald patches. This may be as a result of a habit or tic which the individual needs pointing out to them and may be relatively easy to stop. However, it may also be as a result of some underlying psychopathology possibly related to anxiety.

Patients may deliberately inflict damage to their skin and then consciously try to deceive about the real nature of the lesions—this could be thought of as a form of cutaneous Munchausen syndrome. Those who have true dermatitis artefacta are seemingly unaware of the true nature of their lesions. The lesions in both instances may seem peculiar and not appear like any 'normal' pathological process; however, in some cases, the patient may recreate the symptoms of a previously experience condition. This is a form of self-harm and may be as a result of stressful or anxiety provoking experiences that are occurring in the individual's lives. Referral to a clinical psychologist will be helpful, as they may be able to help the person resolve the experiences leading to the self-harming behaviour.

Delusional parasitosis is extremely difficult to treat as the patient is absolutely convinced that they are infested with insects or worms. They may endeavour to produce 'evidence' of such infestation by digging debris out from under their skin.

Nursing interventions

In this section, the role of the nurse will be considered. The overall objective of the nursing intervention is to provide support to patients who have skin disease, in order to enhance their mental health and thus enable them to cope with their condition as effectively as possible. Nurses will already have a significant skill-set that they

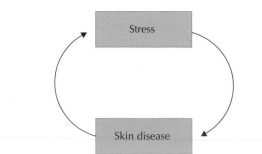

Figure 6.1   Vicious circle of stress and skin disease.

can draw on to achieve this, what is outlined here are ways to develop these skills further. This should not be mistaken as an attempt to train people into being therapists with specific abilities. Instead, communication *skills* will be discussed along with some *techniques* used in cognitive behavioural therapy (CBT). These can be incorporated into developing a set of professional competencies relevant to the area of work. Should a patients needs go beyond the nurses level of competency, referral on to other practitioners e.g. a clinical psychologist, should always be considered. A further exploration of the therapeutic consultation is discussed in Chapter 7.

Active listening

It is easy to assume that listening is a skill that can be done without thinking; however, it is of course possible to listen without hearing, either the words or their meaning. Depending on which studies are considered, only 25–50% of what is heard is actually remembered. Effective communication between two people can only exist when the person receiving the message receives and interprets it in the way that the person doing the sending intended. The likelihood of this occurring is increased if the receiver is engaged in active listening. In other words, their attitude presumes that the person they are listening to is important to them and that they accept the following to be true about that person:

■ what they think
■ what they need
■ how they feel
■ what they want

Active listening has many benefits as it lends itself to developing trust between two people and in turn enhancing the likelihood of arriving at helpful solutions. As well as being a useful skill to have in terms of helping patients, it can be used effectively to resolve conflict and enhance productivity in other work-related situations.

Active listening is by definition active, it cannot be carried out in a passive way, therefore, prior to using active listening skills some preparation is

---

> ### Box 6.1 Setting the environment for active listening
>
> ■ Minimise intrusions or interruptions either from loud noises, telephones or someone in person;
> ■ Room temperature should be neither too hot nor too cold;
> ■ Avoid creating a barrier by the way the desk and chairs are arranged. Sitting facing the patient, but at an angle rather than directly, is best;
> ■ Seating should be comfortable.

needed both of the listener and the environment. Box 6.1 shows some of the environmental factors which need to be taken into consideration.

When first meeting the patient ensure that they are greeted warmly and that introductions are given. Active listening will be taking place in different clinical settings, e.g. a ward environment or a clinic. Wherever it occurs, the principles around establishing the right environment remain the same. At the beginning, it is important that they know the amount of time available and the purpose of the discussion. These may seem like obvious things to explain, but it is worth ensuring that both parties agree the same reason for meeting to prevent misunderstanding. When the patient knows how much time they have got, it means they stop worrying about external factors and prioritise the questions they want to ask, without feeling rushed at the end when the consultation is brought to a close. Once the patient is settled, they need to be given the opportunity to be listened to in a non-judgemental, non-critical manner. Further acknowledgement of what is being said can be given by leaning forward, nodding and responding with appropriate facial expressions, i.e. those that match the patients' feelings. Responses and questions should be paced so as to encourage further disclosure. Finally, the patient will feel listened to and understood, if you summarise and paraphrase what they have said.

The body language that is adopted during active listening is also a vital component of its success. The listener must have an open posture and maintain eye contact with the speaker. When communicating, the words are not necessarily the most important part of the communication. Classic studies carried out by Albert Mehrabian in the 1960s suggested that 7.8% of the impact is through the words and what is actually said, 38% is the tone of the voice, pitch and the way the message sounds and 55% of the impact of a communication is through the movement of the body, facial expressions and hand gestures (Mehrabian & Ferris, 1967; Mehrabian & Wiener, 1967). These studies have been criticised methodologically, but the important findings emphasise two key things. Firstly there are three elements of face-to-face communication (words, tone and body language) and tone and body language are particularly important for expressing feelings and attitude. Secondly when words and body language disagree, it is the body language that is believed. SOLER is a useful mnemonic to act as a reminder of good body language:

Squarely face the person
Open your posture
Lean towards the speaker
Eye contact maintained
Relax while attending

Active listening in a clinical situation will have some slightly different features from active listening within a counselling or mediation situation. In these scenarios, an active listener is expected not to give advice, or try and solve the other person's problems for them. However, in a clinical situation, the reason that an individual has come to see a nurse will be to receive advice and support. Thus advice giving is permissible. However, often individuals with chronic skin conditions have considerable experience of how to manage their condition, and the giving of advice must be in the context of listening to and understanding how they currently manage and what their priorities for treatment are.

Barriers to active listening

There will always be barriers to active listening some of which it may be possible to change,

others whilst important to be aware of, may not be amenable to change. In a clinical situation, time is likely to be at a premium and it may not be possible to have the ideal amount of it with a patient to cover all the issues. If this is the case, it needs to be acknowledged and arrangements made to see the patient again. Some of the things listed in the table on environmental factors may also create barriers to effective communication, but these should be possible to change. Issues that are harder to change are the internal barriers that we all have due to our own experiences and background. These may lead us to hear what we want to hear rather than what is being said. On a simple level if there are concerns in our minds, for example the pressures of other things that need doing, it may be difficult to be focused enough to engage in active listening. It is particularly important to acknowledge the impact of emotions on our listening especially when the topics are ones that touch 'hot buttons'. 'Hot buttons' can be described as topics that have a particular emotional resonance and make active listening difficult or even impossible. An example may be if a patient is talking about bereavement and the listener has recently experienced such circumstances themselves, this may trigger a whole range of emotions that are difficult to control.

The impact of active listening on the listener should also be considered. The process is more likely to expose them to higher levels of emotional energy from the patient and this could make coping with the daily pressures of confronting patient difficulties, harder. In order to deal with this, it is important to ensure that adequate training is in place and that supervision is available to support the health care professional.

Consciously incorporating active listening into consultations with patients will make them more effective from two perspectives. Firstly, it is more likely that psychological difficulties will be expressed by the patients, and secondly, a thorough assessment of the patient's physical problems and how they want to resolve them, will be possible. Table 6.3 summarises some techniques that might be useful when engaged in active listening. The next section considers the assessment process.

Table 6.3 Techniques to promote active listening.

Action	What is it	What is its purpose	Comments
Paraphrasing	Restating a message, usually with fewer words	To test the understanding of what has been heard. To communicate that the listener is trying to understand what is being said	The listener should try and understand: (a) what is the speaker's *thinking* message (b) what is the speaker's *feeling* message
Clarifying	The process of bringing vague communications into sharper focus	To ensure the listener has not misinterpreted what the speaker has said. To get more information	For example, the listener could say: 'I'm confused, let me try to state what I think you are trying to say'
Perception checking	The listener asks the speaker to verify the former's perceptions of the conversation	To give and receive feedback. To check out the listener's perceptions	For example, the listener could say 'You said that you are fed up with having swollen legs, but the stockings you have to wear are too uncomfortable'
Summarising	The listener pulls together, organises and integrates the main aspects of the dialogue	To provide a sense of movement and achievement. To establish a basis for further discussion	It is important to pay attention to the various themes touched upon and emotional overtones, putting key ideas and feelings into broad statements. No new information should be introduced
Empathy	Reflection of content and feeling	For the listener to show understanding of the speaker's experience. This allows the speaker to evaluate their own feelings having heard them expressed by someone else	Empathy should not be confused with sympathy. Empathy is 'I hear what you are saying' while sympathy is 'I share your feelings'. Sympathy immediately means an emotional involvement with the speaker which is best avoided.

Assessing psychological needs

During consultation, there needs to be a focus on assessing the physical and psychological needs of the patient. Although it is unlikely that these two areas of someone's life will neatly be assessed independently of one another, in this section some specific techniques to assess psychological needs through active listening will be considered.

Using the five 'W's is a useful way of thoroughly exploring the impact that a psychological problem is laden with. Consider the following scenario:

A patient with vitiligo comes to see you. They are expressing feelings of anxiety about going out to the shops because they feel they are being stared at, because of the depigmented patches affecting their arms. Using the five 'W's, the following might be explored (see Box 6.2).

This assessment can be further refined by getting the patient to say how often the problem occurs, the intensity of the level of anxiety (on a scale of 0–8), the number of times it occurs and how long it lasts for.

Cognitive behavioural therapy (CBT)

What is CBT?

As the name suggests, CBT is a form of therapy that aims to change thoughts and behaviours in order to improve mental health well-being. It is known as a talking therapy that focuses on the 'here and now' rather than trying to make links

---

Box 6.2   **An example of using the five 'W's to assess psychological need**

1. What is the problem?
   That I have vitiligo and that I get very anxious because of it.
2. Where does the problem occur?
   On my arms.
3. When does the problem occur?
   Only when I am by myself doing the shopping, I don't get so anxious if there is someone with me.
4. Why does the problem occur, the feared consequences?
   I hate being stared at and I am scared that someone will say something rude to me and I won't know what to say or that they will refuse to serve me.
5. With whom is the problem better or worse?
   The problem is significantly worse if I by myself and/or am with people that I don't know, if I have a friend with me I don't feel anywhere near as anxious.

---

between current problems and the past. Its basic tenet is that by changing thought and behavioural patterns, a powerful effect may be seen on a person's emotions. By identifying and analysing counterproductive thoughts and behaviours, an individual can be helped to alleviate feelings of anxiety and depression. CBT is seen as a collaborative relationship between therapist and patient and is most effective with motivated people who want to help themselves feel better (Beck, 1995). It is most successfully used in cases of depression, anxiety, obsessive/compulsive disorder and post-traumatic stress disorders. It is the therapy of preference in many of these instances because it has good scientific evidence to back up its efficacy, unlike many of the other talking therapies. It is recommended in the National Institute for Health and Clinical Excellence guidelines that pertain to mental disorders such as anxiety,

(National Institute for Health and Clinical Excellence, 2007).

Using CBT skills

To practise as a CBT practitioner requires prolonged training; however, some understanding of the fundamental principles of the therapy can be useful when using active listening skills within a consultation situation.

In essence, CBT works through making sense of problems which at the time seem overwhelming to an individual. Thus, an individual will respond to a situation by having thoughts, emotions, physical feelings and actions. All these various components will have an effect on one another, e.g. how someone thinks about a problem will affect how they feel about it emotionally and physically. Helping an individual to pass through a process of appraisal is a useful place to start. Within the context of CBT, this involves appraising the personal meaning and significance of an event and then appraising the capacity of an individual to cope with the event. For each situation, there are helpful and unhelpful ways of responding (see Box 6.3 for an example).

Persistently having negative thoughts about situations leads to uncomfortable feelings, including rejection and sadness, as well as unhelpful behaviour, such as not returning to the gym. Helping patients involves reframing their experiences, so that rather than producing unhelpful emotions the individual feels more comfortable in specific situations. This may simply involve drawing the person's attention to the fact that they view situations negatively and help them to view things more positively. It may be easier for people to do this if they understand the direct connection between thoughts and feelings, i.e. having more positive thoughts is more likely to lead to more positive feelings.

As part of this process, it is useful to help patients to learn that physical/bodily feelings can be changed. This can be done through deep breathing exercises or progressive muscle relaxation achieved by consciously tensing and relaxing muscles. Slow deep breathing is one of the quickest ways to counteract the effects of the sympathetic nervous system which stimulates the 'flight

Box 6.3 Helpful and unhelpful ways of responding to a situation

A young professional man with eczema on his face tells you that he was at the gym and the young female instructor who had been friendly and spent half an hour with him before, barely acknowledged his presence.

An unhelpful cycle would be:

Appraisal
She ignored me because I have eczema on my face
Thought
I hate my eczema
Emotion
Feelings of rejection and sadness
Behaviour
Not going back to the gym
A helpful cycle would be:
Appraisal
She ignored me because she is very busy
Thought
I will come when the gym is less busy
Emotion
Feelings of hope and expectation
Behaviour
Going back to the gym at a less busy time

or fight' response. When fear or stress takes over, breathing tends to be shallow and limited to the chest. Deep breaths which fill the lungs and expand the abdomen will invoke a greater feeling of well-being and relaxation. Yoga and T'ai Chi use slow, steady breathing and movement to support a steady central nervous system response (Pick, 2009).

Changing people's habitual responses to a situation takes time and as has already been mentioned, it requires the patient to be motivated towards those changes. For those with skin disease, there is the added challenge of coping with the physical discomfort of the problem. But using some of these CBT principles may help to reduce the level of psychological anxiety associated with the conditions.

In summary, particular focus should be paid to three key areas:

(1) Helping patients to cope with their disease by providing information about it and how to treat it effectively;
(2) Promoting relaxation and anxiety management, using some of the techniques discussed here;
(3) Using appraisal to work with patients to develop helpful rather than unhelpful patterns of thought.

A programme that used all three of these elements successfully showed that people who enrolled showed significantly greater improvements in disease severity, anxiety, depression, psoriasis-related stress and disability, than those who just had conventional treatment (Fortune *et al.*, 2002).

Measuring impact of skin disease

There are a number of ways by which it is possible to measure the impact that skin disease has on the individual. One way of doing this is to consider disease severity, which assumes that the more severe the disease, the more impact it will have on the patient's life. Some disease severity scores are illustrated in the Appendices of the book. It is also possible to use well-established inventories to assess specific aspects of mental health, for example the Beck Anxiety Inventory or the Penn State Worry Questionnaire, although specific training may be needed to use these effectively. There are also a number of dermatology-specific measures, many of which focus on the concept of quality of life, but others assess the level of disability that is caused by a specific condition.

Put simply, quality of life can be defined as the person's ability to enjoy normal life activities which can include health, personal relationships, environment, quality of working life, social life and leisure time. In dermatology, quality of life is used to measure the impact of a combined effect of psychological and social impacts. They may be used to assess the level of impact that a condition has on the individual at the start of a treatment episode and then re-employed as treatment progresses, to see how effective that treatment has been in improving quality of life. A British Association of Dermatologists (BAD) survey showed, however, that in outpatient notes, only 5% had a quality of life index 'always recorded' or 'well recorded' going down to 3% when inpatient notes were considered (Eedy *et al.*, 2008).

Quality of life measures in dermatology are of particular importance because disease severity is not always directly related to the level of impact that the disease has on the individual (Hon *et al.*, 2006). Thus, someone with severe disease may have a relatively good quality of life, while someone with mild or moderate disease, a dreadful quality of life. Assumptions cannot be made dependent on disease severity. What has also been shown is that health care professionals' perceptions (in this case, doctors) of treatment efficacy and clearance were perceived in a very different way from that of patients (Ersser *et al.*, 2002). Specifically, patients tended to talk about resolution of symptoms whereas doctors were more interested in disease clearance. Richards *et al.* (2004) showed that dermatologists were poor at assessing the psychological distress experienced by patients with psoriasis, and even when this was noted generally nothing was done about it.

What these two studies along with the BAD survey describe, is that health care professionals often assume that they understand how a skin disease impacts on an individual. These assumptions are not always be correct and it is therefore essential to have objective measures available to help with the assessment of the impact that a skin disease has. Quality of life measurement is one that is commonly used, however, as the examples below show there are other validated tools which help health care professionals to understand the impact of a skin disease.

There are a number of different quality of life indices for patients with dermatological conditions. Some of these are disease-specific while some are generic. Here the most commonly used generic score for both adults and children is examined in more detail along with a disease-specific score for psoriasis and one for acne. The advantage of using the quality of life scores that are outlined here is that they have been tested for reliability and validity, i.e. they will consistently measure what they set out to measure.

Dermatology Life Quality Index (DLQI)

This is probably the most well-established and commonly used quality of life tool in British dermatology, it has the advantage of being relatively short and therefore practical to use within the clinical environment. It has been translated into a number of languages. It is completed by the patient on their own and they are asked to answer all questions bearing in mind how they have felt over the last week. The responses either 'very much', 'a lot', 'a little' or 'not at all' are then scored with points of 3, 2, 1 and 0 respectively (Finlay & Khan, 1994). When totalled up the scores are interpreted as follows (see Box 6.4):

However, what is also useful about this score is that it enables the practitioner to get a sense for how certain areas of the individual's life are most affected. This is because the questions can be grouped into themes (see Box 6.5).

Once the score has been completed it becomes a useful part of the assessment process and can guide questioning around the areas that seem to be most affected in the patient's life. The tool with related guidance is available at www.dermatology.org.uk and can be used free of charge in clinical situations.

Box 6.4   Interpreting DLQI scores

0–1: no effect at all on the patient's life
2–5: small effect on the patient's life
6–10: moderate effect on the patient's life
11–20: very large effect on the patient's life
21–30: extremely large effect on the patient's life

Box 6.5   Break down of the DLQI score

Questions 1 and 2 relate to symptoms and feelings with a maximum score of 6
Questions 3 and 4 relate to daily activities with a maximum score of 6
Questions 5 and 6 relate to leisure with a maximum score of 6
Question 7 relates to work and school with a maximum score of 3
Question 8 and 9 relate to personal relationships with a maximum score of 6
Question 10 relates to treatment with a maximum score of 3

Box 6.6   Break down of CDLQI score

Questions 1 and 2 relate to symptoms and feelings with a maximum score of 6
Questions 4, 5 and 6 relate to leisure with a maximum score of 9
Question 7 relates to school and holidays with a maximum score of 3
Question 3 and 8 relate to personal relationships with a maximum score of 6
Question 9 relates to sleep with a maximum score of 3
Question 10 relates to treatment with a maximum score of 3

Children's Dermatology Life Quality Index (CDLQI)

This score is in many ways similar to the DLQI, but it is designed for use in children, i.e. those between the ages of 5 and 16. It is available in both text and cartoon versions, and can be completed by the child with the help of their parent or guardian. The scoring is slightly different from the DLQI in that the score is expressed as a percentage of the total score of 30, the higher the score, the more affected is the quality of life (Lewis-Jones & Finlay, 1995). An Infant DLQI is also available for completion by parents or carers, devised by the same authors (Lewis-Jones *et al.*, 2001).

Once again, more detailed analysis of the scoring can be gained by looking at the themes (see Box 6.6)

The CDLQI assessment tool is available at www.dermatology.org.uk and can be used free of charge in clinical situations. Further discussion is given in Chapter 9.

Family Dermatology Life Quality Index

This score is to be used on adults over the age of 16 and aims to represent the impact that having a family member with a skin disease has on an individual (Basra *et al.*, 2007). It uses the same basic structure as the DLQI and the CDLQI and is available at the same website.

Salford Psoriasis Index (SPI)

This score is a composite tool and is not called a quality of life score; however, it does include consideration of the psychological impact. The index is divided into three sections. Firstly, the Psoriasis Area Severity Index (PASI) is completed (see Chapter 3 and Appendix 1). Once a score is reached, it is then given a SPI score as per Table 6.4. Secondly, the psychological impact is measured by asking the patient to mark on a visual analogue score. The patient is asked 'about the extent to which they perceive that their psoriasis is affecting their day-to-day life at the time of the assessment'. The score is from 0 to 10 with 0 being not at all affected and 10 being completely affected (Kirby *et al.*, 2000). The third and final section of the Index is calculated according to how much treatment the patient has undergone (see Box 6.7).

Once each individual score has been calculated, the total score is then expressed as a ratio. The first number represents the SPI, the second psychological impact and the third the amount of treatment received. Therefore, a ratio of **1:1:0** shows that the individual has very little psoriasis, which is having a minimal psychological impact with no systemic treatment or hospital admissions. A ratio of **10:10:6** shows very severe psoriasis which is having a major psychological

Table 6.4 SPI scores in relation to PASI scores.

PASI	SPI extent
0	0
0.1–3	1
3.1–5	2
5.1–8	3
8.1–11	4
11.1–14	5
14.1–18	6
18.1–23	7
23.1–29	8
29.1–36	9
36+	10

Box 6.7   Points for the amount of treatment received

1 point for each individual systemic treatment including PUVA (Psoralen plus ultraviolet light A).
1 extra point for each treatment received for > one year.
1 extra point if patient has received > 200 treatments or > 1000J/cm² of PUVA.
1 point for every hospital admission for the treatment of psoriasis.
1 point for every episode of erythema.

---

impact and there is a significant history of systemic treatments and/or hospital admissions.

The Cardiff Acne Disability Index

This short questionnaire of five questions asks teenagers and young adults to rate the impact that their acne is having on them on a scale of 0–3, the total maximum score being 15. This is a quick and practical tool that can be given to a patient to complete in clinic and then used as a basis for

discussion about the impact of the disease as well as being used as a tool to monitor the effectiveness of treatment (Motley & Finlay, 1992).

This tool is available at www.dermatology.org.uk and can be used free of charge in clinical situations.

Conclusion

This chapter has sought to explore the social and psychological aspects of skin care. It has done this by considering how society can influence individuals and how they feel about their skin condition. The influence of the brain on the skin and how experiencing a skin disease affects human psychology has also been explored. Whilst lip service may be given to the psychological impact of skin disease, the services and skills are often not in place to help patients in improving their mental well-being. Nurses have a significant role to play here by refining and using skills that they already have. Various tools are available to assess the psychological and social impact of skin disease; these notably include dermatology-specific and some age-specific measures that can be employed in clinical practice.

References

Allen, R., Ed. (2000). *The New Penguin Dictionary*. London: Penguin Book.

Altemus, M., B. Rao *et al.* (2001). Stress induced changes in skin barrier function in healthy women. *Journal of Investigative Dermatology*, **117**(2): 309–317.

Arck, P., A. Slominski *et al.* (2006). Neuroimmunology of stress: Skin takes centre stage. *Journal of Investigative Dermatology*, **126**: 1697–1704.

Bandura, A. (1997). *Self-Efficacy: The Exercise of Control*. New York: Freeman Press.

Basra, M., R. Su-Ho *et al.* (2007). Family Dermatology Life Quality Index: Measuring the secondary impact of skin disease. *British Journal of Dermatology*, **156**(3): 528–538.

Beck, J. (1995). *Cognitive Therapy: Basics and Beyond*. New York: The Guild Press.

Choi, E., B. Brown *et al.* (2005). Mechanisms by which psychologic stress alters cutaneous permeability barrier homeostasis and stratum corneum integrity. *Journal of Investigative Dermatology*, **124**(3): 587–595.

Eedy, D., S. Burge *et al.* (2008). An audit of the provision of dermatology services in secondary care in the UK with a focus on the care of people with psoriasis. *The British Association of Dermatologists and The Royal College of Physicians*, London.

Ersser, S., H. Surridge *et al.* (2002). What criteria do patients use when judging the effectiveness of psoriasis treatment. *Journal of Evaluation in Clinical Practice*, **8**(4): 367–376.

Finlay, A. and G. Khan (1994). Dermatology Life Quality Index (DLQI) – a simple practical measure for routine clinical use. *Clinical and Experimental Dermatology*, **19**(3): 210–216.

Fortune, D., H. Richards *et al.* (2002). A cognitive-behavioural symptom management programme as an adjunct in psoriasis therapy. *British Journal of Dermatology*, **146**(3): 458.

Gilchrest, B. (1982). Pruritus: Pathogenesis, therapy and significance in systemic disease states. *Archives of Internal Medicine*, **142**: 101–105.

Ginsburg, I. and B. Link (1989). Feelings of stigmatization in patients with psoriasis. *International Journal of Dermatology*, **20**(1): 53–63.

Gupta, M., A. Gupta *et al.* (1994). Depression modulate pruritus perception: A study of pruritus in psoriasis atopic dermatitis and chronic ideopathic urticaria. *Psychosomatic Medicine*, **56**: 36–40.

Gupta, M., A. Gupta *et al.* (1998). Perceived deprivation of social touch in psoriasis is associated with greater psychologic morbidity: An index of the stigma experience in dermatologic disorders. *Cutis*, **61**(6): 339–342.

Hon, K., W. Kam *et al.* (2006). CDLQI, SCORAD and NESS: Are they correlated? *Quality of Life Research*, **15**(10): 1551–1558.

Hong, J., B. Koo *et al.* (2008). The psychosocial and occupational impact of chronic skin disease. *Dermatologic Therapy*, **21**: 54–59.

Johnson, M. and J. Jones (1985). Prevalence of dermatologic disease in the United States: A review of the national health and nutrition examination survey, 1971–74. *American Journal of Industrial Medicine*, **8**(4–5): 451–460.

Jowett, S. and T. Ryan (1985). Skin disease and handicap: An analysis of the impact of skin conditions. *Social Science and Medicine*, **20**(4): 425–429.

Kennaway, G. (2008). *Sunbathing Naked*. Edinburgh: Canongate.

Kirby, B., D. Fortune *et al.* (2000). The Salford Psoriasis Index: An holistic measure of psoriasis severity. *British Journal of Dermatology*, **142**(4): 728–732.

Lewis-Jones, M. and A. Finlay (1995). The Children's Dermatology Life Quality Index (CDLQI): Initial validation and practical use. *British Journal of Dermatology*, **132**(6): 942–949.

Lewis-Jones, M., A. Finlay *et al.* (2001). The Infants' Dermatology Quality of Life Index. *British Journal of Dermatology*, **144**(1): 104–110.

Mehrabian, A. and S. Ferris (1967). Inference of attitudes from non-verbal communication in two channels. *Journal of Consulting Psychology*, **31**(3): 248–252.

Mehrabian, A. and M. Wiener (1967). Decoding of inconsistent communications. *Journal of Personality and Social Psychology*, **6**(1): 109–114.

Motley, R. and A. Finlay (1992). Practical use of a disability index in the routine management of acne. *Clinical and Experimental Dermatology*, **17**(1): 1–3.

National Institute for Health and Clinical Excellence (2007). *Anxiety: anxiety (panic disorder with or without agoraphobia, and generalised anxiety disorder): Management of anxiety in adults in primary, secondary and community care*. London: NICE Open University (2006) Models of disability, Retrieved 3rd December 2009, http://www.open.ac.uk/inclusiveteaching/pages/

understanding-and-awareness/models-of-disability.php.

Papadopoulus, L. and R. Bor (1999). Open University (2006). *Psychological Approaches to Dermatology.* London: Wiley.

Pavlovsky, L. and A. Friedman (2007). Pathogenesis of stress-associated skin disorders: Exploring the brain–skin axis. *Current Problems in Dermatology*, **35**: 136–145.

Pick, M. (2009). Deep Breathing – The Truly Essential Exercise. Retrieved 17 April 2009, from http://www.womentowomen.com/fatigueandstress/deepbreathing.aspx.

Richards, H., D. Fortune *et al.* (2004). Detection of psychological distress in patients with psoriasis: Low consensus between dermatologist and patient. *British Journal of Dermatology*, **151**: 1227–1233.

Richards, H., D. Ray *et al.* (2005). Response of the hypothalamic–pituitary–adrenal axis to psychological stress in patients with psoriasis. *British Journal of Dermatology*, **153**: 1114–1120.

Williams, H.C. (1997). *Dermatology Health Care Needs Assessment.* Oxford: Radcliffe Medical Press.

World Health Organisation (2009). Mental Disorder. Retrieved 15 April 2009, from http://www.who.int/topics/mental_disorders/en/.

Helping patients make the most of their treatment

7

Steven J. Ersser

Introduction

A key challenge for people living with chronic skin conditions is the need to ensure that they use their treatment to optimal effect. Despite the efforts to determine the effective treatment plan, a crucial concern is how the individual interprets and engages with the plan, since there are multiple factors that may interfere with their ability to utilise the treatment in an effective way. Treatment effectiveness depends not only on having evidence of beneficial treatments and making discerning clinical judgements but also on the patient's interpretation of the treatment plan, their motivation and understanding of it and how in practice they apply it to their lifestyle. Therefore, effective treatment fundamentally depends on people taking an active role in learning about their therapy and knowing how to utilise it correctly. This chapter focuses on ways of supporting patients to self-manage their condition effectively through playing an active role in treatment decisions and application.

Dermatologists have been accused of thinking that they are the only people who know about skin diseases and that they are the only people sufficiently qualified to treat them. How true is this, and is it likely that dermatologists are going to be the major sources of advice on dermatological matters in the new millennium? *(Prof. Robin Marks, University of Melbourne/Former President, International League of Dermatological Societies; Marks (2000))*

Self-management and patient support

The management of a chronic illness requires a number of factors to sustain effective health behaviour; this includes knowledge, skills and confidence in managing a condition long term. These areas require education and psychological support that is systematically assessed and planned. A key aspect of this support is emotional support to help individuals to cope with their long-term condition and their treatment regimens and recognition of their impact on their lifestyle. Awareness is also needed of specific issues that may affect some people, such as low self-esteem, poor motivation and a lack of social confidence. Educational and support needs reflect aspects of the person's care that can be unmet or poorly met because their management is not necessarily systematically planned for in the same way as treatment regimens.

Chronic illness management relies on a person changing their health behaviour, and specifically adaptive self-management, which in turn requires the patient to understand their condition and treatment to maintain health and improve their quality of life. Professional support is required to achieve this. An editorial in the *British Medical Journal* (Bodenheimer *et al.*, 2005) has highlighted the potential key role of *Nurses as leaders in chronic care*, reflecting the need to combine treatment with education and support, which nurses are well placed to provide.

People living with long-term conditions are high demand users of health services. There is a strong policy context urging the need to address the needs of this group, improve chronic disease management through helping to improve self-care and the individual's contribution to their care (Department of Health, 2004, 2005a, b).

Therefore, a key challenge for the majority living with chronic conditions is to engage in effective self-management and self-care support. The Department of Health (2005a) highlighted the different levels of need for this group to which the service needed to respond (Figure 7.1). For those living with long-term conditions that are at high risk of deterioration, disease management is required to reduce risk, maintain health and reduce the need for hospital admission. A key target group are those living with complex conditions. This includes patients with multiple conditions, such as a person with psoriasis who also has active psoriatic arthropathy and other chronic conditions, e.g. diabetes. Intervention to maintain and promote the health of people living with long-term conditions requires a foundation of support to ensure that they can effectively do self-management.

If people with chronic conditions are to be expected to engage in a degree of self-management, it is necessary to be clear about the expectations of the person and their carers. This provides the basis for instigating an effective plan of care and treatment and determining where support is needed to prepare the person

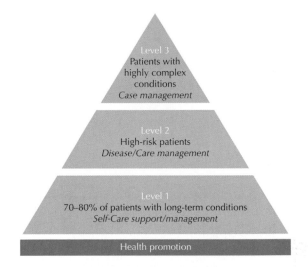

Figure 7.1 Levels of need for people with long-term conditions. (Source: Department of Health, 2005a. Reproduced under the terms of the Click-Use licence.)

and their family. It will also reflect where there are unmet or poorly met educational and support needs and then, where intervention is required, when there are limits to self-management or the process of self-care fails.

Table 7.1 illustrates some of the complexity of helping patients to use their treatment optimally and the educational and support challenges for health professionals. These areas of health care need present nurses and other health professionals with significant therapeutic opportunities to enable or empower the person and their family to engage actively in self-management. Each area of knowledge and skill also requires a degree of confidence for the person trying to apply these.

Educational and support needs are both common and individual. As such, rigorous patient surveys can provide an indication of patterns of need that practitioners can plan to address (Krueger *et al.*, 2001; Beresford, 2002). These needs are reflected in Table 7.1. They convey a need to understand their condition, those factors that adversely affect and improve it and their treatment. Dissatisfaction with the effectiveness of treatments is a theme running through the findings. This has been validated through recent qualitative evidence, reflecting self-management needs (Ersser and Cowdell, 2009).

Table 7.1 An illustration of common areas educational and psychological needs supporting self-management for those with chronic skin conditions.

Self-management competence	Knowledge required	Skill required
Managing symptoms	Understanding and beliefs about their condition	
	Symptoms and their triggers	Effective applications of topical treatments
	Treatment beliefs and understanding	Adapting treatment to change in condition
Communicate effectively with health professionals	Understanding and beliefs about their condition	
	Treatment beliefs and understanding	Ways of adapting their treatment to their lifestyle, whilst maintaining effectiveness
	Treatment choices	Exercising treatment choices adapted to preferences/lifestyle
Managing medication	Treatment beliefs and understanding	Adapting treatment to changes in their condition (e.g. during acute episodes of a chronic skin condition)
	Effectively judge when treatment is not working	Judging the limits of self-management and when to seek help
	Recognising and reporting common side-effects	The ability to recognise common side-effects is important where patients are using or changing treatments on a long-term basis

Educational resources and strategies

It is important to maintain awareness of the range of educational resources available for supporting those living with chronic conditions and their quality. Some key sources are illustrated in Table 7.2.

The task of identifying reliable information sources of quality information is a challenge for patients who can become bombarded with information sources. This may include sources such as internet sites originating from patients, voluntary groups and health professionals as structured educational information of widely varying quality to social networking exchange. A systematic review of studies reviewing health-related websites found that 70% concluded that quality of information was a problem (Eysenbach and Till, 2001). Information also comes in the form of pamphlets from charities and industry, articles in magazines, the media and friends and family. Indeed, Surridge's ongoing study (Surridge, 2005) highlighted the complexity of the process by which parents need to establish whether the source of information is reliable and beneficial or not in helping them to manage their child's eczema.

On account of the high volumes of educational material of variable quality, careful attention is needed to the ways in which patients are guided to information sources and how best to utilise resources. This should be based upon an assessment of their educational needs, preferred methods of learning and the means of access (e.g. internet) and the level and complexity of information required. Indiscriminate handing out of generic information leaflets is invariably ineffective and may well be misleading since it may lack necessary modification for the individual. There is a need to assess the effectiveness of the source material given and evaluate it as part of a package of care. This may be done in follow-up clinics or possibly telephone consultations to review learning, remaining areas of help needed and changing educational needs.

Educational opportunities need to be planned and tailored to individuals; however, consideration

Table 7.2 Educational resources related to managing chronic skin care: examples.

Websites	*Dermatology professionals*: British Association of Dermatologists information sheets www.bad.org.uk/public/leaflets/
	Dermatology sites (advanced): www.dermnet.org.nz/
	Generic sites: NHS Direct www.nhsdirect.nhs.uk/
	Condition specific sites: National Eczema Society*: www.eczema.org/abouteczema.html Psoriasis Association*: www.psoriasis-association.org.uk/ National Psoriasis Foundation: www.psoriasis.org/home/ Ichthyosis: www.ichthyosis.org.uk/
Printed materials	*Dermatology professionals*: American Academy of Dermatology: www.aad.org/forms/pamphlets/default.aspx
	Patient groups: materials can be ordered from many organisations (see above *)
	Pharmaceutical companies: these make some materials and so may have commercial influences; as such, these require careful review before use. However, useful unbiased resources can still be found, e.g. *Dermol* produce some useful tear off pads depicting and explaining the maintenance of the skin barrier using emollients.
Audiovisual materials	These are limited. Again, pharmaceutical companies make some materials and so may have commercial influences.
	Podcasts – these are under-developed at present; however, they are likely to expand: e.g. now available from the Psoriasis Association: www.psoriasis-association.org.uk/ (November 2008)

needs to be given to common learning needs that can be efficiently delivered in a group context. This can provide the added benefit of group support and vicarious learning from others and how they adapt to their condition and treatment. Group support and learning may apply to adults with a chronic skin condition, teenagers with severe acne and those with special needs, such as people living with psoriatic arthropathy or to carers, including parents of children with eczema. To ensure time is used efficiently, learning needs should be identified. Educational aids require consideration, such as the appropriate use of a DVD, discussion time and time for practical demonstrations and for questions.

Systematic methods of education and psychological support have received limited attention in dermatology, although there are a growing number of studies developing and testing interventions to support the management of specific dermatology conditions – some of which are subject to systematic reviews. One such example is a Cochrane review of psychological and educational interventions to manage childhood atopic eczema (Ersser *et al.*, 2007). For the purposes of this chapter, the findings will be briefly summarised related to educational intervention. Following a highly systematic search of the literature and the exclusion of studies which failed to meet quality criteria for effective randomised controlled trial (RCT) methodology, only four educational studies met the inclusion criteria. RCTs' meeting the inclusion criteria included: Chinn *et al.* (2002); Niebel *et al.* (2000); Staab *et al.* (2002) and Staab *et al.* (2006). In each case, the intervention was an adjunct to conventional therapy, not a substitute for it. It was not possible to synthesise the data due to the variation in the type of data available (heterogeneity). However, it was possible to provide an extensive critical appraisal of the included studies.

In summary, the studies by Niebel *et al.* (2000) and Staab *et al.* (2002, 2006) identified that education can lead to an improvement in clinical severity and in parental quality of life (Staab *et al.*, 2006), but only marginal improvement was seen in the latter within the study of Chinn *et al.* (2002). In each case, a systematic approach to education was implemented using one of two models of service delivery: (1) eczema schools – multi-disciplinary approach (more typical in Germany) and (2) nurse-led clinics (more typical in the UK). Each of the four educational studies was directed towards parental education. It was observed in the Cochrane review that the Eczema School model was more resource-intensive compared to the nurse-led clinic model (Ersser *et al.*, 2007), although no comparative studies have been undertaken as yet of their relative effectiveness. Delivery of education was demonstrated in both hospital outpatient settings (Niebel and Staab studies) and in primary care (Chinn) and with and without the use of technology. For example, Niebel's study revealed that video-assisted education was more effective in improving severity than direct education and the control (discussion) ($p < 0.001$). The most rigorous study found to date was that of Staab *et al.* (2006), which evaluated long-term outcomes. This found significant improvements in both disease severity (3 months to 7 years, $p = 0.0002$; 8–12 years, $p = 0.003$; 13–18 years, $p = 0.0001$) and parental quality of life (3 months to 7 years, $p = 0.0001$; 8–12 years, $p = 0.002$), for children with atopic eczema.

Chapter 4 outlines specific methods of psychological intervention which have an educational basis, such as the use of behavioural management (habit reversal) to manage problematic symptoms, for those living with eczema.

Theory supporting effective intervention: Social learning theory and the self-efficacy concept

(There is a need to) '...increase an individual's confidence and belief to take control over their life'. (Department of Health 2002, p. 25: *Expert Patient Programme*)

Supporting effective self-management can be a complex process for the patient and their family. The person living with a chronic condition needs to have confidence in their ability to exercise self-management. Self-efficacy is an important and related concept which is similar to but distinct from that of confidence. It may be regarded as a key motivational force which health professionals need to support. Self-efficacy is defined as: 'an individual's belief in their capacity to successfully execute a health related behaviour' (Bandura, 1977, 1989). It reflects a positive perception or belief set. The concept is based on Albert Bandura's *Social Learning Theory* (Bandura, 1977, 1997) which indicates that people learn by observing the behaviour of others within a social context. Furthermore, they

are more likely to engage in certain behaviours when they believe they are capable of carrying them out successfully; i.e. when they have high self-efficacy. Belief in one's efficacy to exercise control is viewed by Bandura as a common pathway through which psychosocial influences affect health functioning. Self-efficacy reflects a degree of mastery or control achieved through the development of behavioural or cognitive skills, social skills, life knowledge and skills, all of which are directly relevant to managing a chronic skin condition.

So much of chronic illness management is about behavioural adaptation to ensure that lifestyle is adapted to enduring illness, with people managing their illness in the context of their daily lives. Its application has been seen in work with a wide range of groups living with long-term conditions, including those with diabetes mellitus (Shortridge-Baggett and van der Bijl, 1996; Shui, 2006) and end-stage renal disease (Tsay, 2003).

Self-efficacy is directly relevant to a person's agency; this refers to their capacity to make choices and to bring about actions and influences arising from these choices, which are a key facet of such adaptation. However, it is important to note that learning may or may not result in behavioural change. For example, a person may be taught to apply their topical treatments; however, they may not have the confidence to apply them or, say, the skill to effectively apply a wrapping bandage. It is fundamental for a change of behaviour for the person, or indeed the carer, to have sufficient degree of self-belief by the person in their capacity to act, as well as knowledge, skill and indeed motivation. Enhancing a person's capacity to make choices is fundamental to helping them adapt to and effectively self-manage with a chronic illness; as such, this is a fundamental area of facilitative competence that requires development. Self-efficacy is a significant quality for those living with chronic skin conditions because it has been demonstrated to be important to a health-promoting lifestyle (Gillis, 1993). Self-efficacy is recognised as a key basis for effective self-care ability for those with chronic conditions. Principles of self-efficacy have been used to develop self-management skills; extensive testing revealed relief of debility and chronic pain in arthritis (Holman and Lorig, 1992). Perceived self-efficacy has been identified as a predictor of functional disability regardless of the level of pain or disease duration (Schiaffino and Revenson, 1992).

Social learning can be an important route to health promotion since people learn through vicarious experience (Bandura, 2004). Health professionals need to take account of this when working with patients to plan their care. Nurses can use self-efficacy–orientated education to support patient (and family) empowerment and achieve health improvement. The focus for support using the self-efficacy concept may be on the patient, carer or the parent (de Montigny and Lacharite, 2005). Parental self-efficacy is very relevant to the care of the child with conditions such as eczema, since effective management is highly dependent on the parent's effective engagement in the treatment plan. Work has been undertaken to examine parental self-efficacy in other related contexts, such as childhood asthma self-management (Hanson, 1998; Grus *et al.*, 2001).

There is a distinction between the concepts of self-efficacy and locus of control, which requires consideration when planning patient education. Self-efficacy reflects beliefs in control over *action* (such as the belief in your ability to manage your child's eczema symptoms), whereas the locus of control conveys beliefs in control over *outcomes* (such as the parent's ability to improve their child's eczema symptoms). These are distinct but interrelated ideas.

Application of self-efficacy theory to the dermatology clinic

As a basis for informing the development of interventions to enhance self-efficacy, the following strategies to enhance or provide sources of self-efficacy, as identified by (Bandura, 1997), are summarised:

1. Personal accomplishment
2. Vicarious experience (learning through the experience of others; this may be powerfully modelled by patients or carers in a similar situation or health professionals)

3. Verbal persuasion
4. Regulate emotional behaviour (primarily, the management of stress and anxiety which may impair learning)

Their practical application will now be illustrated within the context of a dermatology consultation.

- *Personal accomplishment and verbal persuasion*: Personal accomplishment can lead to stronger efficacy beliefs than other strategies of influence. This involves reinforcing (acknowledging and encouraging) instances when patients effectively engage in successful health behaviour, such as managing to apply topical medications in the correct order. It is important to assess the patient's self-management ability and to give them performance feedback, including verbal persuasion to encourage them to build on what they are already doing well.
- *Vicarious experience:* This refers to social modelling, where opportunities are provided to help the patient learn from others. This may include health professionals demonstrating effective practices, such as a wet-wrapping technique by a parent, or creating group-learning opportunities where there is sharing of good practice by a patient or parental carer with others in a similar social learning situation. Group learning also provides a resource-efficient opportunity for patient or parental carer education; this may include exposure to well-organised patient support groups such as the Psoriasis Association or the National Eczema Society.
- *Regulation of emotional behaviour*: Bandura (1997) highlights how emotional and physical arousal may interfere with the performance of a desired behaviour. Supporting the patient to regulate such emotions involves examining the patient's mood state and emotional responses to their condition and exploring coping strategies that suit them. This may involve, for example, triggering an opportunity to raise awareness for discussion, such as using a quality-of-life

questionnaire as a basis for discussing the psychosocial impact of their condition or of their usual coping methods, adaptive and maladaptive, such as exercise or excessive alcohol intake, respectively. The patient can be directed to strategies to help them manage stress and anxiety more effectively through pursuing relaxation opportunities, such as returning to social hobbies which have been curtailed due to a lack of self-esteem or engaging them in the use of relaxation methods such as progressive relaxation, yoga or mindfulness-based stress reduction techniques (a training technique to focus attention in the present moment) (Kabat-Zinn *et al.*, 1998).

There is a need to promote active engagement with health promotion materials reflection, clarification and interpretation of the person's knowledge, attitudes and beliefs as well as their involvement in health-related decision-making (Kettunen *et al.*, 2001). In practice, this will require exploration at follow-up clinics any questions regarding the information supplied or discussion of priority issues highlighted, such as the sequencing of topical treatments.

Increasingly, interventions are being developed to help improve chronic illness management and treatment adherence, which incorporates a range of educational measures based on theory. This is well illustrated in the asthma field, with studies such as that by Schaffer and Tian (2004) utilising an audio tape and booklet alone and combined, with the tape based on Protection Motivation Theory (Rogers and Prentice-Dunn, 1997). Others include the use of individual action planning based on Bandura's self-cognitive theory (van der Palen *et al.*, 2001). Wangberg (2008) study utilised an internet-based diabetes self-care intervention tailored to enhance self-efficacy. This highlights the scope to devise systematic interventions, based on theory related to motivation or self-efficacy or coping, that may enhance the likelihood of effective learning and behavioural change related to self-management.

The challenge of promoting treatment adherence

Evidence-based health care may identify treatments that are potentially effective for groups of patients; however, these are fundamentally dependent on the patient's behaviour to ensure the method of application. A major problem for many people living with chronic illness, including those with skin conditions, is that they are on a number of medications and they fail to utilise their treatment effectively; this may be due to a lack of knowledge, skill, confidence or motivation.

One example of the problem is illustrated by psoriasis, with research evidence of the problems of treatment adherence. A study by Richards *et al.* (1999) reported high levels of 'non-compliance' with treatment. Several factors are likely to contribute to this situation. Survey evidence of expectations of treatment highlights the high levels of dissatisfaction (Krueger *et al.*, 2001; Richards *et al.*, 2001; Psoriasis Association and Beresford, 2002), with many giving up their treatment. Such evidence conveys the need for more consistent education, but other studies highlight the time burden of treatment (Finlay and Coles, 1995). These findings are significant since patients' treatment expectations may affect their adherence to therapy.

The reasons for poor treatment adherence are complex. The situation involves a consideration of patient beliefs and behaviour. This is now explored in more detail by examining the process by which the health professional engages with the patient during consultation when outlining the treatment plan.

The importance of the concordance process

Effective adherence to treatment requires more than a traditional expectation of compliance, namely doing what the health professional expects 'should' be done. If adherence is to be improved, the process must involve actively engaging with the person 'based on a *negotiation* about medication between health care professional and patient that respects patients' beliefs and wishes' (Royal Pharmaceutical Society of Great Britain, 1997).

The concordance process requires that both the patient and health care professional participate to reach an agreement on the nature of the problem (illness) and the treatment plan; their agreement needs to draw on the experiences, beliefs and wishes of the patient to decide when, how and why to use medicines (Medicines Partnership, 2003). Both parties need to treat each other as partners and recognise each other's knowledge skills to improve decision-making (Atkins and Ersser, 2008). Patients' views are no less important when making decisions about what is suitable for the patient to ensure a match to their preferences and lifestyle. Through such a process of negotiation, it is more likely that there will be co-operation with and so adherence to the agreed plan. Therefore, some of the strategies for developing a negotiated approach may include the following elements:

- Listening to patient's beliefs and expectations;
- Dealing sensitively with patient's emotions and concerns;
- Helping patients to make informed choices;
- Giving explanations and rationales for treatment options;
- Negotiating outcomes of consultations that both the prescriber and patient are satisfied with;
- Giving clear instructions to patients about their medication;
- Checking the patient's understanding and commitment to treatment.

As an example, treatment adherence problems are a common cause for apparent failure that feature in atopic eczema and this includes factors such as the patient or parental carer having a poor understanding of disease (Fischer, 1996). In this context, there may be a discussion about enhancing the parent's capacity to avoid trigger factors, managing the child's sleep disturbance or finding better ways of communicating with professionals regarding treatment. Related concordance concerns may include the parent's ability to manage successfully topical applications such as emollients, antibiotic and steroid creams. Some studies have attempted to enhance concordance within a dermatology context, for example, with improved adherence to compression therapy for patients with venous leg ulcers (Brooks *et al.*, 2004).

To ensure effective use of treatment, it is necessary to explore what the patient understands by their treatment regimen within the consultation, since it may reveal areas of confusion. Evidence suggests that problems of adherence stem more from a disbelief in their efficacy to use prescribed medication effectively than from disease activity or pain (Taal *et al.*, 1993). Furthermore, common problems arise from the need to manage a number of medications and from trying to sequence topical applications effectively. Also, there can be a lack of understanding of the conditions under which 'as required' drugs can be used appropriately. Practitioners also need to explore expectations of treatments. Qualitative research evidence suggests that dermatology patients may not share precisely the same views with dermatology professionals about what criteria are important in judging effectiveness; as in the case of those living with psoriasis (Ersser *et al.*, 2002). In addition, if a person expects their treatment to work quickly but in practice, the medication is effective only after sustained treatment over a number of weeks, such as coal tar or calcipotriol use in psoriasis, there is a high risk that such treatment may be abandoned prematurely. This may also apply to the situation in which the patient believes their medication is designed to help with one symptom when it is for another, such as in the case when topical steroids may be used with the intention of controlling eczema, but when infected, an antimicrobial agent would be required.

There is a need to give consideration therefore to the range of factors affecting both the patients or carers' treatment choice (preference) and use in practice and to recognise the related educational opportunities. The following discussions will take place within the context of the health care consultation, to which we now turn.

The therapeutic consultation

Over-emphasis on technology tends to overshadow therapeutic modalities that can have real significance. Nurses must recognise that they do not create change in people, rather they participate in the process of change to the extent that they bring knowledge to the situation and recognise that the healing process has the potential for healing beyond that which we recognise today. *(Rogers, 1992, p. 61)*

To help the patient make the most of their treatment, there is a fundamental need for health professionals to create effective opportunities for open communication within the context of the dermatology consultation. The consultation provides the key opportunity for effective education and support. It is paradoxical that within the discussion of evidence-based treatment in dermatology care, very little attention is paid to the quality of the consultation opportunity as a human interaction that can profoundly influence the patient's behaviour, treatment plan and the final outcome of the care. Some attention has been paid to these issues in nursing in general (Ersser, 1997; Kinmouth *et al.*, 1998; Watson, 1999), with limited attention in the dermatology nursing context (with some exceptions, e.g. Courtenay *et al.*, 2009). General practice research has paid attention to consultation issues amongst GPs and nurses (Kinmouth *et al.*, 1998); however, this remains a neglected area within the dermatological literature.

The quality of the consultation and its outcome is directly dependent on the quality of the practitioner–patient relationship and the ability to ensure that they optimise opportunities for education and support. Typically, nurses are well placed to do this should they allow time to assess and plan for patients' support need, although it is also essential for the dermatologist–patient consultation when making crucial decisions about treatment plans. This may also apply to nurse–prescriber–patient consultations in some countries such as the UK.

The literature from the social psychology literature on therapeutic professional relationships

Table 7.3 Features of therapeutic-helping relationships.

Feature	Illustrative supporting references
Self-awareness	Freshwater (2002), Egan (1994), Peplau (1988), Krikoriam and Paulanka (1982)
Being genuine and authentic	Jourard (1971), Truax *et al.* (1974), Mitchell *et al.* (1977)
Committed to patient participation in care	Brearley (1990), Hays and Dimatteo (1984), Roberts *et al.* (1995)
Emotional involvement and closeness	Jourard (1971), Strang (1982)
Empathy	Morse *et al.* (1992), Truax *et al.* (1974), Mitchell *et al.* (1977)
Trust	Watson (1985), Bernado (1984)
Unconditional positive regard/ warmth/caring	Geanellos (2005), Sellick (1991), Stickley and Freshwater (2002), Combs *et al.* (1971), Mitchell *et al.* (1977), Morse *et al.* (1992)

reveals common features which apply to all therapeutic and helping relationships. There is also evidence of the exploration of the distinctive therapeutic opportunities that nurses may have through helping patients with everyday living activities as well as treatments (Ersser, 1997); these are summarised and exemplified in Table 7.3.

Central to all the features of therapeutic relationships is the capacity for self-awareness within the health professional, as a prerequisite for enhancing the therapeutic quality of the consultation (Ersser, 1997; Freshwater, 2002). These features help to create the opportunity for effective patient education and support described previously. Taking the example of the concordance process, this is much more likely to be effective when there is a commitment to patient involvement, empathy to their concerns and preferences, unconditional positive regard and self-awareness regarding the health professional's own preferences and predispositions related to patient care. However, these features of therapeutic relationships cannot be taken for granted as being ever present; for example,

Sellick (1991) found that nurses had a stronger desire to control relationships than other professionals, such as occupational therapists.

Through the nurse–patient relationship, the nurse has scope to meet the patient's expectations for seeking help, including their need to receive support to develop their abilities and independence and play their part in managing their condition.

To achieve this, nurses may contribute as a resource and catalyst for the patient by raising mutual awareness of their needs on their journey from dependence to independence; this is achieved through the formation of an attachment, providing the patient with a basis for support (Ersser and Watkins, 2007). Attachment relationships are common in helping relationships and times of need (Ersser, 1997). Attachment theory is relevant to adults as well as children – and remains an important theory in the social psychology literature (Rholes and Simpson, 2006). It is concerned with adult attachment styles and the psychological underpinnings and how these make an impact on the outcomes of different attachment styles. Dependence and anxiety may be reduced and the patient can explore new coping mechanisms adapted to new awareness and diverted into positive control over the experience of symptoms/illness. McCluskey (2005, pp. 86–87) describes the consequences of an effective attachment as follows: 'The care-seeker has the subjective experience of accessing competence. When this happens, the instinctive system for care-seeking will shut down and the exploratory system within the individual will have more energy to engage with the problems of living.' The appropriate caregiver response to the patient's (or parental carer) need is to put them in touch with their competence to act and reactivate their emotional, physical and intellectual capacity and resources applied to the individual (Ersser and Watkins, 2007).

There is evidence of distinctive therapeutic opportunities for education and support provided within nursing therapeutic or helping relationships. This may include meeting a range of patient needs through the provision of skilled bodily or intimate physical care such as washing and moisturising the skin Lawler, 1991; Ersser, 1997). Furthermore, there is evidence of a recognition of the integrated nature of care of mind and body, with an emphasis on maximising the therapeutic opportunities that exist within ordinary daily care, such as skin hygiene or helping to apply treatments events, which provide therapeutic opportunities to integrate the meeting of both physical and psychological needs (Chapman, 1986; Taylor, 1994).

Therefore, in conclusion, there is a need for the health professional to cultivate an accessible, effective consultation style, building on established psychological principles on therapeutic/ helping relationships, as a basis for helping or empowering the person to be able to engage actively in contributing to the management of their own health.

Prescribing skin-related products and opportunities for medicines education

The prescription and administration of medicines provides a substantial opportunity to help people make the most of their treatment through teaching the patient about how to use their treatment most effectively. Nurses have an established role in drug administration, ensuring that suitable medication is delivered at the right dose, time and by the appropriate route. Therefore, whether through drug administration or prescription, health professionals have substantial opportunities to ensure suitable treatment selection taking into account patient needs and preferences and taking of medicines to improve treatment adherence and effectiveness. Treatment adherence and successful medicine management are dependent on effective education and support, which if planned and delivered effectively nurse prescribers are well placed to provide. Consideration is needed of the value of investing sufficient time to explain effectively intricate treatment regimens to the patient, and in doing so, take account of their lifestyle so that the guidance is adapted to the individual and their level of knowledge. This is likely to improve the effective use of medicines and their

---

> **Box 7.1 Mechanisms available for the prescribing supply and administration of medicines**
>
> - Patient-specific directions
> - Patient group directions
> - Specific exemptions covering supply or administration – as contained in medicines legislation
> - Nurse-independent prescribing
> - Pharmacist-independent prescribing
> - Supplementary prescribing by nurses, pharmacists, optometrists, Physiotherapists, radiographers and chiropodists/podiatrists
>
> *Source*: Department of Health (2006). Reproduced under the terms of the Click-Use licence.

efficacy and reduce the time required to deal with the consequences of poor adherence. Nurse prescribing consultations should prioritise these opportunities for education and support, since invariably their *focus* is not on diagnosis.

The prescribing of treatments within dermatology is no longer confined to medical practitioners in some countries, such as the UK, but now by others such as suitably trained nurses, pharmacists and podiatrists. Membership of the Nurse Prescribing sub-group of the British Dermatological Nursing Group continues to increase rapidly.

The mechanisms available for the prescribing supply and administration of medicines is summarised in Box 7.1 (Department of Health, 2006).

These different mechanisms will now be briefly outlined. Note these are only relevant for countries within the UK.

Patient-specific directions

A patient-specific direction (PSD) is the traditional written instruction, from a doctor, dentist, nurse or pharmacist-independent prescriber,

for medicines to be supplied or administered to a named patient (Department of Health, 2006). The majority of medicines are still supplied or administered using this process. In primary care, this might be a simple instruction in the patient's notes. Examples in secondary care include instructions on a patient's ward drug chart. As a PSD is individually tailored to the needs of a single patient, it should be used in preference to a patient group direction (PGD), wherever appropriate.

Patient group directions

A PGD is a written instruction for the supply or administration of a licensed medicine (or medicines) in an identified clinical situation, where the patient may not be individually identified before presenting for treatment. Patients may or may not be identified, depending on the circumstances (DH, 2006). A PGD is drawn up locally by doctors, pharmacists and other health professionals and must meet certain legal criteria. Each PGD must be signed by a doctor or dentist, as appropriate, and a pharmacist and approved by the organisation in which it is to be used, typically a PCT or NHS Trust. PGDs can only be used by specified registered health care professionals, acting as named individuals, including nurses, health visitors, paramedics and podiatrists. Each PGD has a list of individuals named as competent to supply/administer under the direction.

Independent prescribing

The development of independent prescribing is part of a drive to make better use of nurses' and pharmacists' skills and to make it easier for patients to get access to the medicines that they need. From 1 May 2006, 'Nurse Independent Prescribing' (formerly 'Extended Formulary Nurse Prescribing') was expanded. This allows nurses to prescribe any licensed medicine for any medical condition that a nurse prescriber is competent to treat, including some controlled drugs. It allows virtually any licensed medicine in the British National Formulary (see part XVIIB(ii) of the Drug Tariff) to be prescribed (Department of Health, 2006). Pharmacist-independent prescribing now permits suitably prepared pharmacists to prescribe any licensed medicine for any medical condition that they are competent to treat. In the UK, all first-level registered nurses, registered midwives, registered specialist community public health nurses and registered pharmacists may train to be independent prescribers. Further information on nurse-independent prescribing can be found on the Department of Health (Department of Health, 2008) website, which should be checked regularly for updates.

Supplementary prescribing

Supplementary prescribing was introduced in April 2003 for nurses and pharmacists. It was extended to physiotherapists, chiropodists/podiatrists, radiographers and optometrists in May 2005. Supplementary prescribing is a voluntary prescribing partnership between the independent prescriber (doctor or dentist) and supplementary prescriber, to implement an agreed patient-specific clinical management plan (CMP), with the patient's agreement (Department of Health, 2006). Following agreement of the CMP, the supplementary prescriber may prescribe any medicine for the patient that is referred to in the plan, until the next review by the independent prescriber. There is no formulary for supplementary prescribing and no restrictions on the medical conditions that can be managed under these arrangements. It will also be appropriate in specific situations, for instance, when working within a team where a doctor is accessible or for specific long-term conditions, between medical reviews (Department of Health, 2006).

Supplementary prescribers can prescribe controlled drugs and unlicensed medicines in partnership with a doctor, where the doctor agrees within a patient's CMP. From July 2006, chiropodists/podiatrists physiotherapists, radiographers and optometrists are also able to prescribe controlled drugs as supplementary prescribers, but only where there is a patient need and the doctor has agreed in a patient's CMP.

The training for supplementary prescribing is incorporated into nurse and pharmacist-independent prescribing. All professional groups must register their supplementary prescribing qualification with their regulatory body before beginning to prescribe. Further information can be found on the Department of Health (2003, 2008, 2009) website. See Table 7.4 for more sources of information on non-medical prescribing.

Table 7.4 Sources of information on non-medical prescribing.

1.	**Department of Health (DH) website:** The DH website is regularly updated and has comprehensive information on all aspects of prescribing. A section on 'Non-Medical Prescribing guidance' can be found in the 'Policy and guidance A–Z'. This includes *'Improving Access to Medicines – the DH guide to implementation of nurse- and pharmacists-independent prescribing'* April 2006. www.dh.gov.uk/nonmedicalprescribing
2.	**Clinical Knowledge Summaries (CKS):** CKS guidance on common conditions and symptoms managed in primary care is available in a variety of formats. Full guidance provides concise information to support decision-making in the consultation and more detailed background information for use as a learning resource. CKS Patient Information Leaflets (PILs) provide guidance for people who are not health care professionals and give an overview of the condition, side-effects, advice on self-management, information on treatment options and sources of further help. CKS Drugs – lists the drugs recommended and links them to the condition and situation in which they are recommended www.cks.nhs.uk
3.	**Medicines and Health care products Regulatory Agency (MHRA):** The MHRA website contains information about the legal framework governing the prescribing, supply and administration of medicines (www.mhra.gov.uk).
4.	**Other useful websites** • British National Formulary (BNF): http://bnf.org/bnf/ • Examples of patient group directions (PGDs): www.portal.nelm.nhs.uk • Medicines Partnership Programme: www.medicines-partnership.org

(continued)

Table 7.4   *(continued)*

- National Electronic Library for Health: www .nelh.nhs.uk
- NHS Drug Tariff for England and Wales: http:// www.ppa.org.uk/ppa/edt_intro.htm
- NHS National Practitioner Programme: www .wise.nhs.uk
- National Prescribing Centre: www.npc.co.uk
- Nursing and Midwifery Council: www. nmc-uk.org
- Prescribing news: www.nurse-prescriber.co.uk
- Royal Pharmaceutical Society of Great Britain: www.rpsgb.org

Conclusion

Those living with long-term conditions are required to a degree to self-manage their condition with the support of health professionals to ensure that treatment is utilised effectively. This issue is often highly problematic since many people do not know how to use their treatment to optimum levels, leading to difficulties of treatments being ineffective, due to poor adherence. Optimal treatment adherence is that which has arisen from a planned consultation between the practitioner and patient, embracing education and support, to ensure that treatment and condition beliefs and expectations are understood and acted upon. The systematic assessment of educational needs is a vital component of helping a person to live with their chronic skin condition. A concordance process provides an optimal model for engaging the patient in decisions regarding their treatment. However, there is also a need to recognise the limitations of self-management when the person cannot manage their condition effectively. This needs to be built into the educational process to ensure that the person utilises the health service effectively. Non-medical prescribing is an important strategy for improving access to medicines and promoting education surrounding medicines management – provided by suitably qualified staff who can both prescribe and teach patients about their medication and how to use it for optimum benefit.

References

Atkins, S. and S.J. Ersser (2008). Clinical decision-making and patient-centred care. In: Higgs, J., Jones, M., Loftus, S., Christensen, N. (Eds), *Clinical Reasoning in the Health Professions*. Oxford: Butterworth-Heinemann.

Bandura, A. (1977). *Social Learning Theory*. Englewood Cliffs, NJ: Prentice Hall.

Bandura, A. (1989). Human agency in social cognitive theory. *American Psychologist*, **44**(9): 1174–1184.

Bandura, A. (1997). *Self-efficacy: The Exercise of Control*. New York: Freeman.

Bandura, A. (2004). Health promotion by social cognitive means. *Health Education and Behaviour*, **31**(2): 143–164.

Beresford, A. (2002). *Psoriasis Association Members Questionnaire Survey*. Northampton: Psoriasis Association.

Bernado, M.L. (1984). Developing the professional nursing relationship. *Nursing Forum*, **21**(1): 12–14.

Bodenheimer, T., T. MacGregor *et al.* (2005). Nurses as leaders in chronic care. *British Medical Journal*, **330**: 612–613.

Brearley, S. (1990). *Patient Participation*. London: Royal College of Nursing.

Brooks, J., S.J. Ersser *et al.* (2004). Nurse-led education sets out to improve patient concordance and prevent recurrence of leg ulcers. *Journal of Wound Care*, **13**(3): 111–116.

Chapman, G. (1986). Social action theory and psychosocial nursing. In: Kennedy, R., Heymans, A., Tischler, Y. (Eds), *The Family as In-Patient: Families and Adolescents at the Cassel Hospital*. London: Free Association Books.

Chinn, D.J., T. Poyner *et al.* (2002). Randomized controlled trial of a single dermatology nurse consultation in primary care on the quality of life of children with atopic eczema. *British Journal of Dermatology*, **146**(3): 432–439.

Combs, A.W., D.L. Avila *et al.* (1971). *Helping Relationships: Basic Concepts for the Helping Profession*. Boston: Allyn and Baron.

Courtenay, M., N. Carey *et al.* (2009). Nurse prescriber–patient consultations: A case study in dermatology. *Journal of Advanced Nursing*, **65**(6): 1207–1217.

de Montigny, F. and C. Lacharite (2005). Perceived parental efficacy: Concept analysis. *Journal of Advanced Nursing*, **49**(4): 387–396.

Department of Health (2002). *Expert Patient Programme: A New Approach to Chronic Disease Management for the 21st Century.* London: The Stationery Office.

Department of Health (2003). *Supplementary Prescribing by Nurses and Pharmacists with the NHS in England: A Guide for Implementation.* London: The Stationery Office.

Department of Health (2004). *Improving Chronic Disease Management.* Department of Health.

Department of Health (2005a). *Supporting People with Long Term Conditions.* Department of Health.

Department of Health (2005b). *Self-care – A Real Choice: Self Care Support A Practical Option.* Department of Health.

Department of Health (2006). *Medicine Matters: A Guide to Mechanisms for the Prescribing, Supply and Administration of Medicines. D. o. H. C. P. G. Department of Health National Practitioner Programme,* Department of Health.

Department of Health (2008). Supplementary Prescribing. Retrieved 24 April 2009, from www.dh.gov.uk/en/Healthcare/ Medicinespharmacyandindustry/Prescriptions/ TheNon-MedicalPrescribingProgramme/ Supplementaryprescribing/index.htm.

Department of Health (2009). The Non-Medical Prescribing Programme. Retrieved 254 April 2009, from http://www.dh.gov.uk/en/Healthcare/ Medicinespharmacyandindustry/Prescriptions/ TheNon-MedicalPrescribingProgramme/ index.htm.

Egan, G. (1994). *The Skilled Helper: A Problem Centred Management Approach to Helping.* New York: Brooks/Cole Publishing Company.

Ersser, S.J. (1997). *Nursing as a Therapeutic Activity: An Ethnography.* Aldershot: Avebury Press.

Ersser, S.J. and F. Cowdell (2009). *An Exploratory and Developmental Study of Self-management Needs in Adults with Mild to Moderate Psoriasis.* Bournemouth: Centre for Wellbeing & Quality of Life, Bournemouth University.

Ersser, S.J., S. Latter *et al.* (2007). Psychological and educational interventions for atopic eczema in children. Description: *Cochrane Database of Systematic Reviews*, **3**: CD004054. (DOI: 10.1002/14651858. CD004054.pub2.)

Ersser, S.J., H. Surridge *et al.* (2002). What criteria do patients use when judging the effectiveness of psoriasis management? *Journal of Evaluation in Clinical Practice*, **8**(4): 367–376.

Ersser, S.J. and P. Watkins (2007). Psychosocial interventions in dermatology: An analysis of the nursing contribution. Annual Psychodermatology Meeting. Medical Society of London.

Eysenbach, G. and J. Till (2001). Ethical issues in qualitative research on internet communities. *British Medical Journal*, **323**(7321): 1103–1105.

Finlay, A.Y. and E.C. Coles (1995). The effect of severe psoriasis on the quality of life of 369 patients. *British Journal of Dermatology*, **132**(2): 236–244.

Fischer, G. (1996). Compliance problems in paediatric atopic eczema. *Australasian Journal of Dermatology*, **37**(Suppl 1): S10–13.

Freshwater, D. (2002). *Therapeutic Nursing: Improving Patient Care through Self-Awareness and Reflection.* London: Sage.

Geanellos, R. (2005). Sustaining wellbeing and enabling recovery: The therapeutic effect of nurse friendliness on clients and nursing environments. *Contemporary Nurse*, **19**(1–2): 242–252.

Gillis, A.J. (1993). Determinants of a health promoting lifestyle: An integrative review. *Journal of Advanced Nursing*, **18**: 345–353.

Grus, C.L., C. Lopez-Hernandez *et al.* (2001). Parental self-efficacy and morbidity in pediatric asthma. *Journal of Asthma*, **38**(1): 99–106.

Hanson, J. (1998). Parental self-efficacy and asthma self-management skills. *Journal of the Society of Paediatric Nurses*, 3(4): 146–154

Hays, R. and M.R. Dimatteo (1984). Toward a More Therapeutic Physicians–Patient Relationship. In: Duck, S.W. (Ed.), *Personal Relationships 5: Repairing Personal Relationships*. London: Academic Press.

Holman, H. and K. Lorig (1992). Perceived self-efficacy in self-management of chronic disease. In: Schwarzer, R. (Ed.), *Self-Efficacy: Thought Control of Action*, pp. 305–323. Washington, DC: Hemisphere.

Jourard, S.M. (1971). *The Transparent Self*. New York: Van Nostrand.

Kabat-Zinn, J., E. Wheeler *et al.* (1998). Influence of a mindfulness meditation-based stress reduction intervention on rates of skin clearing in patients with moderate to severe psoriasis undergoing phototherapy (UVB) and photochemotherapy (PUVA). *Psychosomatic Medicine*, 60(5): 625–632.

Kettunen, T., M. Poskiparta *et al.* (2001). Empowering counselling – a case study: Nurse–patient encounter in hospital. *Health Education Research*, 16(2): 227–238.

Kinmouth, A.L., A. Woodcock *et al.* (1998). Randomised controlled trial of patient centred care of diabetes in general practice: Impact on current wellbeing and future disease risk. The Diabetes Care from Diagnosis Research Team. *British Medical Journal*, 317(7167): 1202–1208.

Krikoriam, D.A. and B.J. Paulanka (1982). Self-awareness: The key to a successful nurse–patient relationship. *Journal of Psychosocial Nursing and Mental Health Services*, 20(6): 19–21.

Krueger, G., J. Koo *et al.* (2001). The impact of psoriasis on quality of life – Results of a 1998 National Psoriasis Foundation patient-membership survey. *Archives of Dermatology*, 137(3): 280–284.

Lawler, J. (1991). *Behind the Screens: Nursing, Somology and the Problem of the Body*. Melbourne: Churchill Livingstone.

Marks, R. (2000). Who will advise patients about matters dermatological in the new millennium? *Archives of Dermatology*, 136: 79–80.

McCluskey, U. (2005). *To Be Met as a Person: The Dynamics of Attachment in Professional Encounters*. London: Karnac.

Medicines Partnership (2003). *Medicines Partnership Project Evaluation Toolkit*. London: Medicines Partnership.

Mitchell, K., J. Bozanth *et al.* (1977). A reappraisal of the therapeutic effectiveness of accurate empathy, possessive warmth and genuineness. In: Gurucan, A., Raizin, A. (Eds), *Effective Psychotherapy*. Oxford: Pergamon Press.

Morse, J., J. Bortoff *et al.* (1992). Beyond empathy: Expanding expressions of caring. *Journal of Advanced Nursing*, 17: 809–821.

Niebel, G., C. Kallweit *et al.* (2000). Direct versus video-based parental education in the treatment of atopic eczema in children. A controlled pilot study [Direkte versus videovermittelte Elternschulung bei atopischem Ekzem im Kindesalter als Erganzung facharztlicher Behandlung. Eine Kontrollierte Pilotstudie]. *Hautarzt*, 51: 401–411.

Peplau, H.E. (1988). *Interpersonal Relations in Nursing*. Houndmills: Palgrave Macmillan.

Psoriasis Association (UK) and Beresford, A. (2002) Report of the Psoriasis Association Members Questionnaire Survey, Psoriasis Association and Leo Pharmaceuticals.

Rholes, W.S. and J.A. Simpson (2006). *Adult Attachment*. New York: The Guildford Press.

Richards, H.L., D.G. Fortune *et al.* (2001). The contribution of perceptions of stigmatisation to disability in patients with psoriasis. *Journal of Psychosomatic Research*, 50(1): 11–15.

Richards, H.L., D.G. Fortune *et al.* (1999). Patients with psoriasis and their compliance with medication. *Journal of the American Academy of Dermatology*, 41(4): 581–583.

Roberts, S.J., H.J. Krouse *et al.* (1995). Negotiated and non-negotiated patient interactions: Enhancing perceptions of empowerment. *Clinical Nursing Research*, 4(1): 67–77.

Rogers, M.E. (1992). *Prelude to the 21st Century. Commemorative Edition: Notes on Nursing. F. Nightingale.* Philadelphia: Lippincott, J.B.

Rogers, R.W. and S. Prentice-Dunn (1997). Protection motivation theory. In: Gochman, D.S. (Ed.), *Handbook of Health Behavior Research 1: Personal and Social Determinants,* pp. 113–132. New York: Plenum Press..

Royal Pharmaceutical Society of Great Britain (1997). *From compliance to concordance: Achieving shared goals in medicine taking.* Report of the working group at the Royal Pharmaceutical Society which enquired into the causes of medicine taking problems. London: RPSGB.

Schaffer, S.D. and L. Tian (2004). Promoting adherence: Effects of theory-based asthma education. *Clinical Nursing Research*, **13**(1): 69–89.

Schiaffino, K.M. and T.A. Revenson (1992). The role of perceived self-efficacy, personal control and causal attributions in adaptation of rheumatoid arthritis: Distinguishing mediator from moderator effects. *Personality and Social Psychology Bulletin*, **18**: 709–718.

Sellick, K.J. (1991). Nurses interpersonal behaviours and the development of helping skills. *International Journal of Nursing Studies*, **28**(1): 3–11.

Shortridge-Baggett, L.M. and J.J. van der Bijl (1996). International collaborative research on management self-efficacy in diabetes mellitus. *Journal of the New York State Nurses Association*, **27**(3): 9–14.

Shui, A. (2006). *A case study of the education process for diabetes self-management in a nurse-led centre in Hong Kong.* A Unpublished PhD thesis. University of (Southampton). Southampton: School of Nursing and Midwifery.

Staab, D., T.L. Diepgen *et al.* (2006). Age related, structured educational programmes for the management of atopic dermatitis in children and adolescents: Multicentre, randomised controlled trial. *British Medical Journal*, **332**: 933–938.

Staab, D., U. von Rueden *et al.* (2002). Evaluation of a parental training program for the management of atopic dermatitis. *Pediatric Allergy and Immunology*, **13**: 84–90.

Stickley, T. and D. Freshwater (2002). The art of loving and the therapeutic relationship. *Nursing Inquiry*, **9**(4): 250–256.

Strang, J. (1982). Psychotherapy by nurses – some special characteristics. *Journal of Advanced Nursing*, **7**: 167–171.

Surridge, H.R. (2005). Exploring parental needs and knowledge when caring for a child with eczema. *Patient Magazine of the National Eczema Society*.

Taal, E., E. Rasker *et al.* (1993). Health status, adherence with health recommendations, self-efficacy and social support in patients with rheumatoid arthritis. *Patient Education Counseling*, **20**: 63–76.

Taylor, B.J. (1994). *Being Human: Ordinariness in Nursing.* Edinburgh: Churchill Livingstone.

Truax, C.B., H. Altmann *et al.* (1974). Therapeutic relations provided by various professionals. *Journal of Community Psychology*, **2**(1): 33–36.

Tsay, S.L. (2003). Self-efficacy training for patients with end-stage renal disease. *Journal of Advanced Nursing*, **43**(4): 370–375.

van der Palen, J., J.J. Klein *et al.* (2001). Behavioural effect of self-treatment guidelines in a self-management program for adults with asthma. *Patient Education and Counseling*, **43**(2): 161–169.

Wangberg, S.C. (2008). An internet-based diabetes self-care intervention tailored to self-efficacy. *Health Education Research*, **23**(1): 170–179.

Watson, J. (1985). *Nursing: The Philosophy and Science of Caring.* Colorado: Associated University Press.

Watson, J. (1999). *Postmodern Nursing and Beyond: Redefining Nursing for the 21st Century.* Edinburgh: Churchill Livingstone.

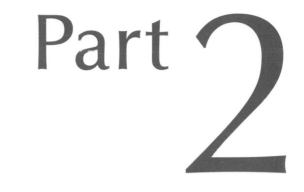

Part 2

Principles of illness management

Psoriasis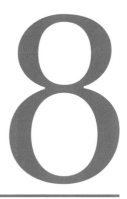

Rebecca Penzer

Introduction

Psoriasis is a chronic inflammatory condition that is thought to affect around 2% of the population in the UK and the USA. It was first distinguished as a unique diagnosis in the 19th century, prior to that it was often mistaken for other conditions such as leprosy (Franklin and Glickman, 1986). Since that time numerous different presentations have been identified with a wide range of morphological features. This has lead to questions about whether all these presentations are indeed the one disease that is called psoriasis, or a range of conditions with some similarities. From a histopathological point of view, it is not always possible to distinguish psoriasis from other chronic inflammatory conditions; this will depend to an extent on the time at which a biopsy is taken. Whilst the very typical clinical appearance allows experienced practitioners to reach the right diagnosis, effective treatment becomes the next challenge. This chapter will consider the biology of psoriasis and explore the various treatment options available and how their efficacy might be enhanced. Specific issues about coping with psoriasis and its impact on quality of life are discussed, with

reference made to Chapter 6 where generic issues of skin disease and mental health are considered in detail.

History of psoriasis

Early references to skin diseases can be found in the Old Testament of the Bible. Translations from Hebrew into English meant that skin diseases became known as leprosy, even though they clearly did not describe the disease we now know as leprosy. In Ancient Greek, the word 'lepra' was used to describe skin that was scaly and rough which relates much more closely to the symptoms of psoriasis than those of leprosy. The word 'psora' was used by the Greeks to describe itchy skin conditions. This is somewhat strange in view of the fact that today some medical textbooks make claim to the fact that psoriasis is not an itchy skin condition.

In the late 18th century two dermatologists Robert Willan and Thomas Bateman described psoriasis as Willan's lepra, a term used to describe the typically dry and scaly lesions. By the mid-19th century an Austrian doctor Ferdinand von Hebra finally labelled the disease by what is now its modern name of psoriasis. The 20th century saw the distinctions made between all the various different types of psoriasis.

Who gets psoriasis?

Exact figures about the proportions of populations that have psoriasis do vary. However in Caucasian populations it is thought that around 2% have psoriasis. The incidence is less in Africans (0.7%), Asians and Native Americans (Camisa, 2004a). It affects men and women equally. The average age of onset is 30; however, psoriasis may be experienced for the first time much earlier than this or indeed much later. There do appear to be two peaks of onset, one in early adulthood and the other in later life (Williams, 1997).

There is little doubt that there is a genetic component to psoriasis; the earlier the psoriasis occurs and the more severe the disease, the stronger the familial association. However, monozygotic twins (i.e. those that come from one fertilised egg that divides) will not always both have psoriasis. This suggests that it is likely that environmental factors play a role in the development of active symptoms.

The understanding of the genetic components of psoriasis is constantly increasing as research allows ever more detailed examination of the human genome. There are a number of chromosomes (e.g. chromosome 6 and 17) which carry genes that seem to increase the likelihood of developing psoriasis, i.e. they are not causative genes but instead they increase the susceptibility of an individual to develop the condition. As there are a number of different genes which code for psoriasis, the way the psoriasis appears, when it appears and how it responds to treatment vary enormously.

Psoriasis, like all chronic skin conditions, is not contagious. This is important to stress to individuals when they are initially diagnosed with the condition as they may worry about passing the disease onto others.

Biology of psoriasis

At a simple level, psoriasis is characterised by an over proliferation of keratinocytes, i.e. skin cells replicating too quickly. The number of proliferative cells in the basal layer doubles and the normal cell cycle (which is around 28 days) is speeded up by seven times, the transit time becoming around 4 days (although this will vary depending on disease severity). Not only does over proliferation occur but incomplete cell development, that is abnormal keratinocyte differentiation, is also seen. The granular layer is either absent or reduced and hyperkeratosis and parakeratosis develop. This hyperproliferation is accompanied by inflammation and vascular changes. Skin cells heap up into plaques and are then shed in noticeable clumps.

Clinically, a typical psoriatic plaque is salmon pink in Caucasian skin and a slightly darker shade of normal skin tone for skin types 4–6. The actual colour of the plaque may be masked by a covering of silvery, white skin scales. Because of the high level of vascular activity within the psoriatic plaques, there is a proliferation of blood vessels near the surface of the plaque. This accounts for the change in colour of the skin and also explains a unique symptom of psoriasis known as Auspitz sign. This describes the symptom of pin-prick bleeding when the skin is scratched or knocked by the slightest trauma. The hyperkeratosis leads to induration or skin thickening so that a plaque is raised from the rest of the skin surface.

The simple description of psoriasis being a hyperproliferative disorder with significant inflammatory components belies a complex cascade of immune stimulated reactions that occur in the skin. Understanding of these processes is increasing, but the picture is still somewhat incomplete. However, it is reasonable to describe psoriasis as an immune-mediated condition in which T-cells play a significant role; indeed, psoriasis is recognised as the most prevalent T-cell-mediated inflammatory condition seen in humans (Kreuger, 2002).

T-cells are a type of lymphocyte (other lymphocytes being B-cells and natural killer cells) and they play an important role in cell-mediated immunity. It is well recognised that T-lymphocytes infiltrate the skin where psoriatic plaques occur and more recently it has been possible to identify the sub-types of these T-cells as $CD4^+$ and $CD8^+$ T-lymphocytes. It is not entirely clear what causes this initial activation of the T-cells; however, once activated they move into the bloodstream and from there into the dermis by 'squeezing' through the blood vessel walls. Here they are reactivated; $CD4^+$ cells into Type 1 helper cells (TH1) and $CD8^+$ cells into Type 1 cytotoxic cells. Reactivation occurs through contact with antigen presenting cells. Together these two types of cells initiate an inflammatory cascade as inflammatory cytokines, whereby interferon gamma (IFN γ) and tumour necrotising factor alpha (TNF-α) are produced. These cytokines incorporate with proinflammatory chemicals which in turn cause the keratinocytes to hyperproliferate. In patients without psoriasis, this inflammatory process is a response to a physical, biological or chemical trigger which threatens (or causes) injury. Once the injury is resolved, the inflammatory process is switched off. In patients with psoriasis, it is thought that the immune system mistakenly recognises the body's cells as foreign, triggering the repair response causing inflammation. This response is not 'switched off' in the way that it is following an actual injury and skin cells continue to proliferate.

Comorbidities associated with psoriasis

There are a number of diseases which are associated with psoriasis; some of which have been recognised for a long time and others which have emerged from more recent research.

The well-recognised comorbidities include psoriatic arthritis (PSA) (which is discussed in the next section), psychological/psychiatric disorders and inflammatory bowel disease, particularly Crohn's disease. Research has confirmed that the associations between psoriasis and these conditions are

well established. Thus up to 30% of those with psoriasis have joint pain (Osborn and Wilke, 2004). The impact on quality of life for those with psoriasis is comparable to those who have cancer, arthritis and depression (Rapp *et al.*, 1999) and patients with inflammatory bowel disease are up to seven times more likely than the normal population to develop psoriasis (Christophers, 2007).

There also appears to be an increased risk of malignancy in those with psoriasis; however, whilst this may be associated with underlying immunological changes in the skin, it is also likely that some treatments (notably PUVA and high-dose methotrexate) lead to an increased risk of malignancy (Gulliver, 2008).

Whilst not strictly speaking comorbidities, there does seem to be a link between psoriasis and certain lifestyle choices, namely smoking and drinking. For example, a study carried out in Italy found that there was a negative effect on the severity of psoriasis (particularly in women) in those who smoked (Fortes *et al.*, 2005). A particularly strong association has been shown between smoking and palmoplantar psoriasis with smokers five times more likely to suffer from the disease than non-smokers (Naldi *et al.*, 2005). The likelihood of alcohol abuse is increased in patients with psoriasis with a German study showing that increased alcohol consumption was seen twice as frequently in patients with moderate to severe psoriasis than in hospital-based controls. It is not clear if psoriasis is a risk factor for tendency to smoking or excessive drinking, but both the behaviours will increase the risk of mortality (Sommer *et al.*, 2006). The direction of the association between psoriasis and drinking and smoking is not clear. It is still not certain whether smoking and drinking are risk factors for developing psoriasis or whether they are behaviours that people develop in order to help them cope with having psoriasis.

More recently research has turned its attention to making connections between diseases which are known to have a chronic inflammatory association and particularly those that are mediated by proinflammatory T-helper type 1 cytokines (as psoriasis is). In a review article,

Gulliver (2008) summarises what he calls the emerging comorbidities: obesity, dyslipidaemia, hypertension and glucose intolerance (otherwise known as metabolic syndrome) all show increased prevalence in people with psoriasis. For obesity and diabetes, at least, it seems there is a greater prevalence in people with severe disease than those with mild disease.

Because of the greater prevalence of cardiovascular risk factors in those with psoriasis, it has been suggested that psoriasis might be an independent risk factor in itself for cardiovascular events including myocardial infarction. In other words just the very fact of having psoriasis makes an individual at higher risk of having cardiovascular events. The evidence here is mixed. However, what does seem clearer is that patients with psoriasis appear to have an increased risk of coronary artery calcification (which predisposes to atherosclerosis) and psoriasis is an independent risk factor for coronary artery calcification. It might therefore be expected that those with psoriasis would have a lower life expectancy than those without, here again the evidence is not wholly clear; however, a study in 2007 indicated that for those with severe disease there was a significantly increased risk of mortality(Gelfand *et al.*, 2007). When comparing those with severe psoriasis to those without psoriasis, the figures from the study indicated that men died 3.5 years earlier and women 4.4 years earlier than the normal population.

Further research is needed in this field to clarify the relationships between psoriasis and the aforementioned comorbidities. The processes which lead to low-grade persistent inflammation as is seen in psoriasis are common to these conditions. Thus obesity is associated with low grade chronic inflammation mediated by levels of circulating TNF-α, IL-2, IL-6 and C-reactive protein. Metabolic syndrome and atherosclerosis show similarities to psoriasis in that Th 1 cytokines drive all three processes.

As there is increased understanding of the importance of the inflammatory process, treatments will increasingly look to tackle the causes of the inflammatory cascades within the skin.

The biological therapies which are discussed later in this chapter will be key in this process. When discussing these associations with patients it is important not to create unwarranted anxiety. Patients need to know that there is a theoretical link between psoriasis and cardiovascular diseases but the evidence is still being collected and analysed. It seems that the links are most important for those with severe disease. Thus 'switching off' the severe inflammatory response quickly may be important not only to reduce the level of psoriasis, but also to decrease the risk of experiencing other inflammatory disease processes.

Clinical variants of psoriasis

Chronic plaque psoriasis

This is the most common form accounting for about 80% of those with psoriasis. Also known as psoriasis vulgaris, where vulgaris means common, it is characterised by well circumscribed, scaly plaques. These plaques can range in shape (although they are usually round or oval) and size from millimetres in diameter to many centimetres (Figure 8.1). The most common sites are extensor surfaces, i.e. elbows and knees, the lower back or sacrum, natal cleft, genitalia and the scalp. More-often-than-not the lesions are symmetrical, i.e. they appear on both knees or both elbows; however, the lesions on each side are not necessarily identical. Psoriasis often occurs on the hairline and can creep down

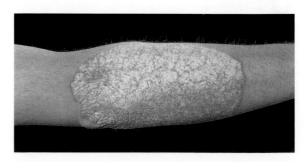

Figure 8.1 Plaque psoriasis. (Source: Reprinted from Graham-Brown and Burns, 2006.)

over the forehead, down the neck and into and around the ears. In reality plaques can occur anywhere, although appearance on the face is considered rare.

If chronic plaque psoriasis (CPP) occurs in flexural areas, the appearance will be quite different from other areas of the body. Because of the heat and occlusive nature of flexures, the scale rubs off leaving a bright red shiny area of skin. There may be a fungal or bacterial infection present along with the psoriasis. This type of psoriasis is sometimes known as inverse psoriasis (Figure 8.2).

CPP on hands and feet (palmar/plantar psoriasis) also has a somewhat different appearance. Individual plaques may not be seen, but thickened fissured skin, often more apparent on the dominant hand, will be in evidence. In order to distinguish this from a contact dermatitis for example, a careful history and an assessment for psoriasis on other parts of the body, for example in the nails, is needed.

When psoriasis occurs in the scalp, the scaling can become particularly thickened as the hair prevents the scale from shedding (Figure 8.3). As the scale develops it can cover the whole scalp which feels tight and uncomfortable; it has been described as feeling like wearing a swimming cap. Although hair loss may seem more extensive than normal, this is not permanent and patients can be reassured that hair will grow back.

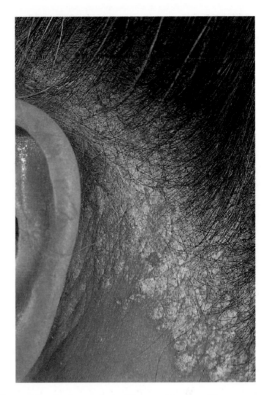

Figure 8.3 Scalp psoriasis. (Source: Reprinted from Graham-Brown and Burns, 2006.)

Guttate psoriasis

The lesions in guttate psoriasis (GP) are generally smaller than those in CPP and appear as if splattered across the body in a rain-drop pattern. The plaques are also generally less indurated and less scaly. GP occurs most commonly on the trunk and proximal areas of extremities, it is also more likely to present on the face (Figure 8.4). This type of psoriasis seems to affect children and young adults predominantly and often occurs after a streptococcal throat infection. It affects around 18% of the psoriasis population. For some, the acute appearance of GP is their only experience with psoriasis. It clears relatively quickly within a 4-week period and they do not experience the condition again. For others, especially those with a strong family history of psoriasis, the guttate form is an initial flare and it then changes into the more chronic form of plaque psoriasis.

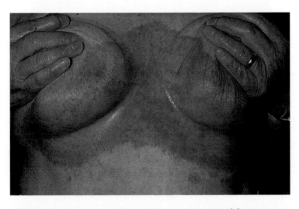

Figure 8.2 Inverse psoriasis. (Source: Reprinted from Weller *et al.*, 2008.)

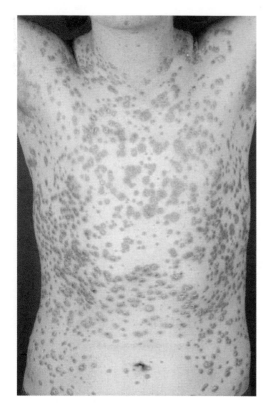

Figure 8.4 Guttate psoriasis. (Source: Reprinted from Graham-Brown and Burns, 2006.)

Nail psoriasis

Psoriasis of the nails is relatively common affecting up to 50% of people who have psoriasis. Both finger and toe nails can be affected, although it would seem that fingernails are more commonly involved (Figure 8.5). The various different apparatus of the nail can be involved. If the nail matrix is affected, the way that the nail grows will be altered; this may be relatively mild with small pits appearing in the nail plate surface. However, more serious effects can be seen when psoriasis affects the nail bed leading to thickened nails; if the hyponichium is also affected, the result is lifting of the nail from the nail bed leading to onycholysis.

Pustular psoriasis

There are two main variants of this type of psoriasis, palmar plantar pustulosis (PPP) and generalised pustular psoriasis (GPP). Some clinicians consider PPP to be a totally different entity from other types of psoriasis. About 70–80% of patients who have PPP will not have any other psoriatic lesions elsewhere on the body (Figure 8.6). It is also worth noting that significantly more women than men suffer with

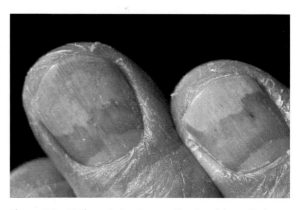

Figure 8.5 Nail psoriasis. (Source: Reprinted from Graham-Brown and Burns, 2006.)

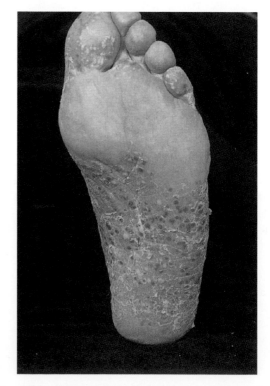

Figure 8.6 Palmar plantar pustulosis. (Source: Reprinted from Graham-Brown and Burns, 2006.)

PPP and that its onset is generally later in life. It is very strongly associated with smoking. Its appearance is of pustules against a background of erythema and scaling. Pustules at different stages will be present at any one time. Initially they are yellowish in colour (although the contents are sterile) and when the pustule breaks, the skin forms brownish macules.

GPP should be considered a dermatological emergency where the patient is generally febrile and unwell. Whilst GPP affects both sexes equally, like PPP it tends to occur later in life (around 50) and can evolve from a pre-existing psoriasis or occur without any psoriasis history. It is relatively rare with only around 2% of the psoriasis population ever experiencing GPP. A strong trigger factor for the development of GPP appears to be commencement on, or withdrawal from, systemic steroids; however, infection or other drug reactions may also cause GPP. GPP can affect any part of the body but seems to have a predilection for flexural areas. There are hundreds of superficial pustules on widespread, irregular patches of bright red skin. These patches tend to have serpiginous or wavy borders which move as the pustules coalesce and then desquamate.

Erythrodermic psoriasis

Erythrodermic psoriasis (EP) is another dermatological emergency; those who experience EP usually have pre-existing CPP. The usual characterstics of CPP disappear as EP progresses; the skin becomes generally inflamed with no noticeable plaques and there is generalised exfoliation (Figure 8.7). Trigger factors include emotional stress, response to systemic illness and alcoholism; however, the most noticeable cause of EP is the inappropriate use of potent steroids (topical, oral and injectable). Like GPP, EP is potentially life threatening and the patient will need to be hospitalised for intensive nursing care.

The various variants of psoriasis may be confused with other skin diagnoses. Table 8.1 lists the common confusions.

Psoriatic arthritis

It is thought that between 6% and 10% of those with psoriasis suffer from inflammatory arthritis known as PSA or psoriatic arthropathy (Figure 8.8). However, it is also thought that the number who suffer from general joint stiffness is more

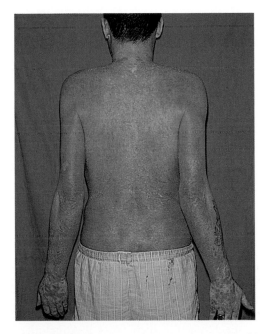

Figure 8.7 Erythrodermic psoriasis. (Source: Reprinted from Weller *et al.*, 2008.)

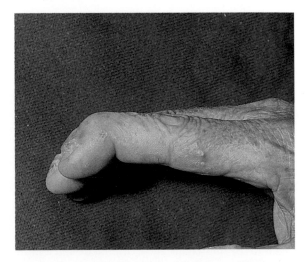

Figure 8.8 Psoriatic arthritis. (Source: Reprinted from Weller *et al.*, 2008.)

Table 8.1 Differential diagnoses for psoriasis.

Type of psoriasis	Key clinical features	May be confused with
Chronic plaque psoriasis	Clear demarcation between psoriatic skin and normal skin Extensive scaling Pin-prick bleeding Appears on extensor surfaces	Nummular eczema Lichen simplex chronicus
Guttate psoriasis	Rain drop type lesions on trunk and arms Often follows a throat infection	Pityriasis rosea
Inverted psoriasis	In flexural areas Bright red Shiney Clear edge	Fungal infection
Nail psoriasis	Pitting of the nail plate Hyperkeratosis of the nail bed leading to thickened nails and lifting of the nail plate	Fungal infection of the nail Ageing nails which will thicken especially if subject to trauma
Erythrodermic psoriasis	Generalised erythema Exfoliation History of chronic plaque psoriasis	Other causes of erythroderma, e.g. drug reaction, eczema

like 33% (Osborn and Wilke, 2004). The pathogenic mechanisms which cause PSA include, like those in the skin, chemical mediators for inflammation and the interaction of T-cells and macrophages. Clinically it may appear as rheumatoid arthritis, although crucially the patient remains seronegative. Those people who have PSA are also very likely to have nail involvement (80%) and that nail involvement is often very destructive. The majority (66%) find that the joint involvement occurs after the lesions appear on the skin; however, for 15% it is around the same time as the cutaneous signs appear and for 15% it is before there are any cutaneous lesions. The different clinical presentations of PSA are outlined in Box 8.1.

Mild to moderate arthritis may be successfully managed using non-steroidal anti-inflammatory drugs. More severe disease is likely to need to be managed by a rheumatologist and will involve systemic treatments similar to those used to treat cutaneous disease.

Physical symptoms that accompany psoriasis

From the description of the clinical symptoms of psoriasis above, it becomes clear what the physical symptoms may be. Like so many chronic skin diseases, psoriasis makes it very difficult for the sufferer to feel comfortable in their own skin. There are a number of constant reminders reflecting the fact that their skin is 'switched on' with a myriad of inflammatory and proliferatory activities taking place.

Scaling

In a multi-centre European study, it was found that nearly 78% of the 330 people in the study found that scaling was a problem related to their condition (de Korte *et al.*, 2005). As has already been described, psoriatic plaques are

---

Box 8.1   Clinical presentations of PSA

Symmetric polyarthritis
- Looks and behaves almost exactly like rheumatoid arthritis;
- Generally affects the proximal joints of the fingers, but can affect any joint;
- Is the most common form of PSA.

Asymmetric oligoarticular arthritis
- Oligo means few, thus this type of arthritis by definition must affect five or fewer joints;
- Dactylis may be seen, this describes the 'sausage' shape of fingers or toes when the distal interphalangeal joint is affected;
- Later onset of oligoarticular arthritis in large joints has the best prognosis.

Distal interphalangeal joint arthritis
- This could be described as the 'classic' appearance of PSA, where only the distal inter-phalangeal joints are affected.
- It affects around 5% of those with PSA.

Arthritis mutilans
- A highly destructive form of PSA, there is osteolysis (dissolution of the bone) in the small joints of the hands;
- Occurs in 1–2% of those with PSA;
- Seems to be linked to early onset disease and has a poor prognosis.

Spondylitis and sacroiliitis
- On X-ray, changes seem to be consistent with ankylosing spondylitis and sacroiliitis; how-ever symptoms may be absent.

---

characterised by over production of keratino-cytes which are shed from the skin in notice-able clumps. This will often limit a person's life in that they restrict activities due to the embarrassment of the 'snowstorm' they create. This may be about restricting the colour of clothing chosen so that white skin scales do not show up against dark coloured clothing, or it may be about limiting holiday choices by not staying in a hotel because of all the skin cells left in sheets or on the floor. In a small unpublished study (Ersser *et al.*, 2000) in which patients were asked to describe how they felt about their psoriasis, one person described it thus:

It is extraordinary how much skin is being produced. When it is like that I mean I think one can get into a mindset of being sort of revolted with one's own body. At home if I'm the last to bed, I get up and there's flakes all over the settee ... I brush it on the floor and then get a hoover so that when people come down in the morning they are not confronted with it. (p. 8)

Related to scaling is the thickness or indu-ration of the plaque. Whilst this symptom seems to be of less importance to the patient than scaling, it is important as a measure of treatment success. A plaque that is resolving becomes flat so that when a finger is run over it there is no change in texture between the normal skin and the plaque. Psoriasis tends to clear from the centre of the plaque outwards, so the patient will not see the plaque decrease in size, instead it will become flat in the middle with an ever decreasing ring around the edge. It is important to feel the skin when looking to see if the plaques are resolving as a plaque coloured mark will remain on the skin for around 2 weeks after the plaque flattens. This is because it takes that time for the superficial blood supply to return to normal (see later for further details).

Inflammation

The over proliferation of skin cells is accompanied by an increased superficial blood supply to the plaques. Because the capillaries run close to the surface of the skin they are easily broken. For the patient this means that the skin can be broken through scratching or knocking it leading to pin-prick bleeding (described earlier). This can be very distressing as it makes a mess of bedding and clothing and also make the plaques more obvious. The redness of the plaques may also be made more obvious by use of treatments and emollients. This is because the superficial white scale on the surface is removed exposing the inflammation of the plaque. Patients with psoriasis will also often complain that their skin feels extremely hot and sensitive; this is probably explained by the inflammation of the plaques.

Pain and pruritus

Psoriasis is not often described as painful, but it can be sore especially if the skin is very dry and cracked and/or scratching has led to damage of the skin surface. It is, however, very often itchy. About 74% in the de Kort study reported itch being a major symptom with only 38% and 12% reporting soreness and pain respectively (de Korte *et al.*, 2005). This is contrary to some dermatological textbooks which report psoriasis

as a non-itchy condition. This may be because unlike in eczema, itch is not one of the key diagnostic clues in psoriasis, but many patients find the itching associated with psoriasis unbearable at some point or other.

> You know terrible itching sort of makes you feel quite nervous. ... and sometimes you can't sleep for itching. I was going to a wedding on Saturday and I was terribly itchy. I couldn't go to the wedding and it was just horrible really. (Ersser *et al.*, 2000, p. 10).

Trigger factors in psoriasis

It is generally agreed that for psoriasis symptoms to manifest themselves there must be a genetic susceptibility (either inherited or spontaneous) along with an external trigger factor. These trigger factors are numerous and varied and science is gradually revealing the pathophysiological mechanisms that make them occur. Some patients will be very clear on what they feel triggers their psoriasis or what makes it feel worse. Others feel that their psoriasis has 'a life of its own' and that it improves and worsens randomly with no easily identifiable trigger factors. Thus, as with so many things about psoriasis, the story is never totally straightforward. Trigger factors will impact upon people in different ways and to different extents.

Koebner phenomenon

One of the classic features of psoriasis is its tendency to Koebnerise, that is to form along the line of injury or trauma. The trauma may be an acute episode such as a surgical incision or a low-grade long-term influence like the constant rubbing of a garment. Where a linear incision is made, the psoriasis is likely to follow the line of the scar rather than forming in its usual oval shape. Patients who are undergoing non-essential surgical interventions should be warned of the possibility of Koebnerisation.

Streptococcal throat infection

It is commonly observed that throat infections, tonsillitis and pharyngitis can trigger GP; this is particularly seen in children and young adults. It is known, therefore, that streptococcal infections can lead to the onset of this specific type of the disease. The mechanism for this is thought to be the effect of superantigens released by the streptococcal bacteria activating T-cells and driving the skin to produce psoriatic lesions.

Drugs

There are certain classes of drugs, which will in some cases trigger an onset or aggravate psoriasis:

- Lithium
- Chloroquine-based anti-malarials
- Beta-blockers

Where possible it is advisable for patients and their health care professionals to seek alternatives to the above systemic medications. For those with severe bipolar disease, lithium is sometimes the only effective treatment, which makes discontinuing it because of worsening psoriasis difficult. A small study in Scotland demonstrated that by introducing the supplement inositol the disease severity of those on lithium could be reduced when compared to those who were given a placebo (Allan *et al.*, 2004). The recommendation from the study was that for patients who could not be withdrawn from lithium, inositol as a supplement is worth considering.

Ultraviolet light exposure

For a small, but not insignificant number of people (around 10%) exposure to ultraviolet (UV) light is an aggravating (rather than therapeutic) factor.

Stress

Psychological stress has for many years been linked with exacerbations of psoriasis. In the last 10 years, there has been a major increase in the amount of scientific evidence which helps to explain the relationship between the brain and the skin – it has been labelled the 'brain-skin axis'. The relationship between the brain and the skin is explored in more detail in Chapter 6. Researchers have looked at the physiological changes that happen when psoriasis sufferers (compared to controls) are subjected to a number of stress tests. It was shown that the patients with psoriasis who were stress-responsive had an abnormal response of the hypothalamus–pituitary–adrenal axis when exposed to stress. It was suggested that this could lead to an upregulation of the inflammatory mediators that lead to the physical manifestations of psoriasis (Richards *et al.*, 2005).

Treatments for psoriasis

Treatments for psoriasis can be divided into topical and systemic. Topical products are generally used to manage mild to moderate psoriasis and systemic therapies the more severe end of the disease spectrum. Topical therapies may be used to treat more severe disease in combination with systemic regimes especially where in-patient or day-care treatment is available, for example coal tar or short-contact dithranol in combination with UV light therapy. There have been relatively few recent breakthroughs for psoriasis therapy, particularly for the treatment of mild to moderate disease. The 21st century has, however, seen major developments in the field of immunologic treatments for severe disease. Camisa (2004a) details a timeline of breakthroughs in psoriasis therapy (p. 3).

Patients seem to have variable results with topical treatments in particular. It does seem to be the case that what will work for one person does not work for another, even though their disease severity and motivation seem to be equivalent. It is true, however, that some people do not have good results from topical therapies because they do not concord. It is vital, therefore, that patients with psoriasis receive support and encouragement when using topical therapies and that their expectations of level of clearance and timescales are realistic. Further information on helping patients to concord with treatment can be found in Chapter 7. There is also a subset of people that, despite their best efforts with a topical product, do not see any positive result. This group should be referred to a Dermatology Department. Further information about referral guidelines is given at the end of this chapter.

Topical therapies

Emollients

As psoriasis is a dry skin condition, a key line of treatment for all types of psoriasis, except perhaps inverse psoriasis, is emollient therapy. Emollients will not resolve plaques, nor will they stop hyperproliferation; however, they do reduce the signs of scaling and they certainly make the skin much more comfortable. Emollients may be applied topically and/or used whilst washing. They are often underutilised in psoriasis care, but should be the first treatment option in all cases. Chapter 5 has further details about selecting and using emollients.

Vitamin D analogues

Vitamin D3 is naturally synthesised in the epidermis. The mechanism involves natural UVB falling on the skin and converting 7-dehydrocholesterol into vitamin D which then binds with vitamin D binding protein. In this form, the vitamin D is transported around the body to the liver and kidneys where it undergoes a number of hydroxylations (addition of oxygen and hydrogen molecules) before becoming the active substance 1,25-dihydroxyvitamin D3, otherwise known as calcitriol. Receptors for the action of calcitriol can be found in human epidermis and also in melanocytes, Langerhans cells, fibroblasts, endothelial cells, T-lymphocytes, macrophages and granulocytes (Camisa, 2004c). Calcitriol has been shown to inhibit cell proliferation and induce terminal differentiation within the epidermis. It also affects calcium homeostasis by stimulating the absorption of both calcium and phosphate through the small intestine and by promoting mineralisation and osteolysis in the bones. The synthetic vitamin D analogues (calcipotriol, tacalcitol and calcitriol) work in the same way as naturally occurring calcitriol, inhibiting cell proliferation and encouraging the skin cells to mature normally.

Calcipotriol is more effective than tacalcitol and calcitriol (Ashcroft *et al.*, 2000) and less calciotrophic (i.e. less likely to impact on calcium levels) than calcitriol. The systematic review undertaken in 2000 showed that calcipotriol was more effective than coal tar, combined coal tar 5%, allatonin 2% and hydrocortisone 0.5% and short-contact dithranol. When measured at 6 weeks it was more effective than potent topical steroids, although this effect was reversed by 8 weeks (Ashcroft *et al.*, 2000). Interestingly in a further study carried out in The Netherlands where calcipotriol treatment was compared with short-contact dithranol treatment in a day-care setting, dithranol treatment was seen as more effective (van de Kerkhof *et al.*, 2006). Thus, where skilled staff are available within a day-care setting, the use of dithranol could be considered as a first line treatment. Its efficacy is significant; however, as is described later in this section, its application and potential side effects are considerable which can make its use outside a clinical setting, undesirable.

Method of application

Vitamin D analogues are designed for use in stable CPP. In practical terms, the vitamin D analogues are relatively easy to apply. They are odourless and come in cream or ointment formulations, so the most appropriate type of product can be selected. Amounts and contraindications are outlined in Table 8.2. Each brand of vitamin D analogue recommends a different quantity per application. Where the manufacturer makes a specific recommendation it is quoted in Table 8.2. The cream or ointment should be applied to the plaque and rubbed in

Table 8.2 Key differences between the vitamin D analogues.

Vitamin D3 analogue	Amount used	Special Instructions
Calcitriol (Silkis™)	• No more than 210 g/week (i.e. 30 g or 60 FTUs per day) • No more than 35% body surface area • Twice-daily application • 'Apply an even layer'	• Use with caution on those who are on treatment that affects calcium levels, e.g. thiazide diuretics • Contraindicated for people with liver or kidney problems and those being treated for calcium homeostasis • Not for use in children • Use of face with caution due to possible irritation
Calcipotriol (Dovonex™ cream and scalp application)	• No more than 100 g/week (adult) (i.e.14 g per day or 28 FTUs) • 75 g/week (children over 12) • 50 g/week (children 6–12) • Twice-daily application • 'Apply cream thickly'	• Avoid use on face • Avoid exposure to natural or artificial sunlight • Contraindicated for patients with known calcium disorders • Can be used in children over 6
Calcipotriol and betamethasone diproprionate (Dovobet™ ointment)	• No more than 100 g/week (i.e.15 g per day or 30 FTUs) • No more than 30% of body surface area • Once-daily application	• As with Calcipotriol • Not to be used in the flexures • Not to be used on infected skin • Not to be used under occlusion • Not for use in children under 18 • Not to be used in conjunction with other steroids • Not to be used for more than 4 weeks at a time
Tacalcitol (Curatoderm™ ointment)	• 70 g/week (i.e. 10 g per day or 20 FTUs) • Once-daily application • 'Apply sparingly'	• Contraindicated for patients with known calcium disorders • Not recommended for use in children

Source: Datapharm (2009).

Note: NB It may be helpful to explain to patients that 1 finger tip unit (FTU) is approximately half a gram, it is then possible to work out how many FTUs it is safe to use per day.

gently; however, if any is left on the skin, clothing should not be worn straight away as this may rub off the product. Side effects include slight stinging or irritation on application which should resolve shortly after application. If calcitriol or calcipotriol get onto sensitive skin, for example the face, they may cause more severe irritation and erythema. However, tacalcitol can be used on the face and in flexures. It is

important that patients are instructed to wash their hands after application of the product so that they do not inadvertently get it onto more sensitive skin.

Calcipotriol is also available as a scalp application. It is in a liquid form which is useful for treating psoriasis once the scale has been removed. Table 8.3 outlines how scalp treatments should be applied.

Table 8.3   Scalp treatments.

Type of scalp psoriasis	Type of treatment	Application technique	Length of time to leave treatment on
Thickened and scaly	Coal tar, salicylic acid and coconut oil	Part hair into sections working around the scalp For each section rub treatment into the scalp. Once whole scalp is covered, gently massage into scalp Use comb gently to loosen any scale. Apply just once daily	Preferably overnight (but if not for at least half an hour). Protect pillow with old pillowcase or wear shower cap; Wash out following morning.
Thin scale but active psoriasis	Calcipotriol lotion	As above but apply morning and evening.	Leave on throughout day and night and then shampoo off
	Calcipotriol/betameth-asone gel	As above but once a day.	
	Clobetasol proprionate shampoo	Apply no more than 7.5 ml to dry scalp and wash off.	Once applied to dry scalp, leave for 15 minutes before adding water lathering and washing off.
Scalp is dry but no active psoriasis	Coconut oil	As per coal tar product	Overnight if possible
Maintenance and/or adjunct to other treatment	Coal tar shampoo	Apply as a regular shampoo 2–3 times per week. Rinse out. May need to use less frequently if being used for maintenance purposes	Leave on scalp for a few minutes before rinsing.

The patient should be warned that it may take up to 4 weeks to see any positive impact of the treatment, that this is normal and that they should persevere.

Calcipotriol and betamethasone diproprionate

A combination treatment containing both a vitamin D analogue and a potent steroid is the most recent addition to the topical treatments for stable plaque psoriasis. It has been shown to be both quicker acting and more effective at reducing disease severity than calcipotriol on its own (Guenther *et al*., 2002). This same study showed that there was no statistical or clinical difference in the outcomes of using the combined product once or twice a day. It has consequently become recommended as a once-daily treatment.

Method of application

This is a once-daily treatment and should be applied in sufficient quantities to cover the plaque and then be gently rubbed in. As with calcipotriol it may not matter if some ointment gets onto unaffected skin, but this should be avoided where possible. Due to the inclusion of potent topical steroids, it is not recommended that the combination treatment should be used for more than 4 weeks. The British National Formulary suggests that further courses may be given after a period of not less than 4 weeks (British Medical Association and Royal Pharmaceutical Society of Great Britain, 2008). The combination calcipotriol/steroid ointment may be helpful for an initial treatment of plaque psoriasis as it seems to be quicker acting; once resolution of the plaques begins this may be maintained by shifting the treatment regime to calcipotriol alone.

Calcipotriol combined with other therapies

When used in conjunction with narrowband UVB, calcipotriol appears to have a UVB sparing effect. A placebo-controlled trial showed that those in the active group (i.e. where calcipotriol was used) needed a significantly lower UVB dosage than those in the control group (Woo and McKenna, 2003). Although there was no significant difference in Psoriasis Area Severity Index (PASI) and quality of life measures between the active and control group at the end of the study, at 8 weeks the PASI had improved to a significantly greater extent in the active group. The UVB sparing effect of calcipotriol could be important in offering an option which decreases the carcinogenicity of the UVB therapy.

A small study involving 40 patients looked at whether combining calcipotriol with acitretin was more effective than acitretin on its own. Their results suggested that calcipotriol may enhance the clinical outcomes when acitretin is used. The duration of treatment and total dose of acitretin required to achieve clearance was slightly lower in the combination group, but this difference did not achieve significance (Rim *et al.*, 2003).

Coal tar

Being one of the oldest treatments for psoriasis, it remains a moderately effective option; however it is rarely popular with patients. Products tend to have a tar smell associated with them, although the weaker strengths have a less potent aroma. The main potential side effects associated with coal tar include skin irritation and folliculitis. It is thought that coal tar works by reducing epidermal thickness and by suppressing epidermal DNA synthesis. It is a complex substance containing some 10,000 different compounds of which only 50% have been identified (Camisa, 2004b). Some researchers are working on identifying which compounds within coal tar are actively anti-psoriatic in the hope that

by distilling these out a more acceptable and yet effective treatment may become available (Arbiser *et al.*, 2006).

A number of studies have been carried out comparing the efficacy of calcipotriol and coal tar. The systematic review carried out in 2000 confirmed that calcipotriol was more effective (Ashcroft *et al.*, 2000). Like calcipotriol, coal tar can be used in combination with UVB; this is known as the Goeckerman regime named after the doctor who first published the use of this methodology in 1925. Coal tar enhances sensitivity to the UVB and may be UVB sparing. Tar and UVB therapy offered within a health care facility (day care) continues to provide treatment that over a period of time improves treatment-resistant psoriasis. In a small study, 100% of patients had 75% improvement in their PASI at the end of a 12-week treatment programme using the Goeckerman regime with narrowband UVB (Lee and Koo, 2005).

There have been some concerns about the carcinogenicity of coal tar. There is no doubt that coal tar does contain some carcinogenic substances as has been demonstrated by animal and occupational studies. There is, however, no research within the dermatological field of the use of coal tar preparations and whether these increase the risk of internal skin tumours (Roelofzen *et al.*, 2007).

Method of application

On a day-to-day basis in primary care, weak coal tar solutions are useful for widespread small plaques of psoriasis as treatment does not need to be accurately applied to the plaques only. They can be applied 2–3 times per day. These weaker solutions will sink into the skin and a patient can get dressed after this. However, there is always a risk of some staining and it may be easier for patients to apply the treatment at a point in time when they can wear 'messy' clothes afterwards. There is no evidence to support the amount that should be used; however enough to cover the areas comfortably is a sensible suggestion. Coal tar preparations should be applied following the lie of the hair in order to reduce the likelihood of folliculitis.

In a health care facility, where stronger strengths of tar may be used, tubular netting bandages can be applied afterwards to keep the tar close to the skin. It is impractical to get dressed during this kind of treatment; some units are therefore advocating 'short contact' coal tar. Where it is left on for 4–6 hours and then washed off and an emollient applied. This is particularly useful in a day-care setting where a patient can come in for a set period of time and then leave.

Tar is particularly helpful for the management of scalp psoriasis. In combination with coconut oil and salicylic acid, it can be successfully used to descale thickened plaques. Tar-based shampoos may be used in conjunction with other treatments or in less severe scalp psoriasis may be sufficient to keep the condition under control without the need for other treatments. Table 8.3 outlines how scalp treatments should be applied.

Dithranol

Also known as anthralin, the active ingredients were originally extracted from the bark of the Brazilian araroba tree. During World War I a synthetic version was synthesised.

Dithranol affects the synthesis of cell DNA and has a pronounced anti-proliferative effect. It also appears to have a rapid effect on the normalisation of epidermal differentiation. In both these ways, it is an effective treatment for psoriasis. However, it does have a number of side effects including irritation and staining, although it has the advantage of being odourless. Its effects may be enhanced by the use of the Ingram regime, which includes UVB as well as topical treatment.

Method of application

In order for dithranol to be most effective, it must be carefully applied. Dithranol in a zinc oxide paste is most commonly used in hospital/day-care facilities. The initial concentration is 0.1% and this in increased every 2–3 days (or according to how well the patient will tolerate

it). Here the preparation is carefully applied to the plaques using a spatula and then 'fixed' using talc which is applied using a makeshift powder puff. This helps to keep the paste in place and minimises smudging onto good skin. This can then be covered with stocking net bandages and left in place for up to 24 hours. Removal of the paste can be difficult if just water is used; cotton wool soaked in a mineral oil is effective at removing the dithranol prior to getting in the bath.

Dithranol can be used on an outpatient basis, but is probably only useful if limited large plaques are present and the patient is well motivated. In this instance, short-contact dithranol can be used. A cream-based product (again starting at 0.1%) is carefully applied to the plaques using a gloved finger or cotton bud and left in place for any period up to an hour. The amount to be applied is sufficient to cover the plaque and be rubbed in, but not excessively or the chance of the product rubbing off onto clothes and furnishing is increased. At the lower strengths, patients might be able to tolerate leaving the product on overnight. Patients should gradually increase the strength of product used and the amount of time it is left on (starting at 10 minutes and working up to an hour). When the strength is increased, the amount of time it is left on should be temporarily decreased. It is possible to use this on the scalp; however as with the skin, the product can stain hair, particularly if blonde.

For both methods of application this is a once-daily treatment. The products should not be applied to sensitive areas, e.g. face or flexures or to sore or pustular psoriasis. Dithranol itself can cause soreness; if this is prolonged, the strength should be reduced or the amount of time left on decreased. If this does not resolve the problem, the treatment has to be stopped.

Corticosteroids

Potent topical steroids on their own are rarely used to treat plaque psoriasis in the UK. In other countries, topical steroids may be more common place. The rationale for not making use of them extensively is the increased chance of rebound and the potential for triggering an episode of GPP. This being said, mild to moderate steroids are commonly used to treat psoriasis in flexural areas, the face and genitalia, as few other products are licensed for treatment in these areas. As shown in Table 8.3, steroids are also used to treat scalp psoriasis.

Vitamin A

Also known as a topical retinoid, its mode of action is not entirely understood. However, it does appear to modulate cell proliferation and increase differentiation. It is marketed as being suitable for mild to moderate plaque psoriasis and should not be used on more than 10% of body surface area. Its main side effect appears to be skin irritation; to help counter this two strengths have been developed, 0.05% and 0.1%.

Method of application
A thin layer should be applied to the plaque only and gently rubbed in. It may be advisable to start at the lower strength first before moving onto the higher strength. One small study suggested that using the product as short contact (product was left on for 20 minutes and then washed off with water) leads to less side effects and equal efficacy (Veraldi *et al*., 2006).

Systemic therapies

Phototherapy

For the majority of people with psoriasis, exposure to ultraviolet radiation improves their condition. There are a small minority of around 10% who have light sensitive psoriasis; for them exposure to UV radiation can cause psoriasis to worsen or develop. The term phototherapy includes therapeutic use of both UVA and UVB light. The principle underpinning both wavelengths of UV radiation is that they suppress the immune response within the skin and thus dampen down the cascade of immunological changes which occur to trigger psoriasis. The most concerning side effect on a long-term basis is the development of skin cancer. For this reason, careful monitoring

of the cumulative doses administered is important and it is usual to limit the course of treatment given to individuals. Other more immediate side effects can include skin dryness and erythema.

There is mixed evidence about whether emollients should be used prior to UVB and PUVA treatments. Because they reduce scaling it is argued that there is improved penetration of the UV radiation; however, it has been shown that a number of emollients have a UV protective capacity (at different parts of the UV spectrum) and thus reduce the efficacy of the light therapy (Otman *et al*., 2006). It is also likely that factors such as plaque thickness, how much emollient is applied and when it is applied will have a role to play. The recommendations by Otman *et al*. (2006) were no more specific than to say that if emollients were to be used prior to UV therapies that they should have minimal UV blocking effects. Box 8.2 shows emollients from the British National Formulary that they found had a sun protection factor of less than 1.2 for UVB, UVA and PUVA. Previous researchers had stated that protection factor of 1.2 or higher represented a reduction in UV transmittance of 17% or more which was thought to be clinically significant (Hudson-Peacock *et al*., 1994).

UVB

Most individuals who have ultraviolet treatment for their psoriasis will be treated with UVB (narrowband) initially. This usually involves three

---

> ### Box 8.2   Emollients that have a SPF of less than 1.2 suitable for use with UV therapy
>
> - Aveeno cream
> - Calmurid cream
> - Dermol 500 lotion
> - Doublebase cream
> - Emulsiderm emollient
> - Emulsifying ointment
> - Oilatum gel

exposures a week which are generally carried out in a Dermatology Department. To ensure the most appropriate starting dose of UVB, a patient's back is exposed to a number of different UVB doses and the dose that produces a small amount of erythema after 24 hours is the dose that the first treatment is calculated upon. This is known as the minimal erythemal dose (MED). The speed at which these doses increase will depend to an extent on the individual's skin type and their response to the therapy. During the administration of the UVB, individuals must wear glasses to protect their eyes and men should protect their genitalia with a jock strap. It is important that the same garment is used for each treatment, otherwise burning may result. If there are no lesions on the face, a full facial shield should be worn as well as goggles.

PUVA

For UVA to be effective, it has to be given in combination with an oral medication called 8 methoxypsoralen (8MOP). Natural psoralens have been used for hundreds of years in India where they have been used to treat vitiligo; their main action is to increase photosensitivity. This then makes the UVA a very effective treatment for psoriasis. Because it must be given in conjunction with an oral medication which can cause a number of side effects listed in Table 8.4, PUVA therapy is usually given if UVB has not been successful. Box 8.3 lists the possible contraindications for giving PUVA. In a similar way to the MED testing for UVB therapy, minimal phototoxic dose (MPD) is calculated for PUVA.

The medication is taken 1–2 hours prior to the treatment being administered. Once the 8 MOP has been taken, the individual must wear eye protection and avoid sun exposure for at least 12 hours. Sunglasses or coated normal glasses must be tested to ensure that they are preventing penetration of UV radiation. Gastrointestinal upsets can be lessened if the medication is taken with a small meal. It is advisable that each time the tablets are taken, the amount of food ingested is more-or-less the same to ensure a consistent serum level of 8 MOP. As with UVB, men

Table 8.4   Possible side effects of PUVA.

Acute side effects	Chronic side effects
Nausea Pruritus Dizziness Flu-like symptoms Headache Erythema (burning)	Skin cancer *Malignant melanoma*: evidence suggests that there is an increase in the long-term, although the risk is not that pronounced. *Squamous cell carcinoma*(SCC): there is a substantial increase in those who have had PUVA. *Basal cell carcinoma*: small increased risk but not as significant as SCC.
	Eye disease Currently there is no clear evidence to link PUVA with increased experience of cataracts where eye protection is used.

Box 8.3   Contraindications for giving PUVA

- Refusal to wear eye protection
- Melanoma and non-melanoma skin cancers
- Photosensitising medication
- Pregnancy
- Cataracts
- Photosensitivity disorders (e.g. lupus, albinism)

---

should wear genital protection. A facial shield should be used if there are no facial lesions.

For those who find that 8MOP induces too many of the below acute side effects, topical PUVA may be helpful. The individual immerses themselves in a bath in which 8MOP solution is dissolved and is then exposed to the UVA in the same way. Exact protocols will vary; however, the UVA can be given immediately after the bath and there is no need to wear eye protection following treatment. Whilst serum levels of 8MOP are lower, the therapeutic benefits appear to be as good if not better during bath PUVA than oral PUVA. There also appear to be fewer side effects (Cooper *et al.*, 2000). Bath PUVA requires more 8 MOP and is therefore more expensive; however, it remains a viable option for those who do not respond to, or who may be excluded from oral PUVA. Cost can be reduced by the use of a polyethylene sheet in the bath which reduces the amount of water that comes into contact with the skin and therefore the amount of psoralen needed to create the correct dilution (Streit *et al.*, 1996).

Topical psoralens can also be applied to localised areas such as hands and feet when the psoriasis just affects these areas. As with bath PUVA, there are none of the acute systemic side effects with this method of treatment (except potential burning). The UVA light is then just directed at those areas using hand and foot PUVA machines.

Methotrexate

Methotrexate is a relatively old treatment which has been used in psoriasis since the late 1960s. There are relatively few randomised controlled trials looking at its efficacy; however, it is considered to be a very useful drug for the management of severe psoriasis. Its downsides are the degree to which it has adverse systemic effects.

It is an anti-proliferative drug, that is it affects cell DNA and stops psoriatic skin cells from developing. It does this by inhibiting folic acid, thus natural levels of folic acid in patients on methotrexate are likely to be lower. For patients with psoriasis, the dosage is kept low and given once a week at the same time. It is usually taken orally (starting at a low dose of 2.5 or 5 mg working up to a maximum dose of 20–25 mg depending on blood results and effect), but can also be given as an intramuscular injection. This latter technique is useful if the patient is particularly affected by nausea. Before commencing a patient on methotrexate, they must be counselled as to the potential side effects (listed in Table 8.5)

Table 8.5 Potential side effects of methotrexate.

Side effects	Notes
Leukopenia and thrombocytopenia	Falling white blood cell and platelet counts indicate bone marrow toxicity and the treatment should be discontinued. Generally occurs 8–11 days after commencement of treatment.
Oral and plaque ulceration	Can indicate toxicity.
Lower levels of folic acid	Can lead to decreases in red blood cells and possible megaloblastic anaemia. A dose of 1–5 mg of folic acid is usually given daily (except on the day when the methotrexate is taken). This does not seem to compromise the therapeutic efficacy of the methotrexate.
Teratogenicity	Some evidence to suggest this, sexually active fertile individuals should take birth control precautions.
Hepatotoxicity	This is a major clinical concern as it is known that prolonged use of methotrexate increases the risk of fibrosis and eventual cirrhosis of the liver. This is made more likely there is a high alcohol intake. Blood tests are helpful to indicate liver function, but they do not indicate fibrosis. For this a liver biopsy is needed which itself carries risks.
Pulmonary toxicity	Is unusual and can present as a non-productive cough with or without fever.

and the likely impact it will have on their lifestyle (e.g. need to reduce alcohol intake). Subsequently regular blood monitoring is needed, particularly to ascertain kidney and liver function. Kidney function is important as the drug is secreted through the kidneys and any decrease in function could increase the likelihood of toxicity.

Ciclosporin

The effectiveness of ciclosporin in psoriasis was first seen as a serendipitous result of treating a patient following a kidney transplant with the drug and seeing the positive effect on the skin. As a relatively modern treatment for psoriasis, there have been randomised controlled trials showing its efficacy at doses between 2.5–5.0 mg/kg/day (Griffiths *et al.*, 2000). Like methotrexate it does have some potent systemic side effects so it is reserved for treating severe psoriasis.

Its therapeutic action is through its effects on the T-cells thus helping to inhibit the stimulation of cytokines which cause cell proliferation seen in psoriasis. Dosing of ciclosporin can be challenging as absorption (through the small intestine) is incomplete (around 30%) and hugely variable (4–89%) (Camisa, 2004d). Thus, the way that the drug is formulated will significantly affect the bioavailability of the drug and patients should not be switched between formulations without careful consideration of this fact.

As with other systemic medications, ciclosporin has a range of side effects, from the relatively mild to the more severe. The side effects of most concern are those related to nephrotoxicity and the resultant kidney function damage and hypertension. The likelihood of a patient experiencing these negative side effects is increased by prolonged time on the drug and higher dosages. Kidney function and blood pressure must be closely monitored. Ciclosporin is also known to interact with a number of drugs; some of which will decrease ciclosporin levels in the blood and others which will increase them (see Table 8.6). More minor side effects are listed in Box 8.4; these usually disappear once the patient has been taken off the ciclosporin.

Table 8.6 Drugs which alter serum levels of ciclosporin.

Drugs which increase ciclosporin levels	Drugs which decrease ciclosporin levels
Bromocriptine	Phenytoin
Danazol	Phenobarbitol
Ketoconazole	Carbamazepine
Fluconazole	Rifampin
Itraconazole	Intravenous trimethaprim
Erythromycin	Sulfamethoxazole
Verapamil	
Nicardipine	
Diltiazem	
Methyltestosterone	
Oral contraceptives	

Box 8.4 Minor symptoms associated with ciclosporin

- Gum hyperplasia
- Tremor
- Hypertrichosis
- Headache
- Nausea
- Paresthesia

Retinoids

This is the generic name given to a range of medications all related to vitamin A. For psoriasis treatment the specific retinoid which is used is known as acitretin. It works by altering keratinisation and epidermal differentiation having anti-proliferative, anti-inflammatory and anti-keratinising effects on the skin (Naldi and Griffiths, 2005). Retinoids are complex drugs with many possible side effects; however, they are effective at treating psoriasis (Griffiths *et al.*, 2000), and as mentioned previously used in conjunction with PUVA their effect may be enhanced thus allowing for a reduced exposure to UV radiation.

Retinoids can affect hepatic function and lead to hyperlipidaemia. It is also highly teratogenic and therefore not suitable for pregnant women or women who are considering becoming pregnant. Women should take contraceptive precautions for 2 years after discontinuing retinoid therapy (Griffiths *et al.*, 2000). Common less severe side effects include dry mucous membranes including eyes, lips and throat (if a patient's lips do not become dry it is reasonable to assume they are not complying with treatment or the dosage is sub-therapeutic) (see Box 8.5 for further common skin related side effects).

Biologics

Biologics represent a new generation of drugs which have been developed to treat chronic immune-mediated inflammatory conditions such as psoriasis (but also rheumatoid arthritis and chronic inflammatory bowel conditions such as Crohn's disease). In common with other systemic drugs, they are reserved for those who have severe disease, and in addition, it is usual for patients to have unsuccessfully tried the other systemic options before being offered biologic drugs. This section briefly considers the three biologic drugs that are currently available for the treatment of plaque psoriasis in the UK. However, new biologic drugs are being developed and this list in unlikely to be exhaustive for very long. For example the National Institute for Health and Clinical Excellence is due to publish its technology appraisal on Ustekinumab (which is a human monoclonal antibody) in September 2009.

The basic principle of biologic drugs is that they interfere with a very specific part of the inflammatory process thus preventing the development of psoriatic lesions. Because the drugs are so targeted it is hoped that the long-term side effects will be less than other systemic medications, but there is no long-term data that categorically confirms this judgement. Some considerable attention is being given, by the British Association of Dermatologists, to collecting data about the effects of biologic drugs thus creating what is called a biologics register (British Association of Dermatologists, 2007).

In April 2009, there were three biologic drugs available for the treatment of severe plaque psoriasis. Table 8.7 outlines what the three drugs are, the dosage and recommendations from NICE as to how and when they should be prescribed. A fourth drug (Efalizumab, Raptiva™) was available until February 2009 when three patients experienced severe adverse effects. As a consequence of this, the European Medicines Agency issued recommendation that the product should not be marketed, that no further prescriptions should be issued and that those already on the drug should talk to their doctor about finding an alternative (European Medicines Agency, 2009).

Box 8.5   Common skin and mucous membrane changes seen with use of acitretin

- Dry mucous membranes including dry lips (cheilitis), dry mouth, dry eyes and dry nasal mucosa
- Altered skin sensation–skin feels sticky
- Dry skin
- Dermatitis
- Flare of psoriasis
- Peeling of finger-tips, palms or soles
- Skin fragility
- Itch
- Hair loss
- Hair texture change
- Nail changes including paronychia

Table 8.7 Biologic drugs and prescribing regimes.

Name	Mode of action	Recommended prescribing regime	Delivery
Etanercept (Enbrel™)	Known as a genetically engineered recombinant protein, it binds to TNF-α molecules preventing them from activating skin cells thus preventing inflammation (Jackson *et al.*, 2007).	Twice weekly doses of 25 mg for up to 24 weeks or until remission occurs, should further treatment be needed the same dose should be followed (i.e. it is an intermittent treatment). Suitable for individuals with PASI[1] of 10 or more and a DLQI[2] of 10 or more Should be discontinued after 12 weeks if the response is inadequate, i.e. there is a less than 75% reduction in PASI or less than 50% reduction in PASI accompanied by a 5 point reduction in DLQI (National Institute for Health and Clinical Excellence, 2006)	Subcutaneous injections
Infliximab (Remicade™)	Known as a monoclonal antibody it binds to all three forms of TNF-α thus affecting the inflammatory process	An initial 5 mg/kg infusion over 2 hours, followed by further 5 mg/kg infusions at 2 and 6 weeks. Subsequent infusions are then given at 8-week intervals Suitable for individuals with PASI of 20 or more and a DLQI of 18 or more Should be discontinued after 10 weeks if the response is inadequate, i.e. there is a less than 75% reduction in PASI or less than 50% reduction in PASI accompanied by a 5 point reduction in DLQI (National Institute for Health and Clinical Excellence, 2008a)	Infusion
Adalimumab (Humira™)	Known as a monoclonal antibody which binds with TNF-α blocking interaction with cell-surface receptors and limiting the promotion of inflammatory pathways	An initial dose of 80 mg followed by 40 mg injections every other week starting 1 week after the initial dose. Suitable for individuals with PASI of 20 or more and a DLQI of 18 or more Should be discontinued after 16 weeks if the response is inadequate, i.e. there is a less than 75% reduction in PASI or less than 50% reduction in PASI accompanied by a 5 point reduction in DLQI (National Institute for Health and Clinical Excellence, 2008b)	Subcutaneous injection

[1]PASI is the Psoriasis Area Severity Index which is a validated method for assessing disease severity. Further details about how to carry out a PASI assessment are given in Appendix 1.
[2]DLQI is the Dermatology Life Quality Index which is a validated questionnaire that assesses the impact that skin disease has on quality of life. It is discussed in further detail in Chapter 6.

Each biologic drug will have its own contraindications which can be found in the British National Formulary (British Medical Association and Royal Pharmaceutical Society of Great Britain, 2008), Electronic Medicines Compendium (Datapharm, 2009) and summarised in the British Association of Dermatologists Guidelines (Smith *et al.*, 2005). However, a concern which is relevant to all biologic drugs is that of infection including risk of tuberculosis. All psoriasis patients being considered for biologic therapies must have a chest X-ray and a Mantoux test, both of which must be negative prior to commencing therapy. If for any reason, there is doubt about the result or an individual can't have a Mantoux test as they are on immunosuppressive therapy they should be referred to a thoracic physician (Smith *et al.*, 2005).

Nursing care

Table 8.8 gives guidelines for a nursing assessment for patients about to undergo biologic therapies. It is modified from an article by Jackson *et al.* (2007).

It is also important that the patient receives full information about the implications of using biologics prior to commencement of treatment. Not only should patients be aware of the potential side effects (see Table 8.9), but they also need to know about the commitment to therapy. All treatments except for etanercept are considered ongoing treatments that will require injections or infusions on a long-term basis.

Other systemic drugs for psoriasis

There are a number of other drugs which may occasionally be used for the treatment of psoriasis particularly when the alternatives explored above are not suitable. In a systematic review (Griffiths *et al.*, 2000), the evidence for the use of these four alternatives was reviewed. In summary their findings were as follows:

Hydroxyurea: One study fulfilled the inclusion criteria and it suggested that hydroxyurea does improve psoriasis in some patients. It was suggested that it may be a helpful drug for individuals who could not take ciclosporin or methotrexate.

Fumaric acid esters (fumarates): These were the drugs for which there was most evidence; they are widely used in German speaking countries. Although initial side effects of gastric upset (up to 66%) and flushing (up to 33%) were reported, these rarely stopped people continuing with the drugs and other more serious side effects were rare. It was concluded that fumarates are helpful in treating moderate to severe psoriasis.

Azathioprine: There were no recent studies relating to this drug and it is rarely used.

Sulphasalazine: One randomised controlled trial showed it was effective, although 25% had side effects bad enough to make them stop taking the drug.

Service provision for those who need treatment for psoriasis

The general rule is that those with mild to moderate disease should be cared for in primary care, whilst those with moderate to severe disease should be referred for specialist care within a hospital environment. The National Institute for Health and Clinical Excellence (NICE) clarified what specialist services should provide (see Box 8.6); at the same time they published referral advice which classified the level of urgency with which someone should be referred (see Box 8.7) (National Institute for Clinical Excellence, 2001).

As well as specialist services within hospitals, there is an ever increasing number of specialist practitioners working in community settings.

Table 8.8   Nursing assessment guide for those about to be prescribed biologics.

Question	Rationale
Are you currently or have you in the past 2 weeks experienced any of the following: • Fever • Night sweats • Sore throat • Runny nose • Face pain • Ear ache • Toothache • Cough • Breathing problems • Painful urination • Blood in urine • Antibiotic use • Headache • Wound complication • Severe fatigue	Any of these could indicate infection
Have you had any recent surgery? • If so were there any complications? • Did you experience any drainage from your incision?	Surgery poses an infection risk which usually requires biologic therapy to be postponed
Have you had a recent flu vaccination or other vaccination?	Live vaccines are contraindicated in people receiving biologic therapy because of the infection risk
Are you taking any other medication?	Possible drug interactions should be considered
Do you have any of the following medical conditions: heart failure, haematological or neurological disease or any malignancies?	These conditions may affect the ability to safely use biologic drugs and must be carefully assessed
Could you be pregnant?	Biologics should be avoided in women who are pregnant, trying to conceive or are breast feeding
Have you gained or lost weight since your previous treatment?	Weight may affect dosing, so changes may need to be made
Did you have any hypersensitivity last time you received your biologic medication?	
What was your response to your previous treatment?	

These may be nurse specialists who provide a range of services across primary care and between hospitals and primary care trusts or General Practitioners with a specialist interest in dermatology. The most commonly seen nursing roles include:

■ Clinical nurse specialists in dermatology will see patients in their own homes or in clinics and generally help with chronic disease management for adults and children. Often they will work in such a way as to improve liaison between dermatological care provided in a

Table 8.9 Potential side effects of biologic drugs.

Name of drug	Very common symptom (≥1/10)	Common symptom (≥1/100 <1/10)
Etanercept	• Bacterial infections (including upper respiratory tract, bronchitis, cystitis and skin infections) • Injection site reaction	• Allergic reactions • Pruritus • Fever
Infliximab		• Viral infection • Serum sickness-like reaction • Headache, vertigo, dizziness • Flushing • Lower respiratory tract infection, upper respiratory tract infection, sinusitis, dyspnoea • Abdominal pain, diarrhoea, nausea, dyspepsia • Increased liver enzymes • Urticaria, rash, pruritus, hyperhidrosis, dry skin • Infusion related (including injection site reaction, chills, oedema, pain)
Adalimumab	• Injection site reaction (including pain, swelling, redness and pruritus)	• Lower and upper respiratory tract infections, viral infections, candidiasis, bacterial infections • Dizziness, vertigo, headache, neurologic sensation disorders • Cough, nasopharangeal pain • Diarrhoea, abdominal pain, stomatitis, mouth ulceration, nausea • Increased hepatic enzymes • Rash, dermatitis, hair loss • Musculoskeletal pain • Pyrexia • Fatigue

hospital and that received in the community. This feature of the role may be emphasised as some are called dermatology liaison nurses. They may or may not be nurse prescribers.

■ Nurse practitioner will do some of the above, but is also likely to have a significant diagnostic role. They are likely to be a nurse prescriber.

Measuring quality of life

Quality of life measures allow health care practitioners to ascertain, using an objective measure, how psoriasis is impacting on an individual. As with many chronic skin conditions, psoriasis can severely impact on the quality of life of an individual. This may not be directly related to the severity of the disease, for example someone with minor disease may be severely affected by it and another person with severe disease may be able to cope with it, thus not allowing it to impact on their quality of life. It is therefore important for health care professionals not to make assumptions about how an individual is affected by their skin condition. These are discussed further in Chapter 6.

Conclusion

Psoriasis is a complex multifactorial immune-mediated inflammatory condition of hyperproliferation. There appears to be a genetic

Box 8.6 What specialist services should be able to provide for patients with psoriasis

Specialist services are in a position to:
- Confirm or establish the diagnosis;
- Provide in-patient and day-care services;
- Provide, in conjunction with other health care professionals, advice on the condition and its treatment, together with social and psychological support;
- Assess and supervise the use of phototherapy and PUVA, as well as oral retinoids, cytotoxic therapy and immunosuppressive therapy;
- Treat psoriasis that is unresponsive to therapies tried in primary care, or to resolve problems where the patient cannot tolerate such treatment;
- Offer acute treatment in patients with severe conditions such as EP or GPP;
- Provide and support specialist nursing services working in primary and secondary care;
- Provide assessment and advice for patients with painful psoriatic arthropathy.

Box 8.7 Referral criteria to specialist services

Referral to specialist services, which may be prompted by features such as sleep disturbance, social exclusion, reduced quality of life or reduced self-esteem is advised if:
- **** The patient has generalised pustular or erythrodermis psoriasis.
- *** The patient's psoriasis is acutely unstable.
- *** The patient has widespread GP (so that he/she can benefit from early phototherapy).
- ** The condition is causing severe social or psychological problems.
- ** The rash is sufficiently extensive to make self-management unpractical.
- ** The rash is in a sensitive area (such as face, hands, feet, genitalia) and the symptoms particularly troublesome.
- ** The rash is leading to time off work or school which is interfering with employment or education.
- ** The patient requires assessment for the management of associated arthropathy.
- * The rash fails to respond to management in general practice. Failure is probably best based on the subjective assessment of the patient. Sometimes failure occurs when patients are unable to apply the treatment themselves.
- **** should be seen immediately (within 1 day)
- *** should be seen urgently (it is recommended that this is within 2 weeks)
- ** should be seen soon (no specific recommendation as to timelines)
- * should be seen as a routine patient (no specific recommendation as to timelines)

susceptibility to the condition which is then triggered by one or more of a number of factors, which are often difficult to determine. There are a number of different clinical variants. The treatments for psoriasis are either topical or systemic. Topical treatments have very variable effects partly due to concordance with treatment issues, but also due to the fact that individuals do seem to respond in an individual manner to topical therapies. For those who do not respond to topical therapies provided in primary care, referral to specialist services is likely to be the next option. Systemic therapies are generally more effective; however, the older ones have significant side effects which can limit their usability. A new generation of biological therapies are now available to those with severe disease who have not responded to other systemic therapies. Health care professionals who work with patients with psoriasis must be aware of the potentially enormous impact that it has on mental health and quality of life issues. Readers are directed to Chapter 6 for further detail on this topic.

References

Allan, S., G. Kavanagh *et al.* (2004). The effect of inositol supplements on the psoriasis of patients taking lithium: A randomized, placebo-controlled trial. *British Journal of Dermatology*, **150**: 966–969.

Arbiser, J., B. Govindarajaran *et al.* (2006). Carbazole is a naturally occurring inhibitor of angiogenesis and inflammation isolated from antipsoriatic coal tar. *Journal of Investigative Dermatology*, **126**(6): 1396–1402.

Ashcroft, D., A. Po *et al.* (2000). Systematic review of comparative efficacy and tolerability of calcipotriol in treating chronic plaque psoriasis. *British Medical Journal*, **320**(7240): 963–967.

British Association of Dermatologists (2007). Biologics Intervention Register. Retrieved 15 April 2009, from www.badbir.org.

British Medical Association and Royal Pharmaceutical Society of Great Britain (2008). British National Formulary 55. Retrieved 17 March 2008, from www.bnf.org.

Camisa, C., Ed. (2004a). The clinical variants of psoriasis. In: *Handbook of Psoriasis*. Malden: Blackwell Publishing.

Camisa, C., Ed. (2004b). UVB phototherapy and coal tar. In: *Handbook of Psoriasis*. Malden: Blackwell Publishing.

Christophers, E. (2007). Comorbidities in psoriasis. *Clinics in Dermatology*, **25**(6).

Cooper, E., R. Herd *et al.* (2000). A comparison of bathwater and oral delivery of 8-methoxypsoralen in PUVA therapy for plaque psoriasis. *Clinical and Experimental Dermatology*, **25**(2): 111–114.

Datapharm (2009). Electronic Medicines Compendium. Retrieved 15 April 2009, from www.emc.medicines.org.

de Korte, J., J. Van Onselen *et al.* (2005). Quality of care in patients with psoriasis: An initial clinical study of an international disease management programme. *Journal of the European Academy of Dermatology and Venereology*, **19**(1): 35–41.

Ersser, S., R. Penzer *et al.* (2000). Research report: Pruritus in psoriasis, School of Nursing and Midwifery, University of Southampton.

European Medicines Agency (2009). Press Release – European Medicines Agency recommends suspension of marketing authorisation of Raptiva (efalizumab). Retrieved 15 April 2009, from http://www.emea.europa.eu/humandocs/PDFs/EPAR/raptiva/2085709en.pdf.

Fortes, C., S. Mastroeni *et al.* (2005). Relationship between smoking and clinical severity of psoriasis. *Archives of Dermatology*, **141**(12): 1580–1584.

Franklin, S. and M. Glickman (1986). Lepra, psora, psoriasis. *Journal of the American Academy of Dermatology*, **14**(5): 863–866.

Gelfand, J., A. Troxel *et al.* (2007). The risk of mortality in patients with psoriasis: Results from a population-based study. *Archives of Dermatology*, **143**: 1493–1499.

Graham-Brown, R. and T. Burns (2006). *Lecture Notes: Dermatology* (9th edition). Oxford: Blackwell Science.

Griffiths, C., C. Clark *et al.* (2000). A systematic review of treatments for psoriasis. *Health Technology Assessment*, **4**(1): 1–125.

Guenther, L., F. Cambazard *et al.* (2002). Efficacy and safety of a new combination of calcipotriol and betamethasone diproprionate (once or twice daily) compared to calcipotriol (twice daily) in the treatment of psoriasis vulgaris: A randomized, double blind, vehicle-controlled clinical trial. *British Journal of Dermatology*, **147**(2): 316–323.

Gulliver, W. (2008). Long-term prognosis in patients with psoriasis. *British Journal of Dermatology*, **159**(Suppl 2): 2–9.

Hudson-Peacock, M., B. Diffey *et al.* (1994). Photoprotective action of emollients in ultraviolet therapy of psoriasis. *British Journal of Dermatology*, **130**(3): 361–365.

Jackson, K., S. Maguire *et al.* (2007). Biologic therapies in psoriasis: The key role of the dermatology nurse specialist. *Dermatological Nursing*, **6**(1): s1–s11.

Kreuger, J. (2002). The immunologic basis for the treatment of psoriasis with new biologic agents. *Journal of the American Academy of Dermatology*, **46**(1): 1–23.

Lee, E. and J. Koo (2005). Modern modified 'ultra' Goeckerman therapy: A PASI assessment of a very effective therapy for psoriasis resistant to both prebiologic and biologic therapies. *Journal of Dermatologic Treatment*, **16**(2): 102–107.

Naldi, L. and C. Griffiths (2005). Traditional therapies in the management of moderate to severe chronic plaque psoriasis: An assessment of the benefits and risks. *British Journal of Dermatology*, **152**: 597–615.

Naldi, L., L. Chatenoud *et al.* (2005). Cigarette smoking, body mass index and stressful life events as risk factors for psoriasis: Results from an Italian case control study. *Journal of Investigative Dermatology*, **125**(1): 61–67.

National Institute for Clinical Excellence (2001). *Referral Advice: A Guide to Appropriate Referral from General to Specialist Services*. London: NICE.

National Institute for Health and Clinical Excellence (2006). *Etanercept and Efalizumab for the Treatment of Adults with Psoriasis: NICE Technology Appraisal*. London: NICE.

National Institute for Health and Clinical Excellence (2008a). *Infliximab for the Treatment of Adults with Psoriasis: Single Technology Appraisal*. London: NICE.

National Institute for Health and Clinical Excellence (2008b). *Adalimumab for the Treatment of Adults with Psoriasis: Single Technology Appraisal*. London: NICE.

Osborn, T. and W. Wilke (2004). Psoriatic arthritis. In: Camisa, C. (Ed.), *Handbook of Psoriasis*. Massachusetts: Blackwell Publishing.

Otman, S., C. Edwards *et al.* (2006). Modulation of ultraviolet (UV) transmission by emollients: Relevance to narrowband UVB phototherapy and psoralen plus UVA photochemotherapy. *British Journal of Dermatology*, **154**(5): 963–968.

Rapp, S., S. Feldman *et al.* (1999). Psoriasis causes as much disability as other major medical diseases. *Journal of the American Academy of Dermatology*, **41**(3(pt1)): 401–407.

Richards, H., D. Ray *et al.* (2005). Response of the hypothalamic–pituitary–adrenal axis to psychological stress in patients with psoriasis. *British Journal of Dermatology*, **153**: 1114–1120.

Rim, J., J. Park *et al.* (2003). The efficacy of calcipotriol + acitretin combination therapy for psoriasis: Comparison with acitretin monotherapy. *American Journal of Clinical Dermatology*, **4**(7): 507–510.

Roelofzen, J., K. Aben *et al.* (2007). Coal tar in dermatology. *Journal of Dermatologic Treatment*, **18**(6): 329–334.

Smith, C., A. Anstey *et al.* (2005). British Association of Dermatologists Guidelines on the use of biological interventions in psoriasis in 2005. *British Journal of Dermatology*, **153**: 486–497.

Sommer, D., S. Jenisch *et al.* (2006). Increased prevalence of the metabolic syndrome in patients with moderate to severe psoriasis. *Archives of Dermatological Research*, **298**(7): 321–328.

Streit, V., O. Wiedow *et al.* (1996). Treatment of psoriasis with polyethylene sheet bath PUVA. *Journal of American Academy of Dermatology*, **35**(2): 208–210.

van de Kerkhof, P., P. van der Valk *et al.* (2006). A comparison of twice-daily calcipotriol ointment with once-daily short-contact dithranol cream therapy: A randomized controlled trial of supervised treatment of psoriasis vulgaris in a day-care setting. *British Journal of Dermatology*, 155(4): 800–807.

Veraldi, S., R. Caputo *et al.* (2006). Short contact therapy with tazarotene in psoriasis vulgaris. *Dermatology*, 212(3): 235–237.

Weller, R., J.A.A. Hunter, J. Savin and M. Dahl (2008). *Clinical Dermatology* (4th edition). Oxford: Wiley-Blackwell.

Williams, H.C. (1997). *Dermatology Health Care Needs Assessment*. Oxford: Radcliffe Medical Press

Woo, W. and K. McKenna (2003). Combination TL01 ultraviolet B phototherapy and topical calcipotriol for psoriasis: A prospective randomized placebo-controlled clinical trial. *British Journal of Dermatology*, 149(1): 146–150.

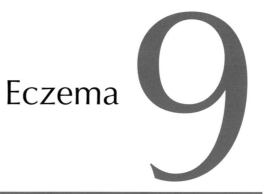

Eczema 9

Steven J. Ersser & Julie Van Onselen

Introduction

This chapter will highlight the different types of eczema and the relevant principles of care that underpin the treatment of people living with eczema. It commences with a review of what eczema is and a brief outline of the variants of the condition. This is followed by an overview of what eczema is commonly mistaken for in a review of the differential diagnosis. The focus is then on the widespread form of eczema, atopic eczema, its features and key principles regarding the care of a child with eczema and related family care. Different treatment options are examined, with due regard to different types of treatment and patterns of their use; this includes topical treatments, occlusive, behavioural and systemic approaches. Other types of eczema are discussed and the related patient care, including seborrhoeic eczema, contact eczema, both irritant and allergic. This is followed by eczemas of adulthood, including those common in older age, such as discoid and varicose eczema, and their related principles of care and treatment.

What is eczema?

Eczema or dermatitis is a type of inflammatory reaction pattern in the skin which may be provoked by a number of external or internal factors (Graham-Brown and Burns, 2006). The term eczema comes from the Greek for 'boiling', which refers to the small vesicles or blisters that are often observed at the early acute stages of the disorder. Eczema and dermatitis are synonymous terms, often used interchangeably.

Eczemas may be categorised as exogenous, due to an external agent, or endogenous, related to a constitutional factor; however, in some cases both causal factors may be present (see Box 9.1).

Some clinical images of eczema can be seen below. Endogenous eczema is exemplified by atopic eczema, which often presents in early childhood – with facial involvement (Figure 9.1). Other images include seborrhoeic eczema (Figure 9.2) and exogenous eczema, such as contact (allergic) dermatitis.

Another useful distinction is that of acute and chronic eczema. Acute eczema is characterised

Box 9.1 Eczema classification

Endogenous
- Atopic eczema (see Figure 9.1)
- Seborrhoeic eczema (see Figure 9.2)
- Discoid eczema
- Varicose eczema
- Endogenous eczema of the palms and soles
- Asteatotic eczema (eczema craquele)

Exogenous
- Primary irritant contact dermatitis
- Allergic contact dermatitis (Figure 9.3)

Source: Reprinted from Graham-Brown and Burns (2006)

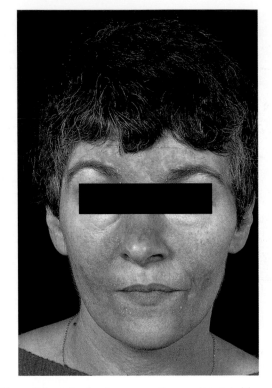

Figure 9.2 Seborrhoeic eczema. (*Source:* Reprinted from Graham-Brown and Burns, 2006.)

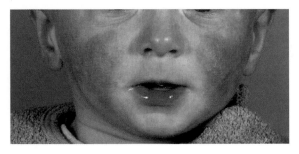

Figure 9.1 Atopic (endogenous) eczema. (*Source:* Reprinted from Buxton and Morris-Jones, 2009.)

this chapter. For people living with a long-term or chronic condition, specific attention is needed to support them and their families with utilising their treatment effectively and appropriately adhering to treatment. Such issues have been examined in Chapter 7.

by weeping crusting, blistering redness, papules, swelling and scaling. Chronic eczema may reveal these changes but it is typically less vascular and exudative, more scaly, pigmented and thickened and more like to fissure and show lichenification (see Figure 9.4). Lichenification describes a state where the skin is dry, leathery and thickened with skin markings secondary to repeated scratching or rubbing (Weller *et al.*, 2008). Chronic eczemas may have acute flare-ups, as in the case of a child with atopic eczema having an eczema flare due to infection. Those living with eczema or their carers need to understand the triggers that may lead to acute flare-ups and their management; these are discussed later in

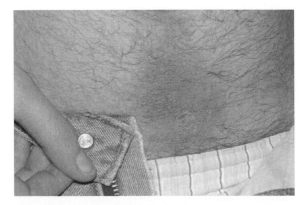

Figure 9.3 Contact dermatitis (allergic) to nickel in a jean stud. (*Source:* Reprinted from Graham-Brown and Burns, 2006.)

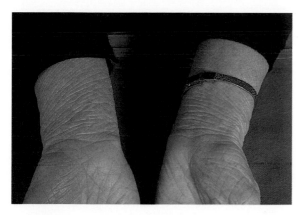

Figure 9.4   Lichenification. (*Source:* Reprinted from Weller *et al.*, 2008.)

Biology and pathophysiology of eczema

Atopic eczema occurs as a result of the interaction of environmental factors with an abnormal immune system in a genetically predisposed individual (Cork, 1997). These genetic changes cause an altered immunological response to antigens and as a result immunoglobulin (Ig) E or IgE is produced. Abnormal T-helper (T_H) lymphocytes play a key role in the disease interacting with Langerhans cells which raises IgE and interleukin levels and reduces interferon levels (INF-γ); this leads to an upregulation of pro-inflammatory cells (Buxton and Morris-Jones, 2009).

In atopic individuals, IgE binds to mast cells and an antigen response causes mast cell degranulation resulting in the release of pro-inflammatory mediators and hence the development of inflamed eczematous lesions (McFadden *et al.*, 1993). In addition, this response can only occur due to the additional genetic alteration of the epidermal barrier, which allows the penetration of antigens (Cork, 1997). The primary defect is the reduced barrier function (e.g. from filaggrin mutations) which allows protein antigens to get into the skin; leucocytes then prime T-helper cells to become T2 helper cells, which then release interleukin 4, 5 and 13, leading to high IgE levels and other effects (Healy, E., University of Southampton, Southampton, pers. comm.). The complex relationship between the epidermal barrier dysfunction in atopic eczema and the interaction between genes and the environment is usefully summarised in (Cork *et al.*, 2006).

The normal skin barrier has lipid lamellae which keep high levels of water within the corneocytes and together with high levels of natural moisturising factors (NMFs), e.g. urea, lactic acid and urocanic acid that maintain the skin's protective features and keep the skin elastic and smooth (Cork, 1999). Skin barrier changes in eczematous skin include the breakdown of lipid lamellae from around the corneocytes and a decrease of up to 80% of the levels of NMF. In addition, genetic changes in atopic eczema of the genes (including filaggrin and protease) responsible for the structure of the skin barrier (stratum corneum) result in decreased levels of NMF within the stratum corneum (Palmer *et al.*, 2006). This results in water loss from the corneocytes, with shrinking and cracking permitting penetration of irritants and allergens and triggering the inflammatory response. The differences between normal skin and eczematous skin barriers are illustrated in Figure 9.5.

The damage to the epidermal skin barrier also results in bacterial colonisation, commonly *Staphylococcus aureus*. People with atopic eczema have a total bacterial skin flora of 90% of *Staphylococcus aureus* compared to 30% in

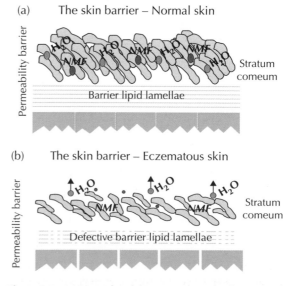

Figure 9.5   (a) Normal and (b) eczematous skin barrier. (Source: Cork, 1999.)

individuals without atopic eczema (Hoare *et al.*, 2000). Even when the skin has not undergone clinical change with overt infection, *Staphylococcus aureus* contributes to disease activity and increases with the severity of atopic eczema (Szakos *et al.*, 2004).

Staphylococcus aureus is an environmental trigger in atopic eczema as it flourishes in eczematous skin. Bacterial colonisation of the skin with *Staphylococcus aureus* will result in active eczema with visible signs of infection, such as weeping, crusting and pustules, present in the skin. Therefore *Staphylococcus aureus* will exacerbate and sustain eczema. There are several mechanisms that support this physiological response in eczema:

(1) Protein A is a constituent of the cell wall of staphylococic (if protein A is injected intradermally, the substance causes initial flare, followed by delayed induration of the skin).
(2) Circulating anti-staphylococcal (IgE) antibodies are found in up to 30% of patients with atopic eczema and can contribute to mast cell degranulation.
(3) *Staphylococcus aureus* produces exotoxins which act as superantigens. These can stimulate T-lymphocytes to release massive amounts of cytokines, thereby contributing hugely to the inflammatory response. This is illustrated in Figure 9.6 (McFadden *et al.*, 1993).

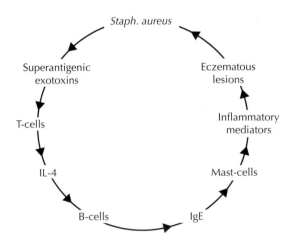

Figure 9.6 Superantigens diagram, illustrating the cycle of events that result from release of superantigenic exotoxins. (*Source:* Reprinted from McFadden *et al.*, 1993.)

Atopic eczema

Clinical features and epidemiology

Atopic eczema, or atopic dermatitis, is an itchy inflammatory skin disease, which usually involves the skin creases (Williams *et al.*, 1995). The diagnostic criteria for atopic eczema are classified by the following clinical picture (Williams *et al.*, 1995) an itchy skin condition, plus three or more of:

■ Past involvement of the skin creases, such as bends of the elbows or behind the knees,
■ A personal or immediate family history of asthma or hay fever,
■ A tendency towards generally dry skin,
■ Onset under the age of 2 year and
■ Visible flexural dermatitis, as defined by photographic protocol.

The risk factors for children developing atopic eczemas include familial factors including genetics (atopy), family size and sibling order; social class (eczema has a higher incidence in more affluent social classes) and concurrent illness/disruption to family life including teething, psychological stress and lack of sleep (National Institute for Health and Clinical Excellence [NICE], 2007).

Clinical signs

Atopic eczema is characterised by inflammation (redness), swelling, crusting, scaling of the skin; intensified by scratching in response to intense itch. It may be acute with oozing and vesicles or it may be chronic with lichenification, altered pigmentation and exaggerated surface markings. Itching is a predominant symptom that can lead to a cycle of scratching, leading to skin damage and in turn more itching (the itch–scratch cycle). A stubborn reverse pattern may occur when the extensor areas (a straight part of the body) as well as the flexural areas (a body part that flexes or bends) are affected, for example, around the elbow (see Figure 9.7).

Atopic eczema is now the commonest inflammatory skin disease of childhood, affecting

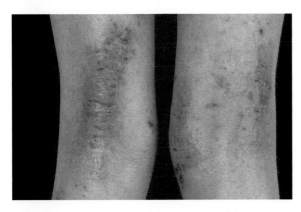

Figure 9.7 Atopic eczema. (Source: Reprinted from Graham-Brown and Burns, 2006.)

around 15–20% of school children in the UK (Herd, 2000). Although only 1–2% of adults are affected by atopic eczema, their disease is often more chronic and severe (Herd *et al.*, 1996). Atopic eczema is more frequent in childhood, especially in the first 5 years of life (Thomas *et al.*, 2008). Young children represent the largest group of individuals with atopic eczema seen by dermatologists, GPs, primary care nurses and nurse specialists. Atopic eczema is the commonest of childhood dermatoses, accounting for 20% of all dermatology referrals (Lewis-Jones *et al.*, 2001). There is reasonable evidence to suggest that the prevalence of atopic eczema has increased two to three-fold over the last 30 years, for reasons which are unclear but possibly due to environmental and lifestyle changes, (Williams, 1992) and in many countries this continues to rise (Asher *et al.*, 2006).

Studies with twins demonstrate that genetic factors are important in atopic eczema but other evidence strongly suggests that environmental factors are critical in disease expression (Williams, 1995). Allergic factors such as exposure to house dust mites may be accountable, but non-allergic factors such as exposure to irritants and infectious agents may also be important. Atopic eczema may be further categorised into extrinsic and intrinsic forms, as highlighted earlier in the chapter. The former denotes individuals with evidence of raised circulating antibodies to common allergens, whereas the latter does not. It is also established that psychological factors, such as stress, play a vital role in the course of

atopic eczema as a trigger or precipitating factor (Buske-Kirschbaum *et al.*, 2001, 2002). Frequent exposure to infections may protect children from expressing atopy; this observation is based on an inverse relationship between prevalence of eczema and family size, leading to the 'hygiene hypothesis' (Strachan, 1989). As referred to in the section on the biology of eczema, atopic eczema is a multifactorial condition that is influenced by the interplay between genetics and the environment; this interplay and its relationship to the skin barrier is discussed in Cork *et al.* (2006). Some of the environmental trigger factors are now discussed.

Trigger factors

Trigger factors need to be identified and managed following clinical assessment; potential factors include (NICE, 2007):

- irritants (e.g. soaps and detergents)
- skin infections
- allergens
  - contact
  - food
  - inhalant

Atopic eczema assessment should consider all the identified trigger factors listed in Table 9.1.

NICE (2007) provides guidance based on a synthesis of evidence, proposing the following considerations. Inhalation allergy may be seen in children with seasonal flares, and those whose eczema is associated with asthma and allergic rhinitis. Allergic contact dermatitis may be seen in children with exacerbations of previously controlled atopic eczema or reactions to topical preparations. Allergy testing on the high street or via the internet should be avoided since there is no evidence of their value. The role of factors such as stress, humidity or temperature extremes have in leading to flares is not known and as such these factors should be avoided where practical.

Health care professionals should consider a diagnosis of food allergy in children with atopic eczema who have previously reacted to food with immediate symptoms. This also applies to

Table 9.1 Trigger factors for atopic eczema.

Potential trigger factor	Source of trigger factor
Irritants	Wool and synthetic clothing, soaps, detergents, disinfectants and chemicals
Contact allergens	Preservations in topical products, perfumes, metals and latex
Food/dietary factors	Cow's milk, eggs, peanuts, wheat
Inhalant allergens	House dust mite, animal dander, tree/grass pollens and mould
Microbial colonisation/infection	*Staphylococcus aureus*, *Streptococcus* species, *Candida albicans*, *Pityrosporum* yeasts and herpes simplex
Climate	Extremes of temperature and humidity and seasonal variation
Environmental factors	Hard water, proximity to traffic, cooking with gas and tobacco smoke

Source: Adapted from NICE (2007).

infants and young children with moderate to severe eczema that has not been controlled by optimum management, particularly if associated with gut dysmobility (including colic, vomiting and altered bowel habit) or failure to thrive (NICE, 2007).

In general there is little evidence to support a diet free of eggs, and milk in unselected patients with atopic eczema nor the use of a few-foods diet. There is, however, some evidence to support the use of an egg-free diet in infants with suspect egg allergy who have positive specific antibodies (IgE) to eggs (Williams *et al.*, 2008). With exclusion, diet consideration also needs to be given to the risks of impaired growth and development in the child. It is not known whether altering a breast feeding mother's diet is effective in reducing the severity of eczema (NICE, 2007). Evidence is currently not available to suggest the optimal feeding regimen in the first year of life for children with established atopic eczema.

Evidence to support the implication of environmental factors increasing the prevalence of atopic eczema in developed countries is outlined by a study showing associations between atopic eczema symptoms and the home environment (McNally *et al.*, 2001). This highlights factors such as dampness in the home environment, the use of radiators in bedrooms (causing nocturnal overheating) and upholstered furniture, bedding and carpets; all these factors encourage house dust mites to thrive. The study concluded that there was an improvement in atopic eczema symptoms by controlling mite allergens through mattress covers and frequent vacuuming. Control of house dust mite by vacuuming is therefore advocated, based on this evidence; a similar principle will apply to damp dusting.

Significance and impact of atopic eczema

Atopic eczema is a significant disease. Children with atopic eczema are a high-priority group for effective intervention. Few individuals experience handicap in adult life with the very chronic form of atopic eczema. However, the onset of disease occurs before the age of 2 years in 90% of newly diagnosed cases. The intractable itch of atopic eczema can cause sleep loss, misery to children and disruption to family life (Williams, 1997). Atopic eczema can be a disfiguring and very burdensome due to the unrelenting itch and desire to scratch. Scratching damages the skin, disturbs sleep, disrupts relationships, triggers mood changes and alters affect (Lewis-Jones *et al.*, 2001). Sleep loss is an important measure of disease intensity in children with atopic eczema (Reid and Lewis-Jones, 1995).

Atopic eczema is the cause of significant emotional difficulties for many sufferers as well as other family members (Elliott and Luker, 1997). The latter study of mothers caring for children with severe atopic eczema highlights the extra burden of normal childcare and the additional housework generated by the disease. Elliott and Luker found that mothers described the major task in keeping their child entertained in order to prevent scratching. This is further compounded by the fact that such children were often found to be irritable and had short concentration spans.

There is a substantial economic cost of eczema to the patient (Kemp, 2003) and the health service (Verboom *et al.*, 2002). Herd *et al.* (1996)

estimated that in 1996 the annual UK personal cost to patients would be £2,297 million, the cost to the service £125 million with a substantial loss of school and working days. The substantial economic impact of the disease is supported by studies such as that from Australia (Kemp, 2003).

Measurement of the impact of skin disease on quality of life is important for our understanding and management of skin diseases. Several studies suggest that atopic eczema has a more profound effect on quality of life than other skin diseases, such as acne and psoriasis (Lewis-Jones and Finlay, 1995).Therefore, it is desirable to measure the impact on quality of life as a potential outcome of intervention. The relationship between the severity of atopic eczema in children and quality of life has been established (Ben-Gashir *et al.*, 2004). Problematic symptoms such as itching can adversely affect quality of life. Itch leads to scratching and these may have a significant impact on a child's sleep, quality of life (Lewis-Jones *et al.*, 2001) and family (Elliott and Luker, 1997).

Due to these various impacts of atopic eczema, it is necessary to measure changes in quality of life impact as well as disease severity as a key outcome measure (further details can be obtained in Chapters 3 and 6). Also, since caregivers, especially parents, are often required to assist with treatments, their ability and confidence are also relevant outcomes to measure. Given that people with atopic eczema require special clothing, bedding, frequent applications of greasy ointments (Reid and Lewis-Jones, 1995), treatment adherence also becomes a relevant clinical outcome to assess. Nurses have a key role in supporting the parents of children with atopic eczema. The challenge for parents is highlighted in the research by Elliott and Luker (1997) and ongoing work by Surridge (2005) on the challenges of appraising knowledge sources to find tolerable solutions to their child's eczema. Parental education is discussed later, but is also highlighted in Chapter 7, on the importance of parental education to make the most of treatment.

What is eczema commonly mistaken for?

Diagnosis of eczema requires identification of its key clinical signs (described earlier) and also differentiation from other skin conditions; the latter is summarised in Table 9.2.

Table 9.2   Common differential diagnoses.

	Eczema variant	Differential diagnosis
Scalp and hair	*Seborrhoeic dermatitis*: Fine scaling (yellow/greasy) on scalp with mild erythema. Tending to confluence.	*Psoriasis*: Thick scaling and erythema extending to hairline and ears. Hair thinning may occur. Tending to discrete paths with clear skin in between.
Face and neck	*Atopic eczema*: Eczematous areas especially of face show erythema, scaling and oozing, but much of non-eczematous skin may be very dry.	*Infantile seborrhoeic eczema*: Greasy yellow-brown scales or crusting on scalp, face and napkin area with mild erythema. May not itch.
	Airborne contact dermatitis: Erythema, blisters and weeping.	*Chronic actinic dermatitis* (*Photosensitivity*): Acute erythema on sun-exposed area.
	Acute eczema: Erythema, vesicles, oozing and crusting. Always itches, hence is scratched.	*Erysipelas/cellulitis*: Intense erythema and oedema.

(continued)

Table 9.2   (*continued*)

	Eczema variant	Differential diagnosis
Palms and soles	*Chronic dermatitis*: Dryness, mild erythema, cracks and fissures.	*Chronic psoriasis*: Thick scaling with silvery scales and erythema, often in discrete patches.
	Pompholyx eczema: Vesicles, bullae and weeping.	*Palmoplantar pustulosis*: Dryness, yellow sterile pustules which resolve to brown macules.
Dorsum hands	*Allergic hand eczema*: Intense erythema, vesicles and blisters.	*Chronic irritant eczema*: Dryness, mild erythema, cracks and fissures.
Generalised	*Discoid eczema*: Circular lesions, dry skin, moderate erythema. Very itchy.	*Psoriasis*: Thick scaling with silvery scales and erythema.
	Atopic eczema: Dryness, erythema, scaling with patchy oozing and marked scratching. Lichenification is increased line markings of the skin and pigmentation due to persistent scratching and rubbing.	*Dermatitis herpetiformis*: Small to medium vesicles on an erythematous and eczematized background – favours shoulder, knees and elbows.
	Acute eczema: Erythema, vesicles, oozing and crusting.	*Bullous pemphigoid*: Large tense bullae on an erythematous and eczematized background.
	Chronic eczema: Dry skin, background of erythema, excoriation and lichenification.	*Tinea* (excluding palms and soles): Erythema, mild scaling with a raised advancing edge and clearing centre.
Flexural/perineal/ genital	*Flexural eczema*: Dryness, erythema, minimal scaling or oozing. Satellite lesions.	*Flexural psoriasis*: Erythema, minimal scaling, plaque forms and bilaterally symmetrical, less likely to be scratched.
		Tinea cruris: Erythema, minimal scaling and unilateral.
Limbs	*Atopic eczema*: Dryness, erythema, scaling and vesicles.	*Keratosis pilaris*: Follicular papules, skin coloured or brown, no erythema.
	Asteatotic eczema (*craquele*): Large dry flaky scales ('crazy-paving appearance'), mild erythema	*Venous eczema*: Erythema, decolourisation (due to haemosiderin) and scaling with associated oedema, ulceration and fibrosis.

Source: Based on Cox and Lawrence (1998).

Eczema severity assessment

NICE (2007) recommends that clinicians should consider using the assessment tools to measure eczema severity, psychological and psychosocial well-being and quality of life. However, the tools used should be easy-to-use validated tools which will aid clinical management. Eczema severity assessment and measurement tools should aid the clinician to ascertain the level of severity of eczema and the effects of treatment. Time-consuming and cumbersome tools may not necessarily be effective in day-to-day clinical practice. A selection of the commonly used tools to assess the impact of atopic eczema in children, recommended by NICE (2007), is outlined in Table 9.3.

The patient-orientated eczema measure (POEM) is a useful tool for adults in self-assessing symptoms and disease severity in atopic eczema. Tools assessing the effects of quality of life for adults with eczema may include the Dermatology Life Quality Index and SCORAD. These assessment tools are discussed in more detail in Chapters 6 and 3 respectively. There is a need for health professionals to adopt a holistic approach to eczema assessment, taking into account of both the severity of atopic eczema, quality of life/everyday activities and psychosocial well-being. NICE (2007) recommends a simple holistic assessment tool outlined in Table 9.4.

Caring for children with eczema

Consultations tend to focus on the physical aspects of the child's problems, neglecting those of a psychosocial nature (Fennessy *et al.*, 2000). The health care professional should include in a holistic assessment the following factors:

- A detailed individualised history of the:
  - □ time, onset, pattern and severity of eczema
  - □ response to previous and current treatments
  - □ possible trigger factors
  - □ the impact of the condition on the child, their parents/carers
  - □ dietary history
  - □ growth and development
  - □ personal and family history of atopic eczema (NICE, 2007)
- Specific problems such as scratching/poor sleep/family impact.

Table 9.3 Eczema severity assessment scales.

Assessment tool	Description
Visual analogue scales	Use a 0–10 scale to capture the child/patient/carer's assessment of severity, itch and sleep loss over the previous 3 days
Patient-Orientated Eczema Measure (POEM)	Patient self-assessment for monitoring symptoms and disease severity
Children's Dermatology Life Quality index (CDLQI)	Impact of eczema on the child
Infants Dermatology Life Quality Index (CDLQI)	Impact of eczema on the infant
Dermatitis Family Impact (DFI) questionnaire	Impact of eczema on the child's parents/carer

Table 9.4 Holistic assessment for atopic eczema recommended by NICE (2007).

Skin/physical assessment		Impact on quality of life and psychosocial well-being	
CLEAR	Normal skin, no evidence of atopic eczema	NONE	No impact on quality of life
MILD	Areas of dry skin, infrequent itching (with or without small areas of redness)	MILD	Little impact on everyday activities, sleep and psychosocial well-being
MODERATE	Areas of dry skin, frequent itching, redness (with or without excoriation and skin thickening)	MODERATE	Moderate impact on everyday activities and psychosocial well-being, frequently disturbed sleep
SEVERE	Widespread area of dry skin, incessant itching, redness (with or without excoriation, extensive skin thickening, bleeding, oozing, cracking and alteration of pigmentation)	SEVERE	Severe limitation of everyday activities and psychosocial functioning, nightly loss of sleep

■ Developmental considerations: It is important to highlight that 10% children with severe atopic eczema display retarded growth. NICE (2007) recommends monitoring growth in children with atopic eczema by regular weight and height measurement, to assess for growth retardation. The reasons for growth retardation in severe atopic eczema are not fully understood, but chronic sleep disturbance and stress may contribute (NICE, 2007). Growth retardation also needs to be assessed with consideration to the child's diet, as children on strict elimination diets (which may not be clinically supervised) often exhibit nutritional deficiencies that may lead to poor growth (Lifschitz, 2008).

■ Parental support/self-efficacy (belief in their ability to manage their child's eczema): managing medication and eczema symptoms and communicating with health care professionals.

■ Challenge of parent and child management of scratching and poor understanding of an effective clinical regimen by parent.

■ Quality of life impact: this is significant in atopic eczema and affects the entire family including:

  □ Sleep disturbance,
  □ Major burden of care causing disruption of family life,
  □ Economic cost and
  □ Treatment adherence: children with eczema are often on multiple medications and parents are given health guidelines that they often struggle to put into practice. Problems of adherence stem more from a disbelief in their ability to use effectively what they are prescribed than from disease activity (Taal *et al.*, 1993).

Other forms of childhood eczema

Seborrhoeic dermatitis

In infancy, seborrhoeic dermatitis is also commonly known as 'cradle cap' (infantile seborrhoeic dermatitis) and occurs on the scalp, face, flexures, nappy area and occasionally can be generalised. It presents with erythema and yellow greasy scales; it is self-limiting, not itchy and generally resolves over several weeks (see Figure 9.2). The aetiology of seborrhoeic dermatitis is unclear but it is believed to be an inflammatory reaction related to the proliferation of a non-pathogenic skin flora, yeast called *Malassezia furfur* (formerly known as *Pityrosporum ovale*). Increased keratinocyte and sebocyte turnover may also play a part.

Juvenile plantar dermatoses

This is a condition mainly affecting school-aged children. It occurs exclusively on the plantar regions of the feet (soles) with glazed erythema and painful fissuring. This is a form of dermatitis which is related to the continual wearing of synthetic footwear (Burns *et al.*, 2004).

Other forms of eczema in adulthood

The following other forms of eczema are more likely to be seen in the middle-aged patient, although these can present in any age group.

Discoid eczema

Discoid eczema describes a type of eczema which presents as disc-shaped, rounded areas of raised eczematous lesions. The lesions have well-defined edges and scale; they are very itchy and occur in asymmetrical patterns all over the body. The cause is unknown.

Lichen simplex

Lichen simplex occurs due to the repeated rubbing or scratching of an irritated or itchy area of skin which becomes a lichenified patch of eczema; scaling and fissuring may also be present. It may appear as a single lesion or occur in multiple sites on any part of the body.

Pompholyx

This is a term given to eczema that typically occurs on the palms, fingers, soles and toes. It presents following severe itching as clear vesicles that are deep seated and may progress to confluent large bullae (blisters). When the bullae resolve, the skin cracks and peels and is painful and susceptible to infection (Figure 9.8) (Burns *et al.*, 2004).

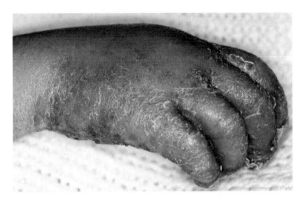

Figure 9.8 Infected eczema. (Source: Reprinted from Buxton and Morris-Jones, 2009.)

The following other forms of eczema are more likely to be seen in the older patient, although these can present in any age group.

Asteatotic eczema

Asteatotic eczema is known as '*eczema craquele*' and describes the crackled crazy paving type appearance of dry, scaled and fissured eczematous skin. It occurs exclusively in the older person, usually in winter and on the lower limbs and trunk. Asteatotic eczema is often associated with the overuse of soaps, overheating and low humidity (see Table 9.2).

Varicose (venous) eczema

Varicose eczema is also known as gravitational, stasis or venous eczema. It occurs in the lower limbs of patients suffering from venous hypertension. An eczematous pattern is present on one or both limbs; the skin is dry, flaky, irritated and inflamed (see Figure 9.9). The skin is fragile and can break down easily, leading to the formation of venous leg ulcers.

It is not uncommon in the community to see a range of erythematous eczema-like lesions affecting the lower leg. Although all are red, eczema is always itchy or sore with broken skin. Superficial thrombo-phlebitis is localised to a vein and tends to be linear and tender, whereas cellulitis is a deep dermal and subcutaneous condition, with painful inflammation and is usually accompanied by a pyrexia and diffuse oedema (Ryan, T., University of Oxford, Oxford, pers. comm.).

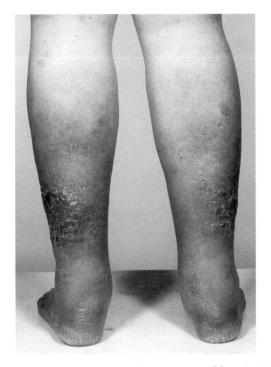

Figure 9.9 Varicose eczema. (Source: Reprinted from Buxton and Morris-Jones, 2009.)

Contact dermatitis

Prevalence and incidence

The majority of occupational dermatoses consist of contact dermatitis. Irritant contact dermatitis is extremely common; it is reported to be as high as 55% in people with certain occupations (e.g. health care workers and those working in catering, cleaning and hairdressing). Contact allergic dermatitis affects 1–2% of the general UK population (English, 1999).

Risk and trigger factors

These include:

- atopic eczema (current or a history of childhood atopic eczema)
- occupations with a high exposure to allergens
- occupations where repeated hand washing is essential

Irritant dermatitis

Irritant dermatitis is inflammation of the skin resulting from a non-immunological reaction to external stimuli due to excessive contact with an irritant (e.g. detergents, soap, acids, alkaline, cement, solvents, chemicals and food). Acute irritant contact dermatitis is often the result of a single overwhelming exposure or a few brief exposures to the irritant or causative agent. Chronic or cumulative contact dermatitis occurs following repeated exposure to irritants (Bourke *et al.*, 2001).

Allergic contact dermatitis

Allergic contact dermatitis is an allergic reaction which only occurs in people whose skin has been exposed to and previously sensitised by an allergen. Subsequent contact with the antigen elicits a specific cell-mediated sensitisation (e.g. nickel, cosmetics, perfumes, hair dye, dyes and plants) of the immune system to a specific allergen/s with resulting dermatitis or exacerbation of pre-existing dermatitis. Phototoxic, photo-allergic and photo-aggravated contact dermatitis occur when allergens are photo-allergens but it is not always easy to distinguish between photo-allergic and phototoxic reactions (Bourke *et al.*, 2001). Phototoxic reactions result from direct damage to tissue caused by light activation of the photosensitising agent. Photo-allergic reactions are a cell-mediated immune response in which the antigen is the light-activated photosensitising agent. Some patients with atopic dermatitis and other chronic inflammatory skin conditions become photosensitive (DermNetNZ, 2009).

Acute dermatitis will follow a single exposure to an irritant or an allergen, and the allergic and eczematous manifestations observed in the skin are defined by Burns *et al.* (2004). The manifestations are as follows:

- Vasodilatation of the dermis causes inflammation;
- Peri-vascular infiltrate of lymphocytes and polymorphs;

- Intra-epidermal vesicles form by accumulation of fluid in cells, and may coalesce to form bullae;
- Vesicles and bullae will rupture to oozing, crusting, scaling and healing.

Patients with allergic contact dermatitis usually present with acute dermatitis at the body site where the allergen has been in direct contact with the skin. Severe allergic contact reactions may extend outside the contact area or it may become generalised.

Diagnosis of irritant and contact dermatitis

The key to diagnosing irritant and/or allergic contact dermatitis is the detection of the irritant sensitising agent respectively. Sensitisation may suddenly occur following years of trouble-free contact with the allergen.

An examination and skin/occupational history will reveal clues and common sites of involvement, e.g.:

- nickel – ear lobes/nape of neck (jewellery)
- leather – wrists (watch straps)
- tanning agents/adhesives – soles of feet (shoes)

Patch testing

Patch testing identifies whether a substance that comes in contact with the skin is causing inflammation of the skin (contact dermatitis) and confirms or excludes an allergen.

The guidelines for managing contact dermatitis (Bourke *et al.*, 2001) recommend that patients with persistent eczematous eruptions should be patch tested. Patch testing should include at least to an extended series of allergens. In addition, patch testing should be undertaken by an individual who has had training in the investigation of contact dermatitis, prescribes the appropriate patch tests and performs patch test readings at day 2 and day 4 for patients undergoing diagnostic patch tests. The dual time sequenced readings allow time for the immunological response to evolve sufficiently.

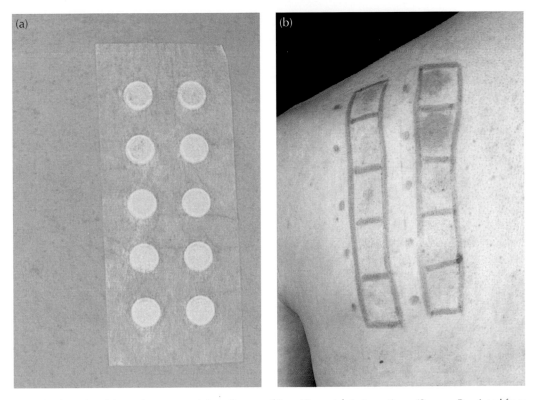

Figure 9.10 Patch testing: (a) metal cups containing allergens; (b) positive patch test reactions. (Source: Reprinted from Graham-Brown and Burns, 2006.)

Patch testing involves testing patients with the suspected substance (prepared allergens) and the European standard battery (the European standard of allergens most widely used in patch testing) plus other likely allergens (English, 1999). The procedure for patch testing is as follows.

(1) Suspected allergens are placed within small metal chambers called Finn chambers and are the placed on the patient's back.
(2) The patch tests are left in place for 48 hours and then removed (the patient is instructed not to wash their back for 5 days).
(3) Results are read at 48 and 96 hours using a four-point scale to score the skin reaction to the patch tests. The scale is as follows:
   - O = no reaction
   - + = a palpable oedematous reaction develops
   - ++ = the reaction becomes vesicular
   - +++ = the reaction is very strong and spreads beyond the boundary of the patch.

(4) The skin reactions from patch testing are interpreted with consideration to the patient's history, lifestyle and occupation. Further details on conducting patch test are illustrated in Radcliffe (1998). Clinical images depicting the process are also given in Figure 9.10.

When photo-allergic dermatitis is suspected, photo-patch testing involves application of the photo allergen series and any other suspected allergens in duplicate on the back. One set of patch tests is irradiated with ultraviolet light ($5 \ J \ cm^{-2}$), and after 48 and 96 hours the patch tests are read in parallel (Bourke *et al.*, 2001).

Treatment options for eczema

Management of eczema aims to relieve symptoms and prevent complications, such as infections, until remission occurs. General principles of eczema management for mild to moderate atopic eczema include emollient therapy and topical therapy, which include topical corticosteroids or immunomodulators, antibacterial and antibiotics and antihistamines. In severe eczema, secondary care referral is required for phototherapy and/or systemic therapy. Severe complex conditions such as atopic eczema require a multidisciplinary approach; a model of international excellence of hospital-based support is illustrated by the National Jewish Medical and Research Center in the USA (Boguniewicz *et al.*, 2008) and specifically nursing advances within (Nicol and Boguniewicz, 2008).

Eczema treatment can only be successful if patients and their carers are fully supported with information, education and practical treatment advice on self-management. Advice on avoiding exacerbating and trigger factors (see Table 9.1) including soaps, detergents, temperature extremes and irritant clothing is important to avoid increasing severity.

Topical treatments

Emollients

There have been no systematic reviews on emollients in atopic eczema (Williams *et al.*, 2008). However, there is overwhelming clinical consensus between dermatology health professionals that emollients are essential in managing eczema in acute and chronic periods. Complete emollient therapy is advocated and every topical preparation that goes onto the skin should be emollient based with soaps and detergents replaced with emollient-based products such as emollient washes, bath and shower products (Cork, 1997; NICE, 2007). For information on emollients, see Chapter 5.

Topical corticosteroids

Topical corticosteroids are highly effective as treatments for inflammatory skin conditions and a mainstay of treatment for eczema. They inhibit the production and action of inflammatory mediators in the skin. It is important for patients to understand that topical corticosteroids relieve symptoms but do not cure eczema.

The appropriate potency for the severity and extent of eczema together with the correct application of topical corticosteroids is essential to reducing the risk of adverse effect. Topical corticosteroids should be used intermittently to control acute eczema exacerbations and reduce inflammation and itching. They are applied in conjunction with emollients but applied at a different time of day to avoid diluting the steroid. The *British National Formulary* (BNF) (British Medical Association and Royal Pharmaceutical Society of Great Britain, 2009) classifies topical corticosteroids as mild, moderately potent, potent or very potent. Examples of topical corticosteroids available for prescription are listed in Table 9.5; details of constituent elements, such as antimicrobials, are given in the current BNF (British Medical Association and Royal Pharmaceutical Society of Great Britain, 2009).

In general, potent and very potent topical corticosteroids should be reserved for recalcitrant dermatoses and avoided on the face and skin flexures and in children (unless prescribed by a dermatology specialist). The least-potent topical corticosteroid that relieves symptoms should be applied (British Medical Association and Royal Pharmaceutical Society of Great Britain, 2009). Mild and moderately potent topical corticosteroids are associated with few side effects. However, particular care is required in the use of potent and very potent topical corticosteroids. As a guide, clinicians should consider the factors outlined in Table 9.6 when prescribing topical corticosteroids and assessing the risk of side effects.

The current recommendation is to apply topical corticosteroids thinly to the affected area; no more frequently than twice daily and use the least-potent formulation which is fully effective (NICE, 2004a; BNF, 2009). We would advocate the use of the Finger-Tip Unit (FTU) here to enable more precise measurement of the topical steroid being used. Further deatils are given later.

Systemic side effects are not common and occur through skin absorption and can rarely cause adrenal suppression and Cushing's syndrome. Absorption is likely to be greatest where skin is thin, broken and in flexural areas. Local side effects are outlined in Box 9.2.

Table 9.5 Topical corticosteroids and their potencies.

Potency	Formulation	Proprietary name
Mild	Hydrocortisone 0.1–2.5%	*Dioderm, Efcortelan, Mildison*
	With antimicrobials	*Canesten HC (e.g. miconazole), Daktacort, Econacort, Fucidin H, Nystaform-HC, Timodine, Vioform-Hydrocortisone*
	With crotamiton	*Eurax-Hydrocortisone*
	Fluocinolone acetonide 0.0025%	*Synalar 1 in 10 dilution*
Moderately potent	eg: Clobetasone butyrate*	*Betnovate-RD, Eumovate*, Haelan, Modrasone, Synalar 1 in 4 dilution, Ultralanum Plain*
	With antimicrobials	*Trimovate*
	With urea	*Alphaderm, Calmurid HC*
Potent	eg: Betamethasone valerate 0.1% eg: Mometasone furoate*	*betamethasone valerate 0.1%, Betacap, Bettamousse, Betnovate, Cutivate, Diprosone, Elocon*, hydrocortisone butyrate, Locoid, Locoid Crelo, Metosyn, Nerisone, Synalar*
	With antimicrobials	*Aureocort, Betnovate-C, Betnovate-N, FuciBET, Locoid C, Lotriderm, Synalar C, Synalar N, Tri-Adcortyl*
	With salicylic acid	*Diprosalic*
Very potent	eg: Clobetasol propionate*	*Dermovate*, Nerisone Forte, Clarelux, Etrivex*

Source: Adapted from the British National Formulary (March 2009). Reproduced from National Collaborating Centre for Women's and Children's Health, *Atopic Eczema in Children: Management of atopic eczema in children from birth up to the age of 12 years*. Clinical Guideline. RCOG Press; 2007. © Royal College of Obstetricians and Gynaecologists; reproduced with permission.

Table 9.6 Factors to consider when prescribing topical corticosteroids for eczema.

Factors to consider	Practical application
Potency	Mild – moderate, children, face and flexures. Potent – for the body. Very potent – for the soles.
Degree of penetration	Occlusion will increase potency. Ointments are better for penetrating dry, scaly lesions. Creams are better for moist, weeping lesions.
Extent of area treated	Single lesion/generalised area.
Daily volume	Grams per day. How long does a tube last?
Age of patient	Children and the older person with fragile skin require lower potencies.

Box 9.2 Potential local side effects from topical corticosteroids

- Spread and worsening of untreated infection
- Thinning of the skin, which may be restored over a period after stopping treatment but the original structure may never return
- Irreversible striae atrophicae and telangiectasia
- Contact dermatitis
- Perioral dermatitis
- Acne, or worsening of acne or rosacea
- Mild depigmentation which may be reversible
- Hypertrichosis also reported

Topical corticosteroid application

A practical measure devised for a practical measurement technique for the application of topical corticosteroids is the Finger Tip Unit (FTU) (Long and Finlay, 1991). One FTU is the amount of cream/ointment squeezed from the tip of an adult index finger to the first crease of the finger tip. One FTU (approximately 500 mg) is sufficient to cover an area that is twice that of the flat adult palm. For treating children, an adult FTU is used but the amount of FTUs are reduced depending on the age of the child (see Figure 9.11). The use of the FTU helps patients to understand how much topical corticosteroid to apply to ensure full therapeutic effectiveness. Current treatment guidelines recommend that topical corticosteroids should be stepped up or down according to severity and clinical response (NICE, 2007). Topical corticosteroids should be used to treat inflamed eczema (flare-ups), and in between flares, periods of using emollients only are advised.

Treatment of atopic eczema

Although there is currently no cure for atopic eczema, various interventions do exist to control symptoms, but the effectiveness of many treatments has not been established (Hoare *et al.*, 2000). Conventional treatment consists of the application of emollients and topical corticosteroids, both of which have been in use for over 30 years (Hanifin and Rajka, 1980; Leung, 2000). NICE (2007) advocates a 'stepped approach' to treatment for atopic eczema in children, which tailors the treatment steps to the severity of atopic eczema. Emollients should always form the basis of eczema treatment and used when there is no visible eczema (see Chapter 5). The use of occlusive techniques, such as wet and dry wrapping,

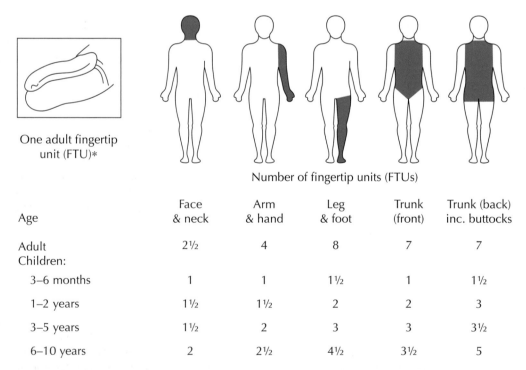

One adult fingertip unit (FTU)*

Number of fingertip units (FTUs)

Age	Face & neck	Arm & hand	Leg & foot	Trunk (front)	Trunk (back) inc. buttocks
Adult	2½	4	8	7	7
Children:					
3–6 months	1	1	1½	1	1½
1–2 years	1½	1½	2	2	3
3–5 years	1½	2	3	3	3½
6–10 years	2	2½	4½	3½	5

* One adult fingertip unit (FTU) is the amount of ointment or cream expressed from a tube with a standard 5 mm diameter nozzle, applied from the distal crease to the tip of the index finger.

Figure 9.11 Diagram of FTU and chart with FTUs for treating adults and children.

Table 9.7 Recommendations for the 'stepped approach' to atopic eczema management.

Mild atopic eczema	Moderate atopic eczema	Severe atopic eczema
Emollients	Emollients	Emollients
Mildly potent topical corticosteroids	Moderately potent topical corticosteroids	Potent topical corticosteroids
	Topical calcineurin inhibitors	Topical calcineurin inhibitors
	Bandages	Bandages
		Phototherapy
		Systemic therapy

Source: NICE (2007).

has been discussed in Chapter 4. The stepped approach is summarised in Table 9.7.

Other treatments include wet wraps, bandaging (damp, occlusive body bandages either impregnated with a therapeutic substance or applied over topical preparations), behavioural management and habit reversal; these have been discussed extensively in Chapter 4. Complementary therapies for atopic eczema, such as medical herbs, are embraced by guidance from NICE (2007) which concludes that there is insufficient evidence to make recommendations for clinical practice. For more severe atopic eczema, secondary care referral for phototherapy and systemic therapies may be employed. The following section discusses other treatment options for acute and severe exacerbations of atopic eczema, including complementary therapies and treatment provided in secondary care settings.

Managing bacterial infection

Atopic eczema is frequently complicated by bacterial infection, commonly, *Staphylococcus aureus*, but infection with *Streptococcus pyogenes* (group A *Streptococcus*) may also occur. NICE (2007) recommends oral antibiotics. Flucloxacillin is active against the common bacterial skin infections and should be the first-line treatment for

Staphylococcus aureus and streptococcal infections. Erythromycin should be used if there is local resistance to Flucloxacillin or in children with a penicillin allergy. NICE (2007) recommends that topical antibiotics and combinations of topical corticosteroids and antibiotics should only be used short term, for no longer than 2 weeks on localised areas of skin infection only. Antiseptics are useful adjunct therapies for reducing bacterial load and are added to some emollients, bath oils, soap substitutes and washes and moisturisers. Bacterial resistance is an ongoing issue; NICE (2007) advises that health professionals should be aware and follow local guidelines for advice on patterns of bacterial resistance to antimicrobials.

Managing viral infection

Viral infections also occur in atopic eczema. The most common viral infections are herpes simplex virus (with the complication eczema herpeticum), molluscum contagiosum, viral warts (and verrucae) and varicella (chicken pox). NICE (2007) recommends the following steps for management of eczema herpeticum: start treatment with oral Aciclovir at first suspicion of eczema herpeticum. For more severe and confirmed infection intravenous Aciclovir may be required.

Managing fungal infections in seborrhoeic eczema

Topical antifungals such as Ketoconazole (cream/shampoo) and Terbinafine are a well-established treatment, based on trial evidence (Picardo and Cameli, 2008). There is limited evidence that oral antifungals are beneficial.

For cradle cap (infant seborrhoeic dermatitis), in addition to scalp being affected, the condition may also affect other areas of the body such as behind the ears, in the creases of the neck, armpits and nappy area. It is treated by regular use of mild baby shampoos and the use of oil to soften the scales, avoiding olive oil which exacerbates the growth of the *Malassezia* yeast. If this is unsuccessful or the rash spreads more extensively, inflamed areas may require a medicated shampoo containing ketoconazole and hydrocortisone cream.

Topical calcineurin inhibitors

Topical calcineurin inhibitors are immunomodulatory treatments, which help modulate the immune system to reduce inflammation. Calcineurin is a protein phosphatase 2B responsible for activating the transcription of interleukin 2 (IL-2), which stimulates the growth and differentiation of T-cell response inhibitors (Hultsch *et al.*, 2005); these are non-steroid drugs. Tacrolimus (Protopic®) and pimecrolimus (Elidel®) are the available topical immunosuppressant agents which may be used as alternative to (topical) steroids topical for eczema. Tacrolimus (Protopic®) for moderate to severe atopic eczema in patients 2 years of age and above, which is not adequately responding to conventional therapies such as topical corticosteroids (Electronic Medicines Compendium [EMC], 2009a). Pimecrolimus (Elidel®) is indicated for treatment of patients aged 2 years and over, with mild or moderate atopic dermatitis where treatment with topical corticosteroids is either inadvisable or not possible (EMC, 2009). NICE recommends that topical calcineurin inhibitors should not be used to treat mild atopic eczema or as 'first-line' treatments (NICE, 2004b). Tacrolimus has also now been licensed in the UK for intermittent use.

Sedating antihistamines

Sedating antihistamines in conjunction with other therapies may help to reduce itching at night, it is the sedating effect that is useful as eczema is not a histamine releasing condition. Paste bandaging and wet wrapping are helpful at night to prevent damage from scratching, reduce itch and help heal the skin (see Chapter 4). Behavioural approaches such as habit reversal techniques can also be useful in chronic atopic eczema.

Behavioural management: habit reversal

Behavioural management, incorporating habit reversal, for the control of damaging itching behaviour has been addressed in Chapter 4.

Secondary care options: phototherapy and oral immunosuppressants

Patients with moderate to severe eczema who are unresponsive to topical therapies in primary care should be referred to secondary care. Phototherapy and other systemic treatments in children should only be initiated after assessment and documentation of disease severity and assessment of quality of life (NICE, 2007). The Primary Care Dermatology Society and the British Association of Dermatologists (PCDS and BAD) have developed referral guidelines for all patients with atopic eczema which are outlined in Box 9.3 (Primary Care Dermatology Society and British Association of Dermatologists, 2006).

Patients with severe eczema should be referred to secondary care for phototherapy and systemic therapies.

Phototherapy

Phototherapy has an immunosuppressive action on the skin and has a particular effect on blocking antigen-presenting Langerhans cells, altering

---

Box 9.3   PCDS–BAD (2006) – Referral guidelines for atopic eczema

Diagnostic doubt

Severe eczema

- Failure to respond to appropriate therapy in primary care
- Eczema not satisfactorily controlled in primary care

Severe infected eczema

- Bacterial infection
- Eczema herpeticum
- Specialist opinion for counselling patients and families with severe social or psychological problems related to eczema.
- Additional advice on treatment application.
- Patch testing for suspected contact dermatitis.
- Consideration for dietary manipulation.

eosinophil functions and altering production of cytokines by keratinocytes (Hoare *et al.*, 2000).

Narrowband UVB (TL01) is the most common form of phototherapy used to treat skin diseases. Narrowband refers to a specific wavelength of ultraviolet (UV) radiation, 311–312 nm. PUVA or photochemotherapy is used for more severe eczema and involves a combination treatment that consists of psoralens (P) and then exposing the skin to UVA (long-wave ultraviolet radiation). Psoralens are compounds found in many plants which make the skin temporarily sensitive to UVA. Medicinal psoralens include methoxsalen (8-methoxypsoralen), 5-methoxypsoralen and trisoralen. Eye protection is required; 24 hours post-oral administration of psoralens. Psoralens can also be applied topically in a bath soak or as lotion for small areas (hands and feet). The amount of UV is carefully monitored for side effects and especially degrees of erythema and burning. A number of protocols exist depending on the individual's skin type, age, skin condition and other factors. Patients will generally attend hospital 2–3 times a week for stepped administration of phototherapy (Hoare *et al.*, 2000).

Oral immunosuppressant therapies

Oral immunosuppressant treatments have been shown to be effective for severe recalcitrant cases of eczema. They act by reducing inflammation and affecting lymphocytes. The only licensed oral therapy for atopic eczema is ciclosporin, an immune suppressant drug which is also used to prevent transplant rejection. In atopic eczema, ciclosporin is indicated for the short-term treatment (8 weeks) of patients with severe atopic eczema in whom conventional therapy is ineffective or inappropriate. The normal dosage is 2.5–5 mg/kg/day given orally in two divided doses for a maximum of 8 weeks. Ciclosporin requires careful monitoring due to side effects; monitoring should be shared between primary and secondary care and involves the following:

■ Blood pressure should be measured once-to twice-weekly for the first month, then monthly thereafter.

■ Kidney function should be tested by blood and urine tests, especially creatinine levels.

■ Other regular tests should include: complete blood count, liver function, fasting lipid levels, uric acid.

Ciclosporin can impair renal and liver function. Close monitoring of serum creatinine and urea is required and dosage adjustment may be necessary. Increases in serum creatinine and urea occurring during the first few weeks of ciclosporin therapy are generally dose-dependent and reversible and usually respond to dosage reduction. Apart from a reduction in renal function, other side effects include hypertension, hirsutism, loss of appetite and nausea, paraesthesia, tremor, sensitive and bleeding gums and an increased risk of infection. Ciclosporin can also increase the risk of developing skin cancer, in particular basal cell and squamous cell carcinoma. The increased risk of developing malignancies and lymphoproliferative disorders (including lymphomas), some with reported fatalities, appears to be related to the degree and duration of immunosuppression (Electronic Medicines Compendium, 2009b).

Other immunosuppressant agents used in severe atopic eczema are prescribed 'off licence' and include: Azathioprine (a thiopurine analogue drug that suppresses the immune system by altering white blood cell function), oral systemic corticosteroids, interferon gamma and intravenous immunoglobulin.

Complementary therapies

NICE (2007) outlines that 60% of children with atopic eczema have tried complementary therapies. However, to date, there is limited evidence of the effectiveness of complementary therapies in atopic eczema, as in the case of medicinal herbs (Sheenan and Atherton, 1994). The National Eczema Society advises patients with eczema, who wish to try a complementary therapy, to go to a properly trained and registered practitioner, always let your health care professional know about the complementary therapy and not to suddenly stop using prescribed eczema treatments (National Eczema Society, 2009).

Safety can also be an important issue. Complementary products sold as 'natural' may have added synthetic ingredients; an example being the addition of steroids within medicinal herbs (Graham-Brown *et al.*, 1994). Furthermore, it cannot always be assumed that natural is safe. An investigation into fraudulent practice with unregistered complementary therapies revealed the addition of potent corticosteroids (All Party Parliamentary Group on Skin [APPGS], 1999). The sound recommendations from NICE (2007) include informing patients on the problems of fraudulent practice and for patients to inform their health care professional.

Treatment options for other forms of eczema

Treatment options for other forms of eczema are summarised in Table 9.8.

Behavioural treatments for eczema: psychological support and educational intervention

Educational and psychological interventions are invariably provided in conjunction with conventional therapy. Such interventions may be directed towards adults or the parent or child

Table 9.8 Treatment options for other forms of eczema.

Type	Treatment options
Irritant dermatitis	Avoidance of the irritating factor(s), liberal use of emollients and topical corticosteroids to reduce inflammation. Napkin rash can be a type of irritant contact dermatitis. Barrier products for treating napkin rash often contain zinc oxide, which has soothing and protective properties.
Contact allergic dermatitis	Topical corticosteroids are used to treat both irritant and allergic contact dermatitis. Oral antibiotics should be prescribed if there are visible signs of infection. Contact dermatitis is considered widespread when greater than 25% of the body is affected and the cause is known and avoidable in future. In adults, oral prednisolone can be prescribed for 2–3 weeks, in reducing doses, when the cause is known and is avoidable in the future.
Seborrhoeic dermatitis	Seborrhoeic dermatitis will require treatment with an antifungal cream for secondary candidal infection. A mild steroid can also be used for up to 1 week to treat inflammation. Antifungal preparations combined with topical corticosteroids are the first-line treatment for adults with seborrhoeic dermatitis.
Juvenile plantar dermatoses	Emollients should be applied liberally, occlusive dressings for deep fissures and potent topical corticosteroids for inflammation. Wearing of trainers should be discouraged.
Discoid eczema	Treatment is with emollients and potent or very potent topical corticosteroids.
Lichen simplex/neurodermatitis	Patches of lichen simplex or neurodermatitis are treated with topical steroids under occlusion, to prevent habitual scratching and rubbing.
Pompholyx	Treatment is with emollients and potent topical corticosteroids. Sedating antihistamines may be required at night as this condition produces intense itch and irritation (Figure 9.12).
Asteatotic eczema	Treatment with emollients; humectants emollients with anti-itch properties may be helpful. Topical corticosteroids will be indicated for reducing mild erythema.
Varicose eczema	Treatment is with emollients and topical corticosteroids (use ointment preparations). Patch testing may be indicated, should contact dermatitis be suspected. Paste bandages may be applied during the acute period. Compression (support) stockings are indicted for chronic periods and long-term prevention. Concordance with compression therapy, leg elevation and ankle movement are also important (Brooks *et al.*, 2004).

Source: Reproduced from National Collaborating Centre for Women's and Children's Health, *Atopic Eczema in Children: Management of atopic eczema in children from birth up to the age of 12 years*. Clinical Guideline. RCOG Press; 2007. © Royal College of Obstetricians and Gynaecologists; reproduced with permission.

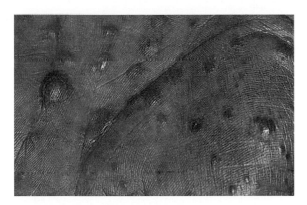

Figure 9.12 Pompholyx. (Source: Reprinted from Buxton and Morris-Jones, 2009.)

with eczema, with parents tending to be the primary focus of the educational approaches and children the main target of psychological interventions. This section builds on principles from Chapter 7 but applies and extends them to the field of eczema, addressing and largely focusing on key issues such as education and support for parents of children with atopic eczema. Such interventions provide considerable scope to nursing staff to approach the assessment and management of educational and support needs in a systematic way.

The importance of education, as a basis for improving adherence to treatment, is highlighted in the NICE (2007) guidance on atopic eczema in children. It highlights the importance of educating both child and parent or carer and reinforced at every consultation, both in written and verbal forms, with practical demonstrations covering:

- how much treatment to use,
- how often to apply treatments,
- when and how to step treatments up and down and
- how to treat infected atopic eczema

Such interventions may be illustrated with the application to children, as in the case of atopic eczema. The suitability of the intervention will depend on the age and developmental stage of the child and, therefore, the child's ability to participate effectively in an educational and psychological intervention will vary.

Since atopic eczema affects children and can be disabling for whole families, it is generally agreed that psychological support and education of the parent/carer are a crucial component of disease management. Little is known, however, of the measurable effects of such interventions and the most recent systematic review of the treatments for atopic eczema to date (Hoare *et al.*, 2000), which found only limited evidence to support psychological treatments or educational interventions, although more recent evidence has been found of the value of some planned educational approaches (Ersser *et al.*, 2007). Psychological interventions are being incorporated into management strategies to reduce scratching behaviours that exacerbate eczema (Horne *et al.*, 1989; Giannini, 1997). Despite the fact that parents are the primary carers for children with atopic eczema, very limited attention has been given to the psychological support of parents (by educational or psychological intervention). As such, the caregiver's ability to manage their child's eczema is an important outcome and therefore the educational or psychological support given to parents is required. It could be argued that the general case for psychosocial intervention to improve clinical outcomes in chronic organic disease such as eczema is established and in related areas such as asthma (Guevara *et al.*, 2003).

The literature refers to a range of psychological interventions that have been used in atopic eczema, such as behavioural management (Noren 1995; Bridgett *et al.*, 1996) and cognitive behavioural therapy (Ehlers *et al.*, 1995). Clinical observations suggest that behavioural techniques can be a useful adjunct to topical therapy and breaking the itch–scratch cycle is argued to be a primary clinical aim (Hagermark and Wahlgren, 1995). However, evaluative research has been limited (Simpson-Dent *et al.*, 1999; Bridgett, 2000), especially with children.

Educational interventions to support eczema management

Educational interventions have also been used to bring about behavioural change through health/patient education or patient teaching for those with eczema (Niebel *et al.*, 2000). These are important since chronic disease management requires a degree of self-management (or caregiver/parental support) and therefore education and behavioural change (Holman and Lorig, 2000). A limited number of evaluative studies have examined the impact of parental education on the management of children with atopic eczema (e.g. Niebel *et al.*, 2000), although some studies have examined the impact of education on adults with eczema; these studies are informative (e.g. Ehlers *et al.*, 1995). The basis for education is highlighted throughout this book, highlighting, for example, key aspects of Chapter 5 on emollient therapy, understanding treatments for eczema – as outlined in this chapter and developing strategies to help patients make the most of their treatment (Chapter 7). These emphasise the need to involve the patient in education, assess educational need systematically and provide education in a planned manner.

A recent systematic review has been undertaken to examine the effectiveness of educational and psychological interventions in changing outcomes for children with atopic eczema (Ersser *et al.*, 2007). This review was published at the time of the production of the NICE (2007) guidance on atopic eczema in children, but provides a more extensive account of the evidence available, information on the typical service delivery models in use and an extensive critique of the evidence available.

Up to this stage the most recent systematic review of the treatments for atopic eczema was a generic review of treatments for atopic eczema (Hoare *et al.*, 2000). Ersser *et al.*'s Cochrane review identified that such interventions have been used as an adjunct to conventional therapy for children with atopic eczema to enhance the effectiveness of topical therapy. The selection criteria for the review included randomised controlled trials (RCTs) of such interventions used to manage children with atopic eczema. Eligibility to enter the trail, assess trial quality and extract data was independently assessed by two reviewers and revealed a limited number of studies that met the quality criteria for inclusion

($n = 5$) and a lack of comparable data prevented data synthesis. Some included that studies required clearer reporting of trial procedures. Rigorous established outcome measures were not always used.

The main results are that five studies (RCTs) met the inclusion criteria; all interventions were adjuncts to conventional therapy, four related to educational intervention (Niebel *et al.*, 2000; Chinn *et al.*, 2002; Staab *et al.*, 2002, 2006). Four focused on intervention directed towards the parents; data synthesis was not possible. Psychological interventions remain virtually unevaluated by studies of robust design; the only included study (Sokel *et al.*, 1993) examined the effect of relaxation techniques (hypnotherapy and biofeedback) on severity. Some educational studies identified significant improvements in disease severity between intervention groups. The largest trial to date, conducted in Germany (Staab *et al.*, 2006) evaluated long-term outcomes and found significant improvements in both disease severity at 1 year (3 months to 7 years, $p = 0.0002$; 8–12 years, $p = 0.003$; 13–18 years, $p = 0.0001$) and parental quality of life (3 months to 7 years, $p = 0.0001$; 8–12 years, $p = 0.002$), for children with atopic eczema. One study by Niebel *et al.* (2002) found that video-based education was more effective in improving severity than direct education and the control (discussion) ($p < 0.001$). The single psychological study found that relaxation techniques improved clinical severity as compared to the control at 20 weeks ($t = 2.13$) but of borderline significance ($p = 0.042$) (Sokel *et al.*, 1993).

In conclusion, the lack of rigorously designed trials (excluding the study by Staab *et al.*, 2006) provides only limited evidence of the effectiveness of educational and psychological interventions in helping to manage the condition of children with atopic eczema. Evidence from included and adult studies (e.g. Ehlers *et al.*, 1995; Gradwell *et al.*, 2002) indicated that different service delivery models were in operation, including multiprofessional eczema schools, which were more common in countries such as Germany and the nurse-led clinic model, which was utilised in the UK. These different models of service delivery require further and comparative evaluation to examine their cost-effectiveness and suitability for different health systems.

Drawing on these two reviews there are indications that there may be considerable scope for developing nurse-led dermatology services, especially targeted at groups such as those with atopic eczema requiring educational support. Indeed the National Eczema Society has issued guidance on developing such clinics (Penzer, 2003). The systematic review by Hoare *et al.* (2000) of treatments for atopic eczema identified the role of specialist nurses as an urgent research priority. An important feature in the development of dermatology services over recent years has been the expansion of nurse-led services. Evidence from a survey conducted of BAD consultants for the BAD Therapy Guidelines and Audit Committee has indicated that there has been a major expansion of nurse-led services in Britain; 69% (*n* = 183) of consultants had nurse-led clinics, which they anticipated to rise by 91% (Cox, 1999); although more recent data is limited in proving new information, the anecdotal evidence on the UK suggests that these have expanded considerably. These developments are consistent with government nursing strategy to identify where the nursing service can expand its role and enhance its contribution to service delivery where health needs are inadequately or poorly addressed (Department of Health, 2000, 2008). Indeed, the NHS plan policy document highlights nurse-led clinics in dermatology as one of '10 key roles for nurses' in the new NHS (Department of Health 2000, p. 83). Despite the rapid expansion of dermatology services over recent years, the evaluation programme for the expansion of these services has fallen behind, especially in settings such as dermatology. There is also limited knowledge of the precise nature of many of these services and their therapeutic impact.

Conclusion

This chapter has outlined the nature of eczema and its management. This includes a summary of its clinical signs, differential diagnosis and its different variants, with reference to its impact on people and their families. This is accompanied by an evidence-based summary of the key treatments and management strategies to control eczema, highlighting the nursing contribution, especially in otherwise neglected areas such as education and behavioural management. The holistic measurement of eczema is also included, as a basis for more rigorous assessment and evaluation.

References

All Party Parliamentary Group on Skin (1999). Report on the enquiry into fraudulent practice in the treatment of skin disease. London: All Party Parliamentary Group on Skin, Portcullis.

Asher, M.I., S. Montefort *et al.* (2006). Worldwide time trends in the prevalence of symptoms of asthma, allergic rhinoconjunctivitis, and eczema in childhood: ISAAC Phase One and Three repeat multicountry cross-sectional surveys. *The Lancet*, **368**: 733–743.

Ben-Gashir, M.A., P.T. Seed *et al.* (2004). Quality of life and disease severity are correlated in children with atopic dermatitis. *British Journal of Dermatology*, **150**(2): 284–290.

Boguniewicz, M., N. Nicol *et al.* (2008). A multidisciplinary approach to evaluation and treatment of atopic dermatitis. *Seminars in Cutaneous Medicine and Surgery*, **27**: 115–127.

Bourke, J., I. Coulson *et al.* (2001). Guidelines for the care of contact dermatitis. *British Journal of Dermatology*, **145**(6): 877–885.

Bridgett, C. (2000). Psychodermatology and atopic skin disease in London 1989–1999 – helping patients to help themselves. *Dermatology and Psychosomatics/ Dermatologie und Psychosomatik*, **1**(4): 183–186.

Bridgett, C., P. Noren *et al.* (1996). *Atopic Skin Disease: A Manual for Practitioners*. Petersfiled: Wrightson Biomedical Publishing Limited.

British Medical Association and Royal Pharmaceutical Society of Great Britain (2009). *British National Formulary*. London, British Medical Journal Publishing Group Ltd and The Royal Pharmaceutical Society of Great Britain.

Brooks, J., S.J. Ersser *et al.* (2004). Nurse-led education sets out to improve patient concordance and prevent recurrence of leg ulcers. *Journal of Wound Care*, **13**(3): 111–116.

Burns, T., S. Breathnagh *et al.* (2004). *Rook's Textbook of Dermatology*. Oxford: Blackwell Publishing Ltd.

Buske-Kirschbaum, A., A. Geiben *et al.* (2001). Psychobiological aspects of atopic dermatitis: An overview. *Psychotherapy and Psychosomatics*, **70**: 6–16.

Buske-Kirschbaum, A., A. Gierens *et al.* (2002). Stress-induced immunomodulation is altered in patients with atopic dermatitis. *Journal of Neuroimmunology*, **129**: 161–167.

Buxton, P.K. and R. Morris-Jones, Eds. (2009). *ABC of Dermatology* (5th edition). Chichester: Wiley-Blackwell and BMJ Books.

Chinn, D.J., T. Poyner *et al.* (2002). Randomized controlled trial of a single dermatology nurse consultation in primary care on the quality of life of children with atopic eczema. *British Journal of Dermatology*, **146**(3): 432–439.

Cork, M.J. (1997). The importance of skin barrier function. *Journal of Dermatological Treatments*, **8**: S7–S13.

Cork, M.J. (1999). Taking the itch out of eczema: How the careful use of emollients can break the itch–scratch cycle of atopic eczema. *The Asthma Journal*, **4**: 116–120.

Cork, M.J., D.A. Robinson *et al.* (2006). New perspectives on epidermal barrier dysfunction in atopic dermatitis: Gene–environment interactions. *Journal of Allergy and Clinical Immunology*, **118**: 3–21.

Cox, N.H. (1999). The expanding role of nurses in surgery and prescribing in British departments of dermatology. *British Journal of Dermatology*, **140**(4): 681–684.

Cox, N.H. and C.M. Lawrence (1998). *Diagnostic Problems in Dermatology*. London: Mosby.

Department of Health (2000). The NHS Plan: A plan for investment, a plan for reform. London: Department of Health, Crown.

Department of Health (2008). Framing the Nursing and Midwifery Contribution: Driving up the quality of care, pp. 1–21. London: Department of Health, Crown.

DermNetNZ. (2009). Photocontact dermatitis. Retrieved 6 May 2009, from http://www.dermnetnz.org/reactions/photocontact-dermatitis.html.

Ehlers, A., U. Gieler *et al.* (1995). Treatment of atopic dermatitis: A comparison of psychological and dermatological approaches to relapse prevention. *Journal of Consulting & Clinical Psychology* **63**(4): 624–635.

Electronic Medicines Compendium. (2009a). Summary of product characteristics (SPC) for Protopic 0.03% and Protopic 0.1%., from http://emc.medicines.org.uk/document.aspx?documentId=8884.

Electronic Medicines Compendium. (2009b). Summary of product characteristics (SPC) for Neoral soft gelatine capsules and neural oral solution. Retrieved 14 April 2009, from http://emc.medicines.org.uk/document.aspx?documentId=4106 and http://emc.medicines.org.uk/document.aspx?documentid=1307.

Elliott, B.E. and K. Luker (1997). The experiences of mothers caring for a child with severe atopic eczema. *Journal of Clinical Nursing*, **6**: 214–217.

English, J. (1999). *A Colour Handbook of Occupational Dermatology*. London: Manson Publishing.

Ersser, S.J., S. Latter *et al.* (2007). Psychological and educational interventions for atopic eczema in children – Description. *Cochrane Database of Systematic Reviews*, **3**: CD004054 (DOI: 10.1002/14651858. CD004054.pub2).

Fennessy, M., S. Coupland *et al.* (2000). The epidemiology and experience of atopic eczema during childhood: A discussion paper on the implications of current knowledge for health care, public health policy and research. *Journal of Epidemiology and Community Health*, **54**(8): 581–589.

Giannini, A.V. (1997). Habit reversal technique and eczema. *Journal of Allergy and Clinical Immunology*, **100**(4): 580.

Gradwell, C., K.S. Thomas *et al.* (2002). A randomized controlled trial of nurse follow-up clinics: Do they help patients and do they free up consultants' time? *British Journal of Dermatology*, **147**: 513–517.

Graham-Brown, R. and T. Burns (2006). *Lecture Notes: Dermatology* (9th edition). Oxford: Blackwell Publishing.

Graham-Brown, R.A.C., J.F. Bourke *et al.* (1994). Letters: Chinese herbal remedies may contain steroids. *British Medical Journal*, **308**: 473.

Guevara, J.P., J.P. Wolf *et al.* (2003). Effects of interventions for self management of asthma in children and adolescents: Systematic review and meta analysis. *British Medical Journal*, **326**: 1308–1309.

Hagermark, O. and C.F. Wahlgren (1995). Treatment of itch. *Seminars in Dermatology*, **14**(4): 320–325.

Hanifin, J.M. and G. Rajka (1980). Diagnostic features of atopic dermatitis. *Acta Dermato Venereologica* (Stockholm), **92**: 44–47.

Herd, R.M. (2000). The morbidity and cost of atopic dermatitis. In: Williams, H.C. (Ed.), *Atopic Dermatitis*, pp. 85–95. Cambridge: Cambridge University Press.

Herd, R., M.J. Tidman *et al.* (1996). Prevalence of atopic eczema in the community: The Lothian atopic dermatitis study. *British Journal of Dermatology*, **135**: 18–19.

Hoare, C., A. Li Wan Po and H. Williams (2000). Systematic review of treatments for atopic eczema. Health Technology Assessment, **4**: 1–19.

Holman, H. and K. Lorig (2000). Patients as partners in managing chronic disease – Partnership is a prerequisite for effective and efficient health care. *British Medical Journal*, **320**(7234): 526–527.

Horne, D.J.D., A.E. White *et al.* (1989). A preliminary study of psychological therapy in the management of atopic eczema. *British Journal of Medical Psychology*, **62**: 241–248.

Hultsch, T., A. Kapp *et al.* (2005). Immunomodulation and safety of topical calcineurin inhibitors for the treatment of atopic dermatitis. *Dermatology*, **211**: 174–187.

Kemp, A.S. (2003). Cost of illness of atopic dermatitis in children: a societal perspective. *Pharmacoeconomics*, **21**: 105–113.

Leung, D.Y.M. (2000). Atopic dermatitis: New insights and opportunities for therapeutic intervention. *Journal of Allergy and Clinical Immunology*, **5**(105): 860–876.

Lewis-Jones, M.S. and A.Y. Finlay (1995). The children's dermatology life quality index (CDLQI): Initial validation and practical use. *British Journal of Dermatology*, **132**: 942–949.

Lewis-Jones, M.S., A.Y. Finlay *et al.* (2001). The infants' dermatitis quality of life index. *British Journal of Dermatology*, **144**: 104–110.

Lifschitz, C. (2008). Is there a consensus in food allergy management. *Journal of Paediatric Gastroenterology Nutrition*, **47**(Suppl 2): S58–S59.

Long, C.C. and A.Y. Finlay (1991). The finger-tip unit – a new practical measure. *Clinical and Experimental Dermatology*, **16**(6): 444–447.

McFadden, J.P., W.C. Noble *et al.* (1993). Superantigenic exotoxin-secreting potential of staphylococci isolated from atopic eczematous skin. *British Journal of Dermatology*, **128**: 631–632.

McNally, N.J., H.C. Williams *et al.* (2001). Atopic eczema and the home environment. *British Journal of Dermatology*, **145**(5): 730–736.

National Eczema Society (2009). Frequently asked questions on eczema: What about complementary therapies? from http://www.eczema.org/faq.php?act=cli.faq_view&id_faq=15&id_domain=0&question=&sql_indx=1&faq_indx=6.

National Institute for Health and Clinical Excellence (NICE) (2004a). Frequency of application of topical corticosteroids for atopic eczema, 34p. London: National Institute for Health and Clinical Excellence (NICE).

National Institute for Health and Clinical Excellence (NICE) (2004b). Tacrolimus and primecrolimus for atopic eczema. London: NICE.

National Institute for Health and Clinical Excellence (NICE) (2007). Atopic eczema in children: Management of atopic eczema in children from birth up to the age of 12 years, from http://www.ncc-wch.org.uk/index.asp?PageID=359.

Nicol, N.H. and M. Boguniewicz (2008). Successful strategies in atopic dermatitis management. *Dermatology Nursing Supplement*: 1–19.

Niebel, G., C. Kallweit *et al.* (2000). Direct versus video-based parental education in the treatment of atopic eczema in children. A controlled pilot study [Direkte versus videovermittelte Elternschulung bei atopischem Ekzem im Kindesalter als Erganzung facharztlicher Behandlung. Eine Kontrollierte Pilotstudie]. *Hautarzt*, **51**: 401–411.

Noren, P. (1995). Habit reversal – a turning point in the treatment of atopic dermatitis. *Clinical and Experimental Dermatology*, **20**(1): 2–5.

Palmer, C.N., A.D. Irvine *et al.* (2006). Common loss-of-function variants of the epidermal barrier protein filaggrin are a major predisposing factor for atopic dermatitis. *Nature Genetics*, **38**: 441–446.

Penzer, R. (2003). How to set up an eczema clinic in primary care. London: National Eczema Society.

Picardo, M. and N. Cameli (2008). Seborrheic dermatitis. In: Williams, H.C., Bigby, M., Diepgen, T. *et al.* (Eds), *Evidence-based Dermatology*, pp. 164–170. Oxford: Blackwell Publishing/BMJ Books.

Primary Care Dermatology Society and British Association of Dermatologists (2006). Guidance for the management of atopic eczema: ECDS & BAD, from http://www.eGuidelines.co.uk/skin, **28**: 372–375.

Radcliffe, J. (1998). How to … conduct a patch test. *British Journal of Dermatological Nursing*, **2**(4): 8–9.

Reid, P. and M.S. Lewis-Jones (1995). Sleep disturbances and their management in pre-schoolers with atopic eczema. *Clinical Experimental Dermatology*, **20**: 38–41.

Sheenan, M.P. and D.J. Atherton (1994). One year follow-up of children treated with Chinese medicinal herbs for atopic eczema. *British Journal of Dermatology*, **130**: 488–493.

Simpson-Dent, S.L., R.C.D. Staughton *et al.* (1999). The combined approach to chronic atopic eczema. A prospective comparison of behavioural modification with standard dermatological treatment against standard treatment alone. Paris: Proceedings of the International Congress of Dermatological Psychiatry.

Sokel, B., D. Christie *et al.* (1993). A comparison of hypnotherapy and biofeedback in the treatment of childhood atopic eczema. *Contemporary Hypnosis*, **10**(3): 145–154.

Staab, D., U. von Rueden *et al.* (2002). Evaluation of a parental training program for the management of atopic dermatitis. *Pediatric Allergy and Immunology*, **13**: 84–90.

Staab, D., T.L. Diepgen *et al.* (2006). Age related, structured educational programmes for the management of atopic dermatitis in children and adolescents: Multicentre, randomised controlled trial. *British Medical Journal*, **332**: 933–938.

Strachan, D.P. (1989). Hayfever, hygiene and household size. *British Medical Journal*, **299**: 1259–1290.

Surridge, H.R. (2005). Exploring parental needs and knowledge when caring for a child with eczema. *Patient Magazine of the National Eczema Society*.

Szakos, E., G. Lakos *et al.* (2004). Relationship between skin bacterial colonization and the occurrence of allergen-specific and non-allergen-specific antibodies in sera of children with atopic eczema/dermatitis syndrome. *Acta Dermato-Venereologica*, **84**(1): 32–36.

Taal, E., E. Rasker *et al.* (1993). Health status, adherence with health recommendations, self-efficacy and social support in patients with rheumatoid arthritis. *Patient Education Counseling*, **20**: 63–76.

Thomas, K., F. Bath-Hextall *et al.* (2008). Atopic eczema. In: Williams, H.C., Bigby, M., Diepgen, T. *et al.* (Eds), *Evidence-based Dermatology*. Oxford: Blackwell Publishing Ltd.

Verboom, P., L. Hakkaart-Van *et al.* (2002). The cost of atopic dermatitis in the Netherlands: An international comparison. *British Journal of Dermatology*, **147**(4): 716–724.

Weller, R., J.A.A. Hunter, J. Savin and M. Dahl (2008). *Clinical Dermatology* (4th edition). Oxford: Blackwell Publishing Ltd.

Williams, H.C. (1992). Is the prevalence of atopic dermatitis increasing? *Clinical and Experimental Dermatology*, **17**(6): 385–391.

Williams, H.C. (1995). Atopic eczema – why we should look at the environment. *British Medical Journal*, **311**: 1241–1242.

Williams, H.C. (1997). *Dermatology: Health Care Needs Assessment*. Oxford: Radcliffe Medical Press.

Williams, H., H. Forsdyke *et al.* (1995). A protocol for recording the sign of visible flexural dermatitis. *British Journal of Dermatology*, **133**: 941–949.

Williams, H., M. Bigby *et al.* (2008). *Evidence-based Dermatology*. Oxford: BMJ Books, Blackwell Publishing.

Acne 10

Rebecca Penzer

Introduction

Acne is a condition of the pilosebaceous gland. Mild acne affects the majority of teenagers at some point, but in one study only 14% of girls and 9% of boys actually consulted their GP and of these 0.3% were referred to see a dermatologist (Rademaker *et al.*, 1989). However, acne is not just a condition affecting teenagers, it can persist into adult years and for a number of people it appears for the first time after teenage years are left well behind. There are also instances in which babies show signs of acne-type lesions (Cunliffe *et al.*, 2001). Acne is a condition which can be effectively treated. In order to make the most of the treatments available, it is helpful for nurses to understand the underlying pathology of the condition. There are a range of treatments available; however, patients need support to ensure that they are used appropriately and effectively.

What is acne?

Acne is a hormonally driven condition which affects the pilosebaceous gland. Sebaceous glands are found on most parts of the human body except for the palms of the hands and the soles and dorsum of the feet. They are found predominantly on the face and scalp, but also exist in relatively large numbers on the chest and back. This explains the tendency for acne to appear in these areas. There is considerable variability in the size of the glands both between individuals and on different anatomical sites on any single individual. Acne lesions and severity assessment have been introduced in Chapter 3.

The sebaceous glands respond to circulating androgens by producing sebum. In acne, sebum production is increased either because the sebaceous gland becomes overly sensitive to circulating androgens or because the levels of circulating androgens are particularly high (O'Connell and Westhoff, 2008). Testosterone is the primary androgen associated with acne. It is produced in the adrenal glands, the ovaries in women and testes in men. Whilst generally thought of as a male hormone, testosterone is present in both males and females and becomes an important factor at puberty when the reproductive organs become active.

There are four key processes which occur to produce acne lesions.

(1) Increased production of sebum;
(2) Hyperkeratinisation within the hair follicle leading to follicular plugging;
(3) Increased bacterial activity within the follicle as there is enhanced colonisation with *Propionibacterium acnes*;
(4) Release of inflammatory mediators (e.g. cytokines, tumour necrosis factor) into the follicle and surrounding dermis causing increased inflammation (Figure 10.1).

Each of these four processes will now be considered in turn.

Increased sebum production

The response of the body to increased circulating androgens (which generally begins to occur at 7–8 years of age) is twofold. Firstly, the androgens drive changes in both sebocytes and follicular keratinocytes which lead to microcomedone formation. Microcomedones are non-inflammatory lesions which are considered the first lesions of acne, i.e. both inflammatory and non-inflammatory acne lesions are preceded by a microcomedone (Gollnick *et al.*, 2003). Secondly, the androgens lead to an increase in sebum production (Gollnick *et al.*, 2003).

Sebum is made up of lipids (triglycerides, waxes, free fatty acids and squalene) and the debris of dead fat-producing cells. As a substance in itself, it is odour free; however, bacterial activity on the sebum does produce a distinctive odour known as body odour. Its purpose is to waterproof the skin and protect it from becoming dry and brittle. Sebum has the unique ability to support the growth of the bacteria *P. acnes* and as such acne cannot occur without the presence of sebum (Thiboutot, 2008). If the amount of sebum produced can be reduced, there is a consequent decrease in *P. acnes* (Leyden and McGinley, 1993). This mechanism is discussed

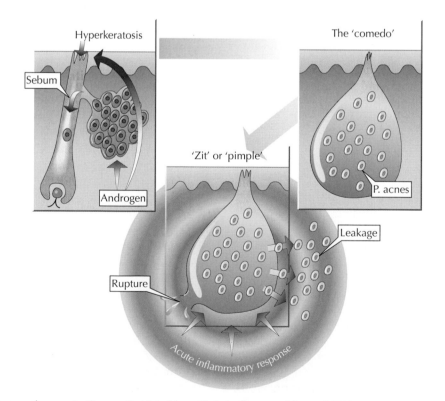

Figure 10.1   Acne pathogenesis. (Source: Reprinted from Graham-Brown and Burns, 2006.)

further in the section on treatments. It seems that the highest density of *P. acnes* is found in areas most rich in sebaceous glands (Leyden and McGinley, 1993).

Follicular plugging

In a normal follicle, the keratinocytes are shed as single cells into the follicular channel and then excreted. It is not fully understood what stimulates the hyperkeratinisation in which the dead keratinocytes remain adherent in the follicular channel leading to blockage, which can be either partial or complete. However, initially these blockages lead to small virtually invisible changes which are the microcomedones. They may take up to 2–3 years before they proceed into more significant acne lesions. As the microcomedone gets bigger and the swelling increases behind the blockage, comedones develop. These are always the precursor lesions to acne.

Comedones can either be open or closed. Open comedones (otherwise known as blackheads) are where the blockage of the follicle is high up and contents of the follicle are pushed through the follicle opening, thus being exposed to the air. The black colour of blackheads is not caused by dirt, although there appears to be disagreement about its origins. Texts vary, with some saying it is due to the presence of melanin (Ashton and Leppard, 2005), others to the way that light is reflected of the tightly compacted horny cells (Leyden and McGinley, 1993) and yet others stating it is caused by the oxidising effect of the air on the contents of the comedone (O'Toole, 1997) (Figure 10.2). Closed comedones (otherwise known as whiteheads) do not have their contents exposed to the air as the blockage is further down the hair follicle. Blackheads and whiteheads are the non-inflammatory stage of acne (Figure 10.3). Acne can resolve spontaneously at this stage never progressing to the inflammatory form of the disease. The blockage within the follicle allows for a build up of sebum which becomes the ideal environment for *P. acnes* to proliferate.

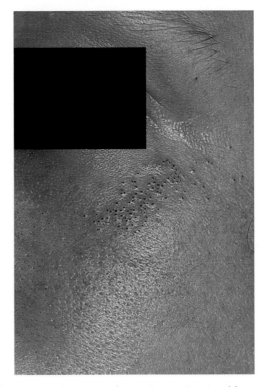

Figure 10.2 Open comedones. (Source: Reprinted from Weller *et al.*, 2008.)

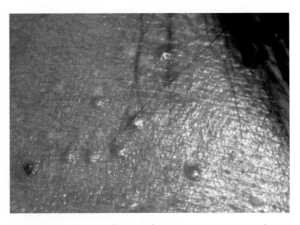

Figure 10.3 Acne with comedones. (Source: Reprinted from Buxton and Morris-Jones, 2009.)

Increased bacterial activity and resulting inflammation

Even where there is no evidence of active acne, *P. acnes* exists on the skin surface; indeed, there does not seem to be any correlation between the levels of *P. acnes* on the skin surface and severity of acne. However, some aspect of the hair follicle itself and the microenvironment found there causes *P. acnes* to proliferate and colonise the hair follicle leading to inflammation. The intensity of the inflammation varies depending on the individual which may, in part, be due to the individual's sensitivity to the inflammatory mediators associated with *P. acnes*. Although the mechanisms are not fully understood, it is thought that the action of the proliferating bacteria causes release of inflammatory cytokines, primarily CD4+ T-lymphocytes. Initially, papules and pustules are seen. Pustules form the typical yellow spot of acne. Because of the inflammatory response, lots of white blood cells are attracted to the area where there are increased levels of bacteria. Pus is formed largely from the dead white blood cells.

As these inflammatory mediators move out into the surrounding dermis, the lesions are more likely to be nodular and/or cystic and there is an increased likelihood of permanent scarring. Nodules are solid and larger than pustules extending deeper into the layers of skin. They are caused when large comedones rupture releasing their inflammatory contents into the surrounding skin. Because they extend deeper into the skin affecting the dermis as well as epidermis, they do lead to scarring. Cysts occur less frequently than nodules but when they do they are even more destructive, leading to greater levels of scarring. They are not as solid as a nodule and will often occur where there are two or three nodules close together (Figure 10.4).

Acne conglobata and acne fulminans

Acne conglobata describes a situation where there is severe nodular acne causing deep abscesses, sinuses in the skin and skin breakdown leading to ulceration. There are also usually large numbers of blackheads affecting the face, neck, upper arms and trunk.

Acne fulminans is a severe form of acne conglobata where the patient becomes systemically unwell. Patients will present with nodular cystic acne plus a number of other symptoms including

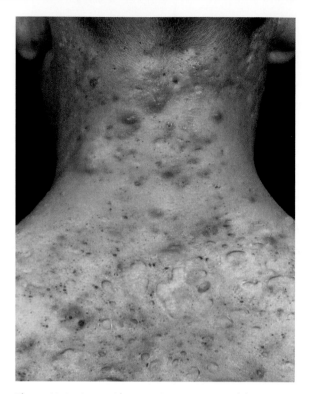

Figure 10.4 Acne with cysts. (Source: Reprinted from Buxton and Morris-Jones, 2009.)

malaise, fever, joint pain and/or swelling. It nearly always affects males and is characterised by an abrupt onset along with the above symptoms and a raised white blood cell count. It may be precipitated by the illegal use of testosterone to boost muscle growth; however, it can just occur spontaneously (New Zealand Dermatological Society Incorporated, 2009). It is considered a dermatological emergency and a patient presenting with acne fulminans must be referred urgently to see a dermatologist (National Institute for Clinical Excellence, 2001).

Acne conglobata and fulminans can present as part of a syndrome known as SAPHO. This syndrome must include any combination of the following:

Synovitis (inflamed joints)
Acne (conglobata or fulminans)
Pustulosis (thick blister containing yellow pus)
Hyperostosis (increase in bone substance)
Osteitis (inflammation of the bones)

Treatment will be multifactorial involving care from dermatologists and rheumatologists in order to treat all of the symptoms.

Scarring

One of the key aims of treatment is to prevent scarring. Should it become evident that scarring is occurring, the patient should be referred for more intensive treatment (National Institute for Clinical Excellence, 2001). Scarring is more likely to occur in patients who have nodules and/or cysts. However, tendency to scar is quite individual and each patient needs to be assessed individually as some people will begin to scar even with relatively mild acne (Figure 10.5).

There are some marks that are left on the face post-acne; these are lesions that are not strictly speaking scars. They are related to pigment changes. The final vestiges of the inflammatory process may appear as small red macules on the skin which will fade over the course of 6 months. Post-inflammatory pigmented lesions describe lesions where melanin has built up in the skin as a result of the inflammation. These may be in evidence for over a year and are often more noticeable in darker skin types.

True scarring can be one of two types. It can either be hypertrophic or atrophic. Hypertrophic scars (sometimes referred to as keloid scars) occur where there is excessive tissue giving the scars a raised up appearance that may extend beyond the margins of the original lesion (Mitchell and Dudley, 2002). The overgrowth of tissue is caused by excessive collagen being laid down in that area. Afro-Caribbean skin seems to be more prone to keloid scarring than other racial groups. Atrophic scars refer to those where there is a loss of tissue, so the lesion appears depressed from the surface of the skin. Different types of atrophic scars include:

- *Ice-pick scars*: Have a well-defined irregular edge and steep sides usually occurring on the cheeks.
- *Atrophic macular scars*: These are flatter on the skin surface and the skin may appear thin and somewhat wrinkled. Although they are generally small on the face, they can be larger on the body; with time, they appear whitish in colour.
- *Follicular macular atrophy*: These scars are so called because they tend to occur around hair follicles on the chest and back following on from severe acne. The elastin fibres in the skin are damaged so that rather than lying smooth and flat they bunch up and cause small lumps to appear in the skin looking rather like white heads. With time, as the elastin repairs, these lesions tend to flatten out (Mitchell and Dudley, 2002).

Treatment for scarring

Patients need to have realistic advice about the likely success of treatment for acne scarring. They should be reassured that hyperpigmentation will gradually fade over time. Skin bleaching creams should be avoided as they are likely to cause hypopigmentation, leaving the patient with a more permanent problem than before. At the current time, there are no treatments for acne scarring that have a good research evidence base. Some options that patients may ask about are listed below.

Camouflage techniques: Special cover-creams can be closely matched to skin tone

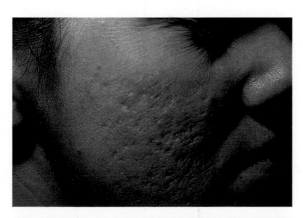

Figure 10.5 Acne scarring. (Source: Reprinted from Weller *et al.*, 2008.)

and applied to the skin to even out colour differences. The creams are fixed with a spray or powder so that they can be left in place for up to a week (Davies, 2007). For patients with acne, this is most effective at covering hyper or hypopigmentation; it is not terrible successful at covering scars. It cannot be used on active inflammatory acne lesions.

Steroid injections for keloid scars: These can be helpful, but small injections should be given over a period of time to get the best results and avoid side effects.

Chemical peels or dermabrasion: These procedures are used for atrophic scarring and aim to remove layers of skin so that the whole skin surface is lowered to the level of the scar tissue. When the new skin grows back, it is smoother and less pitted. Patients should be warned that this can be extremely painful and lead to a prolonged period of sore and damaged facial skin as it heals. The extent of this depends on how severe the treatment is. Those facial peels which do not leave the face feeling sore are unlikely to have much long-term beneficial effect. 'Fillers' may be helpful in lifting shallow depressed scars. Treating scar tissue in these ways requires careful assessment and delivery of the various techniques to obtain the optimal response. In general these treatments are not available on the NHS.

Silicon sheets: These are worn in direct contact with the scar. A systematic review of the evidence for the efficacy of silicon sheets found that there were no good studies which made it difficult to make a judgement about their benefits (O'Brien and Pandit, 2006). They are, however, unlikely to cause any damage.

Lasers: A systematic review of the evidence for the use of lasers in treating acne scarring revealed that the evidence was not sufficiently robust as to determine the efficacy of different laser treatments or in comparison with other treatments. Whilst some case studies suggest there might be a positive effect, the authors of the review felt that the evidence was not strong enough to make recommendations for practice (Jordan *et al.*, 2000).

Who gets acne and distribution

As mentioned earlier, the majority of teenagers will experience acne to some degree. There are, however, other age groups who can also develop acne.

Impact of genetics

As with the majority of inherited skin disorders, the pattern for heritability of acne is not straightforward. However, research carried out on twins does suggest that the severity of acne at all ages and on all sites was influenced by genetic factors (Evans *et al.*, 2005). Monozygotic twins were significantly more likely to have similar severity of acne than dizygotic twins.

Infantile acne

Whilst infantile acne is unusual, it can occur usually between 6 and 18 months. During the first year of life, both boys and girls produce androgens from their adrenal gland; in addition to this, boys also produce testosterone from their testes (this may explain why infantile acne seems more prevalent in boys). In a retrospective study of 29 patients with infantile acne, 24 were boys and 5 were girls (Cunliffe *et al.*, 2001). The same study saw a range of disease severity with 17 having superficial inflammatory lesions and 5 comedonal lesions; it was mild in 7, moderate in 18 and severe in 4. This study highlights the similarities between infantile and teenage acne and indeed the management was the same (although tetracyclines were not used as they should be avoided in children under 12). All responded to therapy, although 11 of the children required 24 months of treatment. In these instances, it is important that the parents and family receive support and reassurance that the lesions will resolve.

Acne in middle age

Although teenagers usually grow out of acne, for some it does persist into middle age, for others acne appears for the first time in middle age.

Treatments

General guidance on using treatment

When deciding on the type of topical treatment to use, assessment of the type of acne the patient is presenting with is important, e.g. is it inflammatory or non-inflammatory or a mixture of the two. It is also important to bear in mind the patient's lifestyle and what sort of treatments they are willing and able to tolerate.

Before discussing with the patient the possible treatment options, it is important that the health care professional ensures that the patient is clear about a number of general issues around acne and its treatment. To start with, patients need to be advised that acne is not caused by any of the mythical causes such as poor hygiene, too much sex, eating chocolate or dietary habits in general. As has been described earlier in the chapter, acne is a complex condition caused by the interplay of a number of different physiological factors. It may be helpful to explain this to patients. Some patients may believe that their acne is contagious and this falsehood must be dispelled. Regardless of which treatments are eventually used, there are some general guidelines about acne management that are worth discussing. These are listed in Box 10.1.

Box 10.1 **General advice on skin care for acne prone skin**

(1) Avoid harsh washing and specifically do not scrub acne affected skin.
(2) It is best for the skin not to squeeze spots. Certainly, if the lesion is red and not pustular it should be left alone. However, for many patients this is difficult to adhere to, so the following guidance is aimed at causing as little permanent damage as possible to the skin:

(a) When trying to express the contents of a pustule, stretch the skin on either side of the lesion using a tissue rather than digging in with the nails and squeezing.
(b) Gentle pressure and squeezing on either side of blackhead is probably the only way to express those lesions. Whiteheads should not be squeezed.
(c) Stop squeezing if blood is seen (Mitchell and Dudley, 2002).
(3) Avoid using oily products on the skin. Moisturisers may be needed as the skin between lesions can become dry and tight (especially if drying topical agents are being used). All products should be labelled oil free and non-comodogenic.
(4) Foundation and cover-up make-up can make acne worse, although lighter non-comodogenic products are likely to be less troublesome.

It is important that patients are aware that there is really no quick treatment option for acne and that results from treatment will only be seen over a prolonged period of time (weeks to months). In addition, due to the number of different processes that are occurring in the development of acne (i.e. increased sebum production, follicular plugging, colonisation by *P. acnes* and the resulting inflammation), it is often necessary to have a combination of treatments which tackle different elements of the disease process. In order to optimise the care of patients with acne (and therefore the results they experience), intervention at an early stage is vital. Often it will be a nurse who has the time and skills to undertake this early care. This will ensure that people with acne understand about the process of the disease, how and why to use treatments and importantly how to recognise if the condition is worsening and more intensive interventions are needed, particularly with the aim of preventing scarring.

Topical treatments

Mild to moderate acne

Topical treatments are the first-line treatment for acne. As has been outlined earlier, non-inflammatory lesions include microcomedones, open and closed comedones. If these types of lesions predominate, with few or no pustules, acne is usually termed mild. In this instance, the first-line treatments are ones that reduce follicular plugging anti-inflammatory properties are less important. There seems to be consensus that in this situation the best treatment options are topical retinoids (Gollnick *et al.*, 2003).

Topical retinoids

Topical retinoids work by reducing the abnormal desquamation of skin cells into the follicular canal thus reducing the plugging. They work on the very earliest of acne lesions, the microcomedone, thus preventing more mature comedones from developing. They also appear to have some anti-inflammatory properties, although these are not their main mode of action. Finally, because of their impact on the follicular microclimate, they appear to enhance the efficacy of antibacterial products such as benzoyl peroxide (BPO) and topical antibiotics (Gollnick *et al.*, 2003). Because of their action on the microcomedone, retinoids can be considered as maintenance therapy once active lesions have been cleared.

Topical retinoids describe a broad group of pharmaceutical products which are derived from vitamin A. Over the years, a number of different 'generations' of retinoids have been developed. Tretinoin and isotretinoin were the first generation; the drawbacks highlighted with these products being skin irritation, delayed and variable responses, photosensitivity and exacerbation of the acne after 2–4 weeks (Naito *et al.*, 2008). In order to get around the problems of skin irritation, a number of different strengths and formulations were developed including the microsphere which was designed to release the tretinoin slowly in a controlled manner (Gollnick *et al.*, 2003). It should be noted that topical isotretinoin has a similar effect to tretinoin, but a very different effect from oral isotretinoin as it has no impact on sebum production.

Adapalene is a newer retinoid (known as third generation) in which the therapeutic action is similar to that of tretinoin, but in which the unwanted side effects of skin irritation and photosensitisation have been reduced. Adapalene also seems to be absorbed into the pilosebaceous duct more effectively than into the rest of the skin surface, thus increasing its efficacy (Naito *et al.*, 2008). As yet there is no Cochrane review giving evidence-based guidance as to which retinoid is best to use; however, there has been a research study indicating that whilst efficacy was similar, adapalene had fewer unwanted side effects than tretinoin microsphere gel 0.1% (Thiboutot *et al.*, 2003).

Topical retinoids can be used in women of child-bearing age; however, they should be advised to avoid pregnancy whilst using them. Should an individual become pregnant whilst using topical retinoids, they should stop the treatment immediately. Whilst it is unlikely for the topical product to have a systemic effect, this is a sensible precaution.

How to apply a retinoid product?

Usually it is best to apply these at night before going to bed. The patient should be encouraged to wash the skin and dry it gently but completely before applying a thin layer of the product to the whole area to be treated, not just the lesions. Retinoids can be applied to any area of the body where acne is present including chest and back. The choice of the formulation of the product, whether a cream or a gel, will usually depend on personal preference. A gel is likely to dry the skin more and may be helpful if the skin surface is very greasy whereas a cream will be more moisturising and may be helpful if the skin surface has a tendency to get dry. After applying the treatment, the patient should wash their hands. The possible side effects of treatment have already been mentioned including redness, soreness and skin peeling and hypersensitivity to sunlight. If the former is a problem, the severity of the symptoms may be reduced by using a weaker formulation, if one is available, or by starting with less than a once-daily application (perhaps alternate days) and then building up to the required once a day. Patients should be advised to avoid overexposure to the sun and to not make use of sunbeds.

Benzoyl peroxide

BPO is a commonly used product for the management of mild to moderate acne. Many teenagers who have acne will purchase over-the-counter products containing BPO, and are likely to have had varying degrees of success with them. BPO works by releasing free radical oxygen within the follicle itself; this has a bactericidal effect thus reducing the bacterial load of *P. acnes* (Tucker, 2008). BPO is therefore an effective antibacterial product and particularly useful when there are inflammatory lesions as well as non-inflammatory lesions. The impact of BPO is enhanced by the use of topical retinoids; they are often used as a combination therapy.

How to use BPO?

Before starting to use the treatment, patients should be made aware that the product can bleach bedding, clothing and even hair, so care should be taken when using it. The main side effect of BPO products is that they cause reddening and soreness of the skin. This is usually mild and can generally be overcome by starting treatments at a low strength and/or using them on alternate days initially. Gradually over time, the frequency can be increased to once or twice daily. If the lower strengths are tolerated and they are not completely clearing the acne, it is worth moving up to the stronger strengths.

The patient should be instructed to wash their skin with a mild cleanser and pat the skin surface completely dry. The product should then be applied all over the affected area, not just to the lesions. The patient should then wash their hands carefully. Another tip if the skin is particularly sensitive is to leave the product on for just a short period of time initially (washing it off after 15 minutes) and then gradually building up increasing amounts of time as the skin tolerates the product.

BPO may be used as part of a combination regime, usually with retinoids. In these instances, BPO should be used in the morning and the topical retinoid in the evening. It is particularly important for the patient to remember to wash their face prior to using each different topical therapy.

Azelaic acid

This has a similar clinical effect to BPO, but causes less irritation and does not have the same tendency to bleach. It has reported antibacterial and comodolytic properties (Strauss *et al.*, 2007). It is available as a 15% gel and 20% cream

How to use azelaic acid?

It should be applied to clean skin twice daily, preferably in the morning and evening. As with BPO, if the skin is particularly sensitive, a gradual introduction of the product might be helpful.

Nicotinamide

This is a physiologically active form of nicotinic acid which is thought to have anti-inflammatory, bacteriostatic effects on *P. acnes* and reduce sebum production. It is therefore most useful if there are inflammatory lesions in evidence.

How to use nicotinamide?

It should be applied to clean skin twice daily, preferably in the morning and evening. It may take up to 12 weeks to have a beneficial effect.

Topical antibiotics

If BPO is not tolerated, topical antibiotics particularly topical clindamycin, erythromycin or tetracycline may be used. There are concerns about antibiotic resistance and it is generally recommended that they should not be used as a monotherapy, but instead be used with a retinoid product. Long term use as a maintenance therapy should also be avoided. They have a slower onset than oral antibiotics and are less effective (Gollnick *et al.*, 2003). Some topical antibiotic products already contain BPO and it has been shown that this combination leads to a reduced potential for developing *P. acnes* resistance (Eady *et al.*, 1996).

How long to use treatment for?

All three of the topical treatments in this section need to have been used for 2 months before assessment as to their success or failure is made. During this prolonged period of time, patients will need to have support and encouragement to continue to use treatments. Concordance will be improved with regular contact to discuss how the treatments are feeling on the skin and whether there are any ongoing problems (see Chapter 7). Ideally, patients should have access to telephone support.

Moderate acne

Moderate acne differs from mild in the number of papular and pustular lesions that are present. These are much greater in number and although there will still be comedones present, the focus of treatment shifts towards managing the high burden of *P. acnes* which leads to significant inflammatory lesions.

Oral antibiotics

Oral antibiotics are a commonly used treatment for acne, and should be considered as appropriate for moderate to severe cases. Typically, the antibiotics of choice are tetracycline or oxytetracycline. Doxycycline may be considered for people who cannot comply with oxytetracycline or tetracycline. Lymecycline is tetracycline which is taken once daily and has the advantage of not needing to be taken on an empty stomach. Erythromycin might be considered if there is no response to the other antibiotic therapies; however, it has been increasingly associated with resistant strains of propionibacteria which may explain its lack of efficacy. It has been suggested that erythromycin is reserved for patients for whom the cyclines are contraindicated, e.g. when breast feeding or when pregnant (Dreno *et al.*, 2004). Trimethoprim is a final option but it is an off-licence use and therefore probably only to be initiated by a specialist. Minocycline has historically been the preferred antibiotic; however, safety concerns including a greater risk of a lupus erythematosus-type reaction and possible permanent skin pigment changes have meant that it is rarely used. A Cochrane review considered the evidence in relation to the efficacy of minocycline in comparison with other oral antibiotics and showed no significant difference (Garner *et al.*, 2003).

An important issue in relation to antibiotic prescribing in acne is that of resistance. It was reported that around 50% of acne sufferers in Europe were colonised with erythromycin- and clindamycin-resistant strains of *P. acnes* and up to 20% were colonised with cycline-resistant strains (Dreno *et al.*, 2004). The same paper states that the longer someone is on oral antibiotics, the more likely it is for resistance to develop; they estimate that at the end of a 6 months course of antibiotics, most people would have developed resistant strains of *P. acnes* (Dreno *et al.*, 2004). Antibiotic resistance should be considered as a possible cause of failure to respond to treatment, especially if they have been given over a prolonged period of time. Box 10.2 summarises the risk factors associated with developing resistant bacteria.

The same article provides a list of recommendations for reducing the likelihood of developing resistant strains of *P. acnes* (see Box 10.3).

Oxytetracycline and tetracycline are given in 500 mg doses twice a day whereas doxycycline is longer acting, thus given as a once-daily treatment at a dose of 100 mg. Lymecyline taken once a day in a dose of 408mg. Treatment should be given for 3 months before an assessment as to whether it is making any improvement or not. If no improvement is seen, the antibiotic should be changed; however, it should be noted that maximum improvement is usually seen at 4–6 months. More severe cases of acne may need oral antibiotics for 2 years or more (but see comments earlier with regards to resistance). Fatty food in particular decreases the absorption of tetracycline

---

> ### Box 10.2 **Risk factors for bacterial resistance**
>
> - Long courses of antibiotics
> - Multiple course of antibiotics
> - Poor compliance with treatment
> - Being close to someone who has resistant acne.
>
> *Source*: Dreno et al. (2004).

thelium which allows more systemic antibiotic
to be transported to where the *P. acnes* resides
(Gollnick *et al.*, 2003).

Hormonal therapies
The combined oral contraceptive pill (containing both oestrogen and progesterone) has been
shown to be effective in reducing both inflammatory and non-inflammatory acne lesions in
women (Strauss *et al.*, 2007). It does not appear
that one particular combined oral contraceptive pill is particularly better than any other.
However, this therapeutic option is recommended for women who have acne but who also
want birth control, and as such this may be a
reasonable choice.

Severe acne

In cases of acne that do not respond to the
above oral therapies, the final option is oral
isotretinoin. Whilst usually reserved for the
severe end of the disease scale, if the acne is
proving to be particularly scarring either physically or psychologically it may be considered
as an option earlier, when the disease is more
moderate.

Isotretinoin
Isotretinoin is a unique therapy because it targets all aspects of the acne disease process. Its
effects are summarised in Box 10.4.

Box 10.3 Recommendations for reducing likelihood of developing resistant bacteria

(1) Do not use antibiotics where other acne treatments can be expected to bring about the same degree of clinical benefit;
(2) Use antibiotics according to clinical need (e.g. should not in general be used for mild acne);
(3) Do not use them as monotherapy;
(4) Stop the treatment when the health care professional and the patient agree that there is no further improvement or the improvement is only slight;
(5) Try to avoid using antibiotics beyond 6 months;
(6) Use BPO either concomitantly or pulsed as an anti-resistance measure;
(7) Do not swap antibiotics without adequate justification (i.e. if a further course of antibiotics is needed, use the same one) (p. 394).

---

and oxytetracycline and to a lesser extent, doxycycline. Patients should be recommended where
possible to take the antibiotics on an empty stomach to maximise their therapeutic value.

The most common side effects of these antibiotics are gastrointestinal disturbances which
patients should be warned of.

It is generally agreed that clearing inflammatory and comedonal lesions is quicker when oral
antibiotics are used in conjunction with topical retinoids and antibacterials (Gollnick *et al.*,
2003). Thus oral treatment is not used instead
of topical treatment, but as an additional therapy. The mechanisms for improved efficacy of
combined therapy is in part due to the different modes of action of the various therapeutic
agents (i.e. they target different aspects of the
disease process). However, it is also thought
that topical retinoids affect skin permeability
thus enhancing topical agent penetration and

Box 10.4 Effects of isotretinoin

- Decreases the size of, and secretions from, the sebaceous glands;
- Normalises the follicular keratinisation thus preventing follicular plugging and comedone formation;
- Alters the microenvironment of the follicle so that it is not conducive to *P. acnes* growth;
- Has an anti-inflammatory effect.

Taking isotretinoin can reduce the sebum production by up to 90%; the effect of this is that *P. acnes* levels decrease significantly (Gollnick *et al.*, 2003). This in turn leads to a significant decrease in inflammatory lesions. Most cases respond to a single 4–6 month course. Pustules clear more rapidly than papules and nodules and those lesions on the face, upper arms and legs clear more quickly than those on the trunk. Beneficial effect may take 1–2 months to notice and occasionally the acne may worsen in this period of time prior to improving. Patients need to be warned of this fact.

Dosing ranges from 0.1–2.0 mg/kg but in reality doses higher than 1.0 mg/kg are rarely used. In order to minimise potential side effects (especially a flare-up of the acne), a starting dose of 0.5 mg/kg/day for the first month may be advisable. If tolerability is not a problem, this dose may be followed by 1 mg/kg per day for the rest of the course. More severe deeper nodular acne may need a longer treatment period.

Side effects

The side effects of oral isotretinoin are significant and require detailed discussion with the patient to ensure full understanding of the implications of taking the drugs. Because one of the therapeutic benefits of isotretinoin is as a drying agent, patients will experience dry skin, chapped lips, dry eyes and a dry mouth. Secondary skin infections with *S. aureus* can also occur and should be treated with oral antibiotics or antiseptics (depending on the level of infection). Less frequently patients may experience muscle and back aches and mild headaches, although these usually resolve as the treatment progresses. Nosebleeds and skin fragility may occur. There may be a rise in serum lipid levels. Certain symptoms should be taken very seriously and warrant discontinuation of the treatment immediately. These include:

- severe headache
- decreased night vision
- signs of adverse psychiatric events

Generally, the unwanted side effects will resolve once treatment is discontinued.

Both brands of isotretinoin available in Britain contain soya oil. Some patients with peanut allergy may have cross-reactivity with soya and this needs to be discussed. The capsules that encase the active ingredients contain gelatine which may make taking the tablets unacceptable to someone on a vegetarian diet.

Monitoring

Serum lipid and liver function tests (LFTs) should be monitored. LFTs should be measured as a baseline prior to the commencement of treatment and then checked at 4 and 8 weeks (although exact timings will vary depending on local clinical practice). If blood levels are normal at 8 weeks, further monitoring is probably not necessary as long as the dose remains the same.

Because isotretinoin is teratogenic (it can seriously adversely affect the unborn child), women of child-bearing age must have a negative blood pregnancy test before commencement of therapy. Once a negative pregnancy test has been received, therapy should be started after the 2nd or 3rd day of the first menstrual period after the test. Current practice requires women to undergo monthly urine pregnancy tests prior to a further prescription of isotretinoin being given. It should be noted in the patient record that contraception and pregnancy avoidance advice have been discussed and understood by the patient. Different countries have different policies on the issue of pregnancy avoidance. Grewal-Fry outlines the policy in the USA (Grewal-Fry, 2007).

Patients may well already be aware of the potential psychological impacts of taking isotretinoin as these have been extensively covered in the popular press. Whilst severe psychiatric changes are unlikely, patients should be counselled about the possibility of mood swings. Acne itself can lead to high levels of anxiety (Aktan *et al.*, 2000) and it is not always possible to categorically identify mental health changes being as a result of isotretinoin. Very occasionally severe psychiatric changes may occur with some reports of depression and suicidal ideation (Gollnick *et al.*, 2003). A more recent study suggested that there is a link between isotretinoin use and depression in those with acne vulgaris (Azoulay *et al.*, 2008). In a commentary on this article, however, the categoric results were debated with the author questioning whether the research methods allowed the conclusions to be drawn (Bigby, 2008). This author states that 'Firm conclusions regarding the risk of depression associated with isotretinoin cannot be drawn' (p. 1199), although he confirms that discussions about the possibility of depression should be had with the patient. It is important, therefore that patients are asked about their mood and warned of depression as a potential side effect.

Relapse

Relapse can occur post-isotretinoin therapy. A large study (17,351 first time isotretinoin users over a 20-year period) looked at the prescriptions given to this cohort. It identified that 41% of the patients required further acne treatments (isotretinoin or other systemic or topical therapy). Twenty six percent required a second dose of isotretinoin (Azoulay *et al.*, 2007). The authors looked for predictive factors for relapsing and noted that male subjects and those under the age of 16 were more likely to require further treatment with anti-acne medications. Those who had lower doses and shorter courses also seemed more at risk of needing subsequent anti-acne treatments. Generally, it seems to be the case that if relapse is going to occur it occurs most frequently in the first year post-treatment (Gollnick *et al.*, 2003).

Supporting patients who are taking isotretinoin

Patients being prescribed isotretinoin need to be supported throughout their course of treatment. They need advice with regards to managing a range of issues (Box 10.5).

It is not possible to totally ameliorate the drying effects of the drug, but certain protective behaviours may help (Box 10.6).

The drug's effect can be significantly enhanced by taking it with food. It is thought that 40% is absorbed if taken with a meal whereas only 20% is absorbed if it is taken on an empty stomach (Gollnick *et al.*, 2003). The drug can be taken as a single dose once a day or divided and taken as two doses at different times of the day. If the drug dose is to be split, it may be helpful for the patient to use a dosing box to ensure that they keep track of their tablets.

Box 10.5   Checklist of topics that need to be discussed with patients on isotretinoin

- Change in mood
- Contraception (in women)
- Dryness: eyes, mouth, lips, nose (nosebleeds), genitalia
- Joint and/or muscle discomfort
- Sun protection/avoidance
- Avoiding Alcohol
- Waxing/exfoliating
- Avoiding planned surgery/cosmetic procedure
- Should not give blood
- Avoid vitamin supplements

Box 10.6   Advice that may help with the drying effects of isotretinoin

- Avoiding activities which dry the skin, e.g. taking hot showers/baths and using soap;
- Using emollients extensively if skin becomes dry;
- Not using exfoliants or topical treatments that will dry the skin further. All topical acne treatments should be stopped;
- Not waxing;
- Having a chapstick handy for dry lips and using this frequently (may need to be hourly);
- Avoiding exposure to UV radiation and not making use of sunbeds. Always using an oil-free sunscreen of at least SPF 15;
- Wearing soft contact lenses or glasses are likely to be more comfortable than hard contact lenses;
- Using hypromellose eye drops;
- Keeping a bottle of water handy at all times, to sip.

Preventing pregnancy is key for female patients who are on isotretinoin. Contraceptive advice should be given to all sexually active patients. Teenagers who attend with parents may be unwilling to admit they are sexually active; however, information should still be given. It is advised that one or preferably two types of contraception are used. Depending on the level of advice needed, the woman may need to be referred to a family planning service to ensure that the most effective and suitable contraception is provided. Contraception must be used for a month prior to the planned start of treatment, during treatment and for 5 weeks after the end of treatment. This is because it takes this length of time for the isotretinoin to be excreted from the body completely.

Although very low levels of isotretinoin may be found in the semen of men on the drug, these are not thought to be sufficient to harm an unborn child or their sexual partner.

Newer treatments with less evidence

Photodynamic therapy

A review carried out in 2008 considered the various uses for photodynamic therapy (PDT) including its potential role in the treatment of acne (Morton *et al.*, 2008). PDT is a type of light therapy in which a photosensitising drug is applied to the skin and then a light source is shone onto the skin in order to alter, in some way, targeted cells. The light source varies and can be a laser, filtered xenon arc and metal halide lamps, fluorescent lamps and light emitting diodes. When used for treating cancerous lesions, for example basal cell carcinomas, the process of applying the light to the sensitised skin is to kill the cancer cells. In acne treatments, the exact mechanism is not wholly understood but it is thought that the treatment has a number of effects:

(1) It has an antimicrobial effect on *P. acnes*.
(2) It causes selective damage to sebaceous glands.
(3) It reduces the keratinocyte shedding and therefore follicular blocking.

A number of studies are reported by Morton *et al.* (2008) showing beneficial results from PDT both immediately after treatment and at various time points after the treatment. Some studies looked at results after one treatment, others after a series of treatments. Some of the studies reported some unpleasant side effects including pain during treatment, severe erythema after treatment, pustular eruptions and epithelial exfoliation. Most of the studies were small. Few trials compare laser light therapy to conventional treatments but in one case where PDT was compared to 1% adapalene gel the results showed that PDT was no better than the gel (Hamilton *et al.*, 2009). The conclusion drawn by Morton *et al.* (2008) was that whilst this looks like a promising treatment for inflammatory acne on both the face and back, further work needs to be done on determining the most effective treatment protocols.

A Cochrane review looked at the evidence in relation to laser therapy and found that trials of blue light, blue–red light and infrared light were more successful than light alone particularly when multiple treatments were used (Hamilton *et al.*, 2009).

Psychological impact

A brief discussion with teenagers with acne will quickly illuminate the degree to which 'spots' can affect their lives. Appearing as it does, during the emotionally turbulent teenage years, responses to acne range from mild annoyance to depression and even suicidal ideation. Not only can acne cause severe psychological hardship, but it can also prevent young people from achieving their full potential as they avoid applying for the job they really want because it means being in the public eye, for example. Whilst some people with acne may require extensive psychological support and intervention, for the majority having someone who takes their problem seriously and works with them to find a treatment regime which works will be all that is required. For this reason, nurses who care for people with acne need to take the time to find out how the disease is impacting on life and work with the person to find a satisfactory therapy. (See Chapter 6 for further information on the psychological impact of skin disease.)

Conclusion

Acne results from a number of pathological processes which have been outlined in this chapter. Treatments need to be matched to the level of disease severity and in particular the type of acne the patient is experiencing. Patients need to have treatments clearly explained to them including descriptions of possible side effects and the length of time they take to have a therapeutic impact.

References

Aktan, S., E. Ozmen *et al.* (2000). Anxiety, depression, and nature of acne vulgaris in adolescents. *International Journal of Dermatology*, **39**(5): 354–357.

Ashton, R. and B. Leppard (2005). *Differential Diagnosis in Dermatology*. Oxford: Radcliffe Publishing Ltd.

Azoulay, L., D. Oraichi *et al.* (2007). Isotretinoin therapy and the incidence of acne relapse: A nested case-controlled study. *British Journal of Dermatology*, **157**(6): 1240–1248.

Azoulay, L., L. Blais *et al.* (2008). Isotretinoin and the risk of depression in patients with acne vulgaris: A case-crossover study. *Journal of Clinical Psychiatry*, **69**(4): 526–532.

Bigby, M. (2008). Does isotretinoin increase the risk of depression. *Archives of Dermatology*, **144**(9): 1197–1199.

Buxton, B.K. and R. Morris-Jones (2009). *ABC of Dermatology* (5th edition). Oxford: Wiley Blackwell.

Cunliffe, W., S. Baron *et al.* (2001). A clinical and therapeutic study of 29 patients with infantile acne. *British Journal of Dermatology*, **145**: 463–466.

Davies, V. (2007). The use of camouflage in skin conditions. *Dermatological Nursing*, **6**(4): 16–20.

Dreno, B., V. Bettoli *et al.* (2004). European recommendations for the use of oral antibiotics for acne. *European Journal of Dermatology*, **14**: 391–399.

Eady, E., J. Cove *et al.* (1996). The effects of acne treatment with a combination of benzoyl peroxide and erythromycin on skin carriage of erythromycin resistant propionibacteria. *British Journal of Dermatology*, **34**(1): 107–113.

Evans, D., K. Kirk *et al.* (2005). Teenage acne is influenced by genetic factors. *British Journal of Dermatology*, **152**: 505–594.

Garner, S., E. Eady *et al.* (2003). Minocycline for acne vulgaris: Efficacy and safety. *Cochrane Database of Systematic Reviews*, (1): Art No. CD002086.

Gollnick, H., W. Cunliffe *et al.* (2003). Management of acne – A report from a global alliance to improve outcomes in acne. *Journal of the American Academy of Dermatology*, **49**(1): S1–S37.

Graham-Brown, R. and T. Burns (2006). *Lecture Notes: Dermatology* (9th edition). Oxford: Blackwells.

Grewal-Fry, R. (2007). The management of patients on isotretinoin in the USA. *Dermatological Nursing*, **6**(2): 26–29.

Hamilton, F., J. Car *et al.* (2009). Laser and other light therapies for the treatment of acne vulgaris: Systematic review. *British Journal of Dermatology*, 160(6): 1273—85.

Jordan, R., C. Cummins *et al.* (2000). Laser resurfacing for facial acne scars. *Cochrane Database of Systematic Reviews* (3): Art No. CD001866.

Leyden, J. and K. McGinley (1993). Coryneform bacteria. In: Noble, W. (Ed.), *The Skin Microflora and Microbial Skin Disease*. Cambridge: University Press.

Mitchell, T. and A. Dudley (2002). *Acne – The 'At Your Fingertips' Guide*. London: Class Publishing.

Morton, C., K. McKenna *et al.* (2008). Guidelines for topical photodynamic therapy: An update. *British Journal of Dermatology*, **159**: 1245–1266.

Naito, A., S. Ovaisi *et al.* (2008). Topical retinoids for acne vulgaris. *Cochrane Database of Systematic Reviews* (3): Art No. CD007299.

National Institute for Clinical Excellence (2001). *Referral Advice: A Guide to Appropriate Referral from General to Specialist Services*. London: NICE.

New Zealand Dermatological Society Incorporated (2009) DermnetNZ. Retrieved 25 March 2009, from www.dermnetnz.org.

O'Brien, L. and A. Pandit (2006). Silicon gel sheeting for preventing and treating hypertrophic and keloid scars. *Cochrane Database of Systematic Reviews* (1).

O'Connell, K. and C. Westhoff (2008). Pharmacology of hormonal contraceptives and acne. *Cutis*, **81**(1 Suppl): 8–12.

O'Toole, M., Ed. (1997). *Miller-Keane Encyclopedia and Dictionary of Medicine, Nursing and Allied Health*. Philadelphia: WB Saunders.

Rademaker, M., J. Garioch *et al.* (1989). Acne in schoolchildren: No longer a concern for dermatologists. *British Medical Journal*, **298**(6682): 1217–1220.

Strauss, J., D. Krowchuk *et al.* (2007). Guidelines of care for acne vulgaris management. *Journal of the American Academy of Dermatology*, **56**(4): 651–663.

Thiboutot, D. (2008). Overview of acne and its treatment. *Cutis*, **81**(1 Suppl): 3–7.

Thiboutot, D., R. Thieroff-Ekerdt *et al.* (2003). Efficacy and safety of azelaic acid (15%) gel as a new treatment for papulopustular rosacea: Results from two vehicle-controlled, randomised phase III studies. *Journal of the American Academy of Dermatology*, **48**(6): 836–845.

Tucker, R. (2008). The use of over-the-counter products in acne vulgaris. *Dermatological Nursing*, **7**(1): 11–18.

Weller, R., J.A.A. Hunter, J. Savin and M. Dahl (2008). *Clinical Dermatology* (4th edition). Oxford: Blackwell Publishing.

Skin cancer and its prevention

11

Rachel Duncan, Julie Van Onselen, Steven J. Ersser

Introduction

Cancer is the commonest cause of death in people aged 50–64; one in four people die of cancer (Office of National Statistics, 2009). Skin cancer is the most frequently diagnosed cancer in the UK, and rates of melanoma have risen faster than any other major cancer (Cancer Research UK, 2009a). The All Party Parliamentary Group on Skin (APPGS, 2003) enquiry into the treatment, management and prevention of skin cancer reports that the incidence of skin cancer has doubled within the last 20 years. The incidence and referral rate for skin cancer is also rising, due to greater public awareness. Lack of education and training in skin cancer by GPs is highlighted in the APPGS (2003) enquiry. The APPGS (2008) highlights the need for emphasis being placed on improving education amongst all those who have contact with people with skin conditions and especially in primary care. Nurses have a key role in skin cancer prevention, detection and in the support and treatment of those who develop skin cancer. Specifically, the APPGS argue for each dermatology unit having a clinical nurse specialist (CNS) in skin cancer at a ratio of one full-time employee per 160,000 of the population (APPGS, 2008).

This chapter introduces the epidemiology of skin cancer and locates this within the UK policy context. Three main sections then follow, embracing key diagnostic groupings of pre- and cancerous skin lesions; these include pre-malignant skin lesions, non-melanoma skin lesions and melanoma. The final section outlines the causation, risk prevention and early detection of skin cancer and the key role nurses and other health professionals can play, especially, in primary care.

Skin cancer epidemiology: the scale of the problem

In UK, around 9000 cases of melanoma are diagnosed annually and, although mortality rates are relatively low, they account for 80% of skin cancer deaths with incidence rising rapidly (Cancer Research UK, 2004, 2009c; Royal College of Physicians [RCP], 2007). Non-melanoma skin cancer (NMSC) is relatively common (approximately 100,000 cases/year (Cancer Research UK, 2009b).

Placed within a policy context, the Department of Health (DH) aims to reduce by 20% the number of deaths from cancer in people below

75 years by 2010 (Department of Health, 2000, 2007). Half of all cancers may be prevented by promoting awareness and changes in lifestyle (DH, 2007); for skin cancer, this is a priority (Health Development Agency, 2002). The new government's *National Awareness and Early Diagnosis Initiative* supports local interventions to raise public awareness of cancer and seek help sooner (Cancer Research UK, 2009d).

Melanoma is a cancer which affects all adult age groups. Incidence rates are highest in people over 75 years, and whilst rare in young people; it is the second most common cancer diagnosed in 20–39 year olds (Cancer Research UK, 2009c). Men and women are often equally affected, but in some countries a slight female preponderance is seen (Karim-Kos *et al.*, 2008).

The incidence of melanoma is small compared to other cancers, with 9,583 new cases recorded in the UK in 2005 (Cancer Research UK, 2009a) but large increases have occurred over the last few decades. The number of people living with melanoma in the UK, known as the prevalence, is estimated to be between 24,500 and 31,000 (Forman *et al.*, 2003). Knowing the prevalence of a disease is important when planning future resources. A substantial number of deaths occur in younger people. It is predicted that the incidence of melanoma will continue to rise steeply, yet mortality rates will remain the same (Mackie, 2003).

Pre-malignant skin lesions

Common types of pre-malignant skin lesions

Actinic keratosis

Actinic keratosis (AK) or solar keratoses are pre-malignant skin lesion showing early changes of increase in keratosis (see Figure 11.1). AKs present as scaly, erythematous, hyperpigmented crusty lesions, predominantly in sun-exposed skin, often the back of the hands, face and scalp. They are very common in older

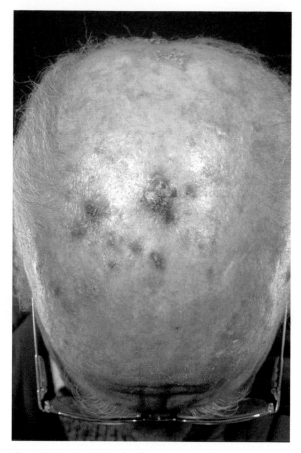

Figure 11.1 Actinic (solar) keratoses. (Source: Reprinted from Graham-Brown and Burns, 2006.)

people, and there is a high prevalence in patients receiving chronic immunosuppression such as organ transplant recipients. Evidence suggests that most AKs are the result of chronic exposure to ultraviolet (UV) light. A small percentage may have the potential to progress to squamous cell carcinoma (SCC) (de Berker *et al.*, 2007).

Bowen's disease

Bowen's disease usually presents as a single erythematous scaly patch or plaque on sun-exposed skin (see Figure 11.2). Bowen's disease is a form of intra-epidermal carcinoma *in situ*, which may progress to an invasive SCC and is also referred to as intra-epidermal SCC (Buchanan and Courtenay, 2006).

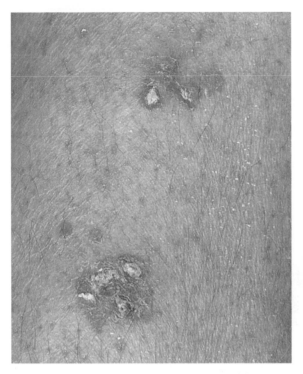

Figure 11.2 Bowen's disease. (Source: Reprinted from Graham-Brown and Burns, 2006.)

Diagnosis of pre-malignant skin lesions

Diagnosis is generally made on clinical examination. Differential diagnosis for AK may include superficial basal cell carcinoma (BCC), Bowen's disease, SCC and amelanotic melanoma. If there is any clinical doubt, a punch biopsy will be performed to confirm diagnosis (de Berker *et al.*, 2007).

Treatment of AK

Actinic keratosis and Bowen's disease are treated with topical or destructive treatment. Topical treatment may include emollients, sun blocks, salicylic acid ointment, topical non-steroidal anti-inflammatory agents (Diclofenac), topical cytostatic preparation (fluorouracil) and topical immune response modulators (Imiquimod). Topical treatment

recommendations from the British Photobiology Group (de Berker et al 2007) are outlined in Table 11.1.

Destructive treatments for AK may include cryotherapy, photodynamic therapy (PDT), surgery, laser chemical peels and dermabrasion.

Table 11.1 British Photobiology Groups recommendations for the topical treatment of AK.

Recommended AK topical therapy	Rationale for AK treatment
No therapy	21% AK respond spontaneously over 12 months.
Emollient therapy	Management of clinical manifestations only. Emollients do not reverse biological process.
Sun block	Long-term application is preventative against further AK development.
Salicylic acid	Removes overlying keratin and does not reverse biological process.
Diclofenac gel (Solaraze®)	Moderate efficacy for AK treatment and clearance of lesions, this treatment is well tolerated with minimal side effects. Application: Apply by smoothing cream into lesion twice daily until clearance (for up to 60–90 days).
Fluorouracil cream (Efudix®)	Good efficacy for AK treatment and clearance of lesions; this treatment is less well tolerated due to side effects of soreness. Application: Apply thinly once or twice a day until clearance.
Imiquimod (Aldara®)	Moderate efficacy for AK treatment and clearance of lesions; this treatment is less well tolerated due to side effects of pruritus and application site pain, burning and irritation. Application: Apply thrice a week, for 4 weeks, leave on skin for 8 hours and then wash off.

Source: Adapted from de Berker *et al.* (2007).

These therapies will be discussed in more detail in the non-melanoma section of this chapter.

Prevention of pre-malignant lesions and reoccurrence of AK

Evidence suggests the regular use of sunscreens reduces the number of AKs. Patients should be advised on sun protection measures and advised to regularly use and apply sunscreens (de Berker *et al.*, 2007).

Non-melanoma skin lesions

Basal cell carcinoma

Basal cell carcinoma (BCC) is also commonly referred to as a rodent ulcer or basalioma. BCC is the most common type of cancer in Europe, Australia and the US Caucasian population but it is rare in Africans, Afro-Caribbean and Asians; and extremely rare in oriental races. BCCs arise due to solar damage and ionising radiation; they also occur in burn scars and vaccination sites (Burns *et al.*, 2004). There is a worldwide increase in the incidence of BCCs, and the significant aetiological factors include a genetic predisposition and exposure to UV radiation (sun exposure in childhood is indicated). Other risk factors include: increasing age, males, fair skin types I and II, immunosuppression and arsenic exposure (Telfer *et al.*, 2008). The tendency to develop multiple BCCs is a feature of Gorlin syndrome (basal cell naevus syndrome).

BCC is defined as a malignant tumour, which rarely metastases and is composed of cells similar to those in the basal area of the epidermis and its appendages (Burns *et al.*, 2004) (see Figure 11.3). BCC is a slow growing but locally invasive tumour which infiltrates tissues through a three-dimensional growth pattern. BCCs will continue to develop and grow and may cause extended local tissue invasion and destruction,

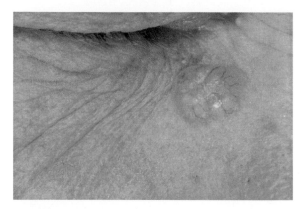

Figure 11.3 Basal cell carcinoma. (Source: Reprinted from Graham-Brown and Burns, 2006.)

particularly, on the face, head and neck (Telfer *et al.*, 2008).

Types of BCC

There are several types of BCC and classically they arise in skin of a normal appearance. They can also vary in size from a few millimetres to several centimetres in diameter. There are several different clinical presentations of BCC, which are outlined in Table 11.2 (DermNet NZ, 2009a).

Diagnosis and definition of high- and low-risk BCCs

BCCs are diagnosed by examining the suspect lesion in good light and with the optional aid of a dermatoscope. If clinical doubt exists, a punch biopsy may be performed. Imaging techniques may also be used where bony involvement is suspected (Telfer *et al.*, 2008). BCCs are treated with either surgery or other non-invasive techniques. The chosen treatment almost always results in a cure; although BCCs can reoccur at the same sites. Metastatic BCC is extremely rare and can be fatal; this involves a BCC that has spread to the lymph glands and other organs.

The British Association of Dermatologists (BAD) guidelines for the management of BCC

(Telfer *et al.*, 2008) recommend that high-risk BCCs, defined as those most likely to reoccur, are excised with predetermined margins or Mohs micrographic surgery is performed. High-risk BCCs also includes previous treatment failure and patients who are immunosuppressed. The features of high-risk BCCs are defined by the factors in Table 11.3.

Table 11.2 Different clinical presentations of BCC.

Nodular BCC	• Most common type on the face • Small, shiny, skin-coloured or pinkish lump • Blood vessels cross its surface • May have a central ulcer so its edges appear rolled • Often bleeds spontaneously then seem to heal over • Cystic BCC is soft, with jelly-like contents • Rodent ulcer is an open sore • Micronodular and microcystic types may infiltrate deeply
Superficial BCC	• Often multiple • Upper trunk and shoulders, or anywhere • Pink or red scaly irregular plaques • Slowly grow over months or years • Bleed or ulcerate easily
Morphoeic BCC	• Also known as sclerosing BCC • Usually found in mid-facial sites • Skin-coloured, waxy, scar-like • Prone to recur after treatment • May infiltrate cutaneous nerves (perineural spread)
Pigmented BCC	• Brown, blue or greyish lesion • Nodular or superficial histology • May resemble melanoma
Basisquamous BCC	• Mixed BCC and SCC • Potentially more aggressive than other forms of BCC

Source: Reproduced from DermNetNZ (2009a).

Table 11.3 Factors affecting the prognosis of BCC.

Tumour size
Tumour site
Tumour type and definition of tumour margins
Growth pattern/histological subtype
Failure of previous treatment (recurrent tumours)
Immunocompromised patients

Source: Reprinted from Telfer *et al.* (2008).

Treatment of BCC

Low-risk BCCs, tumours that do not confer with the features in Table 11.3, are generally treated with a variety of destructive surgery and non-surgical techniques.

Curettage and cautery and cryotherapy procedures may be used. Cryotherapy, although convenient and less expensive than surgery or radiotherapy, has poor cure rates in comparison with surgery and radiotherapy, especially for lesions greater than 2 cm; surgery also provides a better cosmetic effect (Bath-Hextall and Perkins, 2008). Carbon dioxide laser is an uncommon treatment with poor evidence to support its use. Non-surgical techniques include topical immunotherapy, PDT and radiotherapy.

Topical immunotherapy

There is a good evidence for using topical immunotherapy to treat primary and superficial BCC (Telfer *et al.*, 2008). Imiquimod is the only topical immunotherapy licensed for the BCCs but is not indicated for BCCs on the face (Electronic Medicines Compendium [EMC], 2009). Imiquimod cream is applied over the treatment area, including 1 cm of skin surrounding the BCC. Before applying Imiquimod cream, patients should wash the treatment area with mild soap and water and dry thoroughly. Sufficient cream should be applied once a day (at bedtime is ideal) and rubbed into the treatment area until the cream vanishes. Imiquimod cream remains on the skin for approximately 8 hours; showering and bathing should be avoided. After this period it is essential that Imiquimod cream is removed with mild soap and water, and the hands are washed thoroughly (EMC, 2009).

Imiquimod cream can be applied for 12 weeks and treatment response can then be assessed. If the treated tumour shows an incomplete response, a different therapy should be used. A rest period of several days may be taken if the local skin reaction to Imiquimod cream causes excessive discomfort to the patient, or if infection is observed at the treatment site. In the latter case, other appropriate measures should be taken (EMC, 2009).

During therapy and until healed, affected skin is likely to appear noticeably different from normal skin. Local skin reactions, such as pruritus, burning, irritation and pain on application site, are common but these reactions generally decrease in intensity during therapy or resolve after cessation of Imiquimod cream therapy (EMC, 2009).

Photodynamic therapy

Photodynamic therapy (PDT) is a procedure which causes a photochemical reaction within tumour cells due to the reaction with a photosensitising agent (methyl aminolevulinate cream), red light and cellular oxygen. This procedure destroys the targeted tumour cells by apoptosis and necrosis (Buchanan and Courtenay, 2006). PDT is indicated for superficial BCCs, Bowen's disease and AK. A PDT light source is used by a trained clinician within a dermatology clinic. The lesion is prepared by gentle decaling; a photosensitising agent is applied and several hours later (usually between 3 and 6 hours to allow the drug to concentrate in the cancer cells), the lesion is then illuminated with red light. Following treatment, the lesion site will form a scab, which will fall off after 3 weeks. More than one lesion can be treated in a session, and PDT can be repeated after a 4-week interval (National Institute for Health and Clinical Excellence [NICE], 2006b).

Radiotherapy

Radiotherapy is a less commonly used therapy to treat BCCs. It is effective for primary and recurrent BCC and is generally suitable for high-risk older patients who are unable to tolerate surgery. Good cosmetic results are achieved using superficial radiotherapy (generated at up to 170 kV) as once-weekly treatments for several weeks (Telfer *et al.*, 2008).

Prevention of BCC

Advice on sun protection and sunscreens is crucial, as people with BCCs have a high risk of developing further BCCs; also they have an increased risk of developing other skin cancers.

Patients should be advised to complete skin self-examination (SSE) and seek the opinion of a clinician if they have any suspected moles or other skin lesions.

Squamous cell carcinoma

Squamous cell carcinoma is defined as a malignant tumour arising from the keratinocytes of the epidermis (see Figure 11.4). SCC has the potential to metastasise; spread is almost always by the lymphatic route (Burns *et al.*, 2004). Unlike BCCs, SCCs do not often arise in healthy skin and usually present as an indurated nodular keratinising or crusted tumour, or as an ulcer without the evidence of keratinisation. SCC is the second most common skin cancer, and the incidence has been rising since the 1960s (Preston, 1992). Aetiology is usually related to chronic UV light exposure, especially in fair-skinned individuals, those with albinism or xeroderma pigmentosum. SCC may also develop as a result of previous exposure to ionising radiation, arsenic; or within chronic wounds, scars, burns or from pre-existing lesions, such as Bowen's disease (Motley *et al.*, 2002).

Diagnosis of SCC

The diagnosis of SCC is generally established by histology. Punch biopsies will be performed to provide a tissue sample, which will be assessed by histology and a report produced outlining the pathological pattern (e.g. adenoid type),

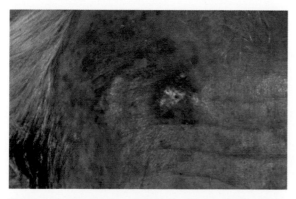

Figure 11.4 Squamous cell carcinoma. (Source: Reprinted from Buxton and Morris-Jones, 2009.)

cell morphology (e.g. spindle cell SCC), degree of differentiation (e.g. poorly or well differentiated) and the histological grade. SCC grading is by Borders' classification system; grades 1, 2 and 3 denote ratios of differentiated to undifferentiated cells (Motley *et al.*, 2002).

Treatment of SCC

The treatment of choice for all resectable SCCs is surgical excision; Mohs surgery is recommended for high risk and recurrent SCCs. Small and well-defined, low-risk SCCs are generally treated by curettage and cautery or cryotherapy. Radiotherapy may be indicated for non-resectable tumours (Motley *et al.*, 2002).

Prevention of SCC

Patients with SCCs require follow-up for recurrent skin cancer. Patients should be instructed in self-examination. Early detection and treatment improves patient survival from recurrent disease. Ninety-five percent of local recurrences and 95% of metastases are detected within 5 years (Motley *et al.*, 2002).

Cutaneous T-cell lymphoma

Lymphomas are generally carcinomas of the lymphatic system; however, lymphomas can occur in the skin with no evidence of disease elsewhere. They are referred to as primary T-cell lymphomas and account for 65% of lymphoma's affecting the skin. Cutaneous T-cell lymphomas (CTCL) refer to a serious but uncommon skin condition in which there is an abnormal neoplastic proliferation of lymphocytes with a 'T' subtype (thymus derived).

Mycosis fungoides

Mycosis fungoides is the most common type of CTCL presenting as patches or lumps composed of white cells called lymphocytes. It generally follows a low-grade clinical course, often persisting slowly over years in a patch stage, then slowly progressing to the tumour stage (DermNet NZ, 2009b) (see Chapter 13 for further detail).

Primary cutaneous CD30+ lymphoproliferative disorders

This is the second most common group of CTCL and accounts for about 30% of all CTCL cases. This group includes primary cutaneous anaplastic large cell lymphoma, which presents as solitary or localised nodules or tumours. Prognosis is usually good but there may be regional lymph node involvement for 10% of patients. The other common type in this group is lymphomatoid papulosis, with lesions occurring predominantly on the trunk and limbs; they clear spontaneously but may scar (DermNet NZ, 2009b).

Sézary syndrome

Sézary syndrome (sometimes referred to as 'red man syndrome') is the name given when T-cell lymphoma affects the skin of the entire body. The skin is also thickened, dry or scaly and usually very itchy. Examination usually reveals the presence of neoplastic T cells (Sézary cells) in skin, lymph nodes and peripheral blood. The prognosis of Sézary syndrome is generally poor with a median survival between 2 and 4 years; infection caused by immunosuppression is the main cause of death (DermNet NZ, 2009b).

Treatment of CTCL

Treatments of CTCL depend on the tumour, site, stage, distribution, age and general health of the patient. Various treatments may include topical steroids, phototherapy, photophoresis, topical nitrogen mustard, chemotherapy, radiotherapy, interferons and oral retinoids.

Introduction to melanoma

Melanoma is a rare type of skin cancer which affects all age groups. Although melanoma is the major cause of skin cancer mortality, it is usually curable if detected and treated at an early stage (Scottish Intercollegiate Guidelines Network [SIGN], 2009).

What is melanoma?

Melanoma occurs after the malignant transformation of melanocytes (Barnhill *et al.*, 1993). The melanocyte is a skin cell, which is found in the epidermis. Its most important physiological function is to produce melanin, one of the pigments responsible for skin colour. This helps to protect the skin from damage caused by UV radiation from the sun. Most melanocytes are found in the skin and it is for this reason that most melanomas are known as cutaneous melanomas (see Figure 11.5).

At first melanomas grow horizontally. The basement membrane, a barrier separating the epidermis from the dermis, acts as a mechanical barrier, preventing the melanoma from invading deeper into the skin. Early stages of melanoma that are limited to the epidermis are called melanoma *in situ* and are curable. If the melanoma cells grow vertically through the basement membrane to the dermis, it is known as an 'invasive' melanoma.

The depth that the melanoma grows into the skin provides important prognostic information. The measurement, known as the Breslow thickness, is taken from the granular layer of the epidermis to the base of the tumour (Roberts *et al.*, 2002) and is measured in millimetres with a small ruler called a micrometer (see Figure 11.6). The greater the Breslow thickness, the greater the chance the cancer may spread to other areas of the body via the lymphatic or blood stream.

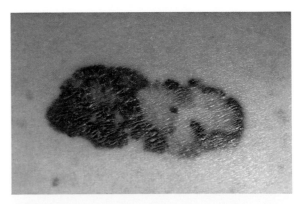

Figure 11.5   Cutaneous melanoma. (Source: Reprinted from Graham-Brown and Burns, 2006.)

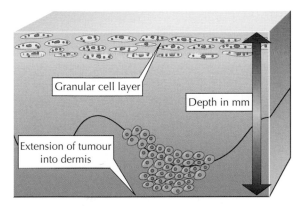

Figure 11.6 Breslow thickness. (Source: Reprinted from Graham-Brown and Burns, 2006.)

Type of melanoma

Melanomas are categorised according to clinical and pathological parameters into four main types: superficial spreading melanoma, nodular melanoma, acral lentiginous melanoma and lentigo maligna melanoma.

Superficial spreading melanoma is the most common type, accounting for approximately 70% (Cancer Research UK, 2009c). This type often grows slowly over a period of months or years and approximately 50% of patients will give a history of a pre-existing apparently benign lesion. The classic clinical presenting features include an irregular lateral margin, irregular multicoloured central pigmentation and a history of growth (Mackie, 2000). They are commonly found on the trunk in men and the leg in women, and patients are often in their fourth or fifth decade of life.

The second most common type is nodular melanoma. These often present as raised lesions which bleed easily and are ulcerated. Although often dark in colour, they may be colourless or amelanotic. Lentigo maligna melanoma tends to occur on the face of elderly patients with extensive chronic sun damage. Lentigo maligna melanoma should not be confused with lentigo maligna, a type of melanoma *in situ*. Acral lentiginous melanoma, whilst rare, is the most common type of melanoma seen in Asians and people with dark skin. It is often found on the palms, soles, under fingernails and toenails and can affect mucous membranes.

Risk factors

Melanoma occurs most commonly in fair-skinned persons, especially those with a history of significant sun exposure. Whilst sun exposure is thought to be a risk factor for melanoma, the relationship is not straightforward. The exact cause of melanoma is not known. Patients often have freckles, red hair and tan poorly. Having multiple naevi is a powerful predictor of risk of melanoma.

Cutaneous melanoma can occur anywhere on the skin. Most frequently it is found on the leg in women (particularly between the knee and ankle) and on the trunk (especially the back) in men. In elderly people, melanomas develop most commonly on the face (Austoker, 1994). Figure 11.7 depicts the distribution of melanoma on parts of the body by sex.

Diagnosis of primary melanoma

As primary melanomas are clearly visible on the surface of the skin, most melanomas are first detected by the patient or a spouse examining the skin and then bought to the attention of the GP. The three major features of melanoma (in terms of diagnostic importance) in a skin lesion are as follows: (1) a change in size of the lesion, (2) the presence of an irregular outline or edge around the lesion and (3) the presence of three or more colours within the lesion. Other minor signs include a lesion with a diameter greater than 7 mm, inflammation, oozing or a change in sensation.

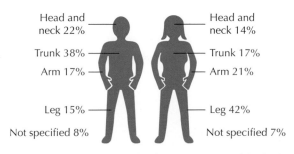

Head and neck 22% Head and neck 14%
Trunk 38% Trunk 17%
Arm 17% Arm 21%
Leg 15% Leg 42%
Not specified 8% Not specified 7%

Figure 11.7 Distribution of melanoma on parts of the body by sex. (Source: Cancer Research UK, 2009a.)

The ABCDE guidance formula is another commonly used clinical guide for the diagnosis of early melanoma; see Box 11.1.

It is recommended that patients with a lesion suspicious of melanoma are referred to a doctor trained in the specialist diagnosis of skin cancer, normally a dermatologist (National Institute for Health and Clinical Excellence, 2006a). In England, it is a requirement for patients to be seen within 2 weeks of referral, as early diagnosis and treatment represents the best chance of cure (Department of Health, 2006). In order to meet this target set out in the National Cancer Plan (2000), most hospitals have designated skin cancer clinics.

At the skin cancer clinic an assessment will be undertaken; a clinical history will be ascertained, and the lesion examined, often with the aid of a dermatoscope (see Chapter 3). Suspicious lesions should be biopsied with a 2 mm margin of skin often using a local rather than general anaesthetic promptly. The National Cancer Plan (Department of Health, 2000) provides details on the referral arrangements.

A record of the patients treatment plan agreed by the multidisciplinary team (MDT) whose core members should include a dermatologist, a plastic surgeon, a histopathologist, a specialist nurse, a radiotherapist and an MDT coordinator (Department of Health, 2000) should be recorded in the patient's notes.

Treatment of primary melanoma

Following a histological examination of the suspicious lesion, the treatment for primary cutaneous melanoma is wide local excision under local or general anaesthetic (Roberts *et al.*, 2002). The purpose of this treatment is to minimise the risk of local recurrence. The excision margins specified in the UK Guidelines (Roberts *et al.*, 2002) are determined by the Breslow thickness of the lesion, as described and depicted earlier (Figure 11.6).

At the same time, a sentinel lymph node biopsy (SLNB) may be performed in patients with thick tumours in order to discover if the melanoma has spread from the skin to the lymph nodes. The sentinel lymph node(s), the first lymph node to which cancer may have metastasised, is identified by injecting a blue dye or a radioactive material, or both, into the skin at the site of the primary melanoma. The surgeon then uses a scanner to find the lymph node(s) containing the radioactive substance or looks for the lymph node(s) stained with dye. The lymph nodes are surgically removed and examined histologically. If the sentinel lymph node contains metastatic melanoma, then the surrounding lymph nodes are often removed during a subsequent procedure known as a lymphadenectomy. Whilst there is no proof to date that SLNB leads to an overall survival benefit for all patients, it is an accepted staging procedure. Its availability to patients is not standardised across the UK.

Adjuvant treatments

Adjuvant treatment can be defined as any treatment in addition to surgery which may reduce the risk of recurrence. There is currently none of proven benefit (Roberts *et al.*, 2002) but patients should be referred for entry into clinical trials, examples of which include bevacizumab (AVAST-M).

Follow-up

It is recommended that patients are followed up 'to reduce morbidity and mortality through the detection of metastatic disease and other primary melanomas' (Sober *et al.*, 2001, p. 6). It is estimated that 4–8% of patients diagnosed

---

Box 11.1   ABCDE guidance to the recognition of melanoma

- A = Asymmetry
- B= Border
- C= Colour
- D= Diverse structure
- E= Elevation

with a primary melanoma may develop a further primary melanoma within the first 3–5 years following diagnosis (Levi *et al.*, 2005). It is suggested that 'all patients with invasive melanoma should be followed up at three monthly intervals, for three years. Thereafter patients with melanomas less than 1.0 mm thick may be discharged but others should be reviewed 6 monthly for a further two years' (Roberts *et al.*, 2002).

Physical examination, by a health professional, is the mainstay of follow-up interventions. The site of the primary tumour and the adjacent skin should be examined for local recurrences and local metastatic disease; the draining lymph node basins should be examined for lymphadenopathy; and the remaining skin should be examined for other suspicious lesions such as other primary melanoma (Roberts *et al.*, 2002). Routine investigations, such as blood tests and X-rays, contribute little to recurrence detection (Kersey *et al.*, 1995), as most melanoma recurrences produce symptoms or can be found by physical examination.

Metastatic melanoma

Melanoma can spread to virtually any organ or tissue such as the skin, subcutaneous tissue, lymph nodes, lung, gastrointestinal tract, liver, bone and brain (Essner, 2001). The majority occurs in the first 3 years after diagnosis (Shumate *et al.*, 1995; Poo-Hwu *et al.*, 1999). Many of the first metastases, after treatment of the primary tumour, develop in the regional lymph nodes or in the skin close to or at the site of the primary tumour (McCarthy *et al.*, 1988; Dickers *et al.*, 1999).

Skin metastases often present as nodules but they may be inflammatory, cicatrical or bullous lesions (Lookingbill *et al.*, 1993). They are normally flesh coloured, although they may be red, purple, brown or black and about a third are pigmented or ulcerated (Evans *et al.*, 2003). Often round or oval in appearance, they can be non-tender, non-painful, solid, firm or rubbery in texture (Strohl, 1998). They can be moveable or fixed and vary in size and may present as single or multiple nodules in the skin (Strohl,

1998). Skin metastases can be found by palpation and visual examination, and diagnosis is most commonly confirmed by histological analysis following a biopsy: needle, incisional or excisional (Balch *et al.*, 1994).

Lymph nodes are oval- or bean-shaped structures, found scattered throughout the body in groups, located along the length of the lymphatic system (Tortora and Derrickson, 2005). Lymph nodes containing metastatic melanoma are generally more firm and rubbery, and are non-tender compared with inflammatory nodes, which are usually softer, more resilient and tender (Balch *et al.*, 1994). Lymph nodes can therefore be found by palpation but diagnosis is confirmed by histological analysis following a biopsy: needle, incisional or excisional (Balch *et al.*, 1994).

The signs and symptoms of distant metastases to the lungs, liver, bone or brain depend on the site of relapse and on whether they are at single or multiple sites. Metastatic disease remains relatively resistant to current treatments with dacarbazine (an alkylating agent) being the current single chemotherapy agent of choice (Roberts and Crosby 2008).

Survival

To allow the health professional to identify those patients most at risk of developing metastases, offer prognostic information to patients and their families and to compare treatment results, the American Joint Committee on Cancer (AJCC) melanoma staging system classifies patients' disease into tumour (T), regional lymph nodes (N) and distant metastases (M) (Kim *et al.*, 2002). From this classification, melanomas are grouped into four stages, stages I–IV.

In Stage I and II, patients have a primary tumour but there is no evidence that the cancer has spread to the lymph nodes or distantly. Patients have favourable overall survival outcomes of up to 95% (Kim *et al.*, 2002) (AJCC). Although patient age, site of the primary melanoma, level of invasion of the tumour and gender have been identified as prognostic factors, tumour thickness and the presence of ulceration of the lesion are the most powerful predictors of survival in patients in Stage I and II (Balsh *et al.*, 2001). The 7th edition of the AJCC melanoma staging system will be published in the spring of 2009 and it is likely that the number of mitoses per square millimetre will also be included as an independent prognostic predictor.

The strongest indicator of survival is tumour thickness: the thinner the Breslow thickness, the better the prognosis (Table 11.4). Most patients diagnosed with melanoma have thin tumours. A total of 57.8% of patients in the South Australian Cancer registry from 1994 to 2000 had tumours ≤0.75 mm in thickness (Luke *et al.*, 2003). Ulceration of the primary tumour carries a worse prognosis compared to non-ulcerated lesions.

In Stage III, patients have developed a lymph node metastasis or intransit/satellite lesion but have no distant metastases. The number of metastatic nodes, tumour burden and the presence and absence of melanoma ulceration are the most powerful predictors of survival in Stage III disease patients. In Stage IV disease, patients have developed distant metastases with the anatomic site of these metastases being the most significant predictor of survival (Kim *et al.*, 2002). Patients with metastases in visceral sites have a poorer prognosis compared with those with metastases at non-visceral sites (i.e. skin, subcutaneous and distant lymph nodes) (Kim *et al.*, 2002).

Psychological impact of a diagnosis of skin cancer and the role of the CNS

A diagnosis of cancer can be one of the most devastating events of a person's life (Buckman, 1996). An individual's emotional response to hearing that they have cancer may be complex and include an array of emotions such as anxiety, shock, anger, denial, fear and uncertainty (Van der Molen, 1999). Until recently, little has been known about the specific impact of the diagnosis of skin cancer and the specific needs of this client group, but an audit undertaken through the use of focus groups of patients with melanoma found that many patients reported feelings of shock and blankness when learning of the diagnosis (Wright *et al.*, 2004). The way in which the diagnosis is communicated can affect the individual's adjustment to the disease and his or her attitude to treatment (Buckman, 1996). It is therefore recommended that health professionals, including the CNS who should be present during this consultation, who inform patients that they have skin cancer have attended a communication skills course (National Institute for Health and Clinical Excellence, 2006a).

Table 11.4 Illustration of a 5-year survival rates for patients diagnosed with cutaneous melanoma at each stage.

	IA	IB	IIA	IIB	IIC	IIIA	IIIB	IIIC
Ta: Non-ulcerated melanoma	T1a 95%	T2a 92%	T3a 79%	T4a 67%		N1a N2a 67%	N1b N2b 54%	N3 28%
Tb: Ulcerated melanoma		T1b 91%	T2b 77%	T3b 63%	T4b 45%		N1a N2a 52%	N1b N2b N3 24%

Source: Kim *et al.* (2002) and American Joint Committee on Cancer (2002).

The CNS plays a vital role in supporting patients with skin cancer; a role recognised by NICE (National Institute for Health and Clinical Excellence, 2006a) in the *Manual for Improving Outcomes for People with Skin Tumours including Melanoma*. Often the CNS will be designated the patient's 'key worker' who co-ordinates their care across many disciplines and thus acts as a permanent fixture in their journey. To help the CNS identify the most 'at risk' patients and provide the appropriate intervention, Perkins (1993) describes four psychosocial phases. The first two are important at the time of diagnosis. During psychosocial Phase 1, known as the existential crisis, acute anxiety is often experienced due to a poor knowledge of melanoma and 'anticipatory grief due to the fear of dying'. During this phase, the CNS may reduce the patient's anxiety by providing information. The need for information appears greatest at the time of diagnosis. Whilst the type of information required varies according to the stage of the patient (Bonevski *et al.*, 1999), information pertaining to diagnosis, test results and treatment, risk of recurrence, life expectancy, effect of the disease on work and family life is most desired (Bonevski *et al.*, 1999; Schofield *et al.*, 2001).

Nationally produced written materials by 'Cancerbacup' (Macmillan Cancer Support, 2009), Cancer Research UK (Cancer Help; Cancer Research UK, 2009e), 'Marc's Line' (Melanoma and Related Cancers of the Skin) (Wessex Cancer Trust, 2004) and the British Association of Dermatologists (2009) provide generic information. However, information outlining local services, including names of key personnel and contact details, and relevant and local and national support groups should be provided (National Institute for Health and Clinical Excellence, 2006a). The offer and acceptance of written information should always be recorded in the patient's notes. In addition, a permanent record of the consultation at which treatment options were discussed should be offered (NICE, 2006a). Whilst it is recommended that patients should receive targeted information throughout their cancer journey (SIGN, 2003), this can be difficult to achieve since patients with skin cancer make few visits for diagnosis and treatment, many of which are brief outpatient visits. An alternative means of providing information may be via structured information programmes whereby patients diagnosed with melanoma are invited to participate in a group meeting such as that described by Brandberg *et al.* (1996).

To help patients to deal with 'anticipatory grief due to the fear of dying' suggested by Perkins (1993), the CNS may help by offering simple interventions such as signposting patients to relevant self-help groups, facilitate emotional disclosure, listening and responding to their worries and concerns and helping them to normalise their experiences (Thompson, 2009). The CNS should ascertain individual patient's coping styles and teach appropriate coping strategies if appropriately trained to do so. A randomized control trial of patients with melanoma found that a 6-week structured, psychiatric group intervention improved outcomes in terms of affective states and coping style at 6 weeks follow-up and at 6 months follow-up (Fawzy *et al.*, 1990). A later study by Fawzy *et al.* (2003) found that a 6-week structured, psychiatric group intervention which included health education was associated with a survival advantage, after adjusting for gender and Breslow thickness.

In the second psychosocial phase (Phase 2), referred to as accommodation and mitigation, 'patients feel physically healthy, yet are constantly living with the fear that the disease may return' (Perkins, 1993, p. 162). Nationally organised support, specific to patients with a diagnosis of melanoma, is limited to a telephone support, 'Marc's Line' and therefore many patients rely on the CNS whom they are likely to have established a good report with. Those who are identified as struggling to come to terms with their diagnosis should be referred to an appropriate individual within the extended skin cancer team such as the clinical psychologist.

Surgery

Surgical excision is the recommended treatment for all primary melanoma and most NMSC, although various non-surgical treatments are appropriate for some NMSC subtypes. Pre-operative assessment should include whether the patient has allergies to latex and whether they are on medications, such as anticoagulants, steroids or aspirin.

Written consent prior to the procedure is essential. Most common post-operative complications include bleeding, infection and scarring. Surgery is most often carried out using a local rather than a general anaesthetic most often as day case by trained dermatologists or plastic surgeons, although occasionally, very complex surgery as an in-patient may be required. Primary surgery for melanoma involves a number of stages. Initially, a biopsy including a narrow margin of normal skin is taken and the resulting defect can almost always be closed directly. After analysis of the biopsy, a wider excision may need to be performed according to the thickness of the tumour in the biopsy and the resulting defect can often be closed directly but the size or anatomical site of some defects may dictate the use of skin flaps or skin grafts. Increasingly, sentinel node biopsy, a procedure whereby the first draining lymph gland is removed, is performed at the same time as wider excision of a melanoma in order to provide extra prognostic information about the patient. This is performed by specifically trained surgeons only and usually as part of a clinical trial.

The same reconstructive ladder applies to NMSC and these tumours are most commonly treated at a single operation. Following the procedure, patients need to be provided with written instructions to assist them in caring for their wound, provide them with information about suture removal and care of grafts and flaps in post-operative period. A number of patients will have surgery that will result in disfigurement particularly if it involves the head and neck area. Sustained psychological support is essential both before and after the treatment to enable patients to adjust psychologically and socially to their disfigurement and to develop coping strategies (NICE, 2006a). After the surgery, patients may need access to prosthetic, camouflage and lymphoedema services.

Causation, risk prevention and early detection

The Department of Health (DH) aims to reduce cancer deaths in patients below 75 years by 20% by 2010 (Department of Health, 1999, 2000b, 2007). At least half of all cancers are preventable by promoting awareness and changing lifestyle (DH, 2007), especially skin cancer (Health Development Agency, 2002).

The International Cancer (International Cancer Research Funding Organisations, 2008) highlights US educational prevention research with young people. Although childhood sun exposure is an important preventable factor, since risk develops in childhood (Armstrong and Kricker, 2001) through genetic mutation and learnt risk behaviour, educating this group remains problematic. Adolescents continue to seek exposure to secure a tan (e.g. Melia *et al.*, 2000; Cokkinides *et al.*, 2002). Recent qualitative evidence suggests that in young women sun-related behaviours are complex but their activities in the sun are directed towards meeting their physical and psychological comfort needs and not health protection (Norton, 2008). A review argues that prevention is also valuable later in life, especially for those with high childhood sun exposure (Armstrong and Kricker, 2001). Achieving attitude and UV-protective behaviour in adults, who may be parents, may result in good practice being passed to children (parental risk-behaviour predicts that by young people; Cokkinides *et al.*, 2002). However, adults received limited attention in preventive studies.

Attitudes and behavioural change

Limited knowledge and unsafe sun practices continue in the UK (Miles *et al.*, 2005; Office of National Statistics, 2009). Research is required to promote and evaluate behavioural change to prevent cancer and promote early detection (National Cancer Research Institute, 2005). The *SunSmart* campaign aims to achieve this by 'action ... to inform and empower patients so that they can play an active role in decisions', but delivery models other than UV-awareness campaigns are not detailed (Department of Health, 2007; Cancer Research UK, 2009f). A review of evidence of primary care prevention proposes due caution when drawing from US/Australian strategies (Melia *et al.*, 2000). Melanoma prevention guidelines advise sun-avoidance and effective sunscreen/clothing use (Royal College of Physicians, 2007).

Using theory on effective behaviour change is likely to maximise the effectiveness of lifestyle interventions (Berwick *et al.*, 2000; National Institute for Health and Clinical Excellence, 2007). Research applying the *Self-efficacy Theory* (Bandura, 1996, 1997) highlights it as an important predictor of healthy behaviours (Havas *et al.*, 1998; Rosal *et al.*, 1998; Clark and Dodge, 1999). Ajzen's *Theory of Planned Behaviour* (Ajzen, 1991, 2001) is the most widely applied model of beliefs, attitudes and intentions that precede action (Connor and Sparks, 2005).

Nursing intervention and promoting self-examination

Evidence suggests primary care nurses can reduce cancer risk by promoting early detection/ referral (Austoker, 1994; Taylor and Roberts, 1997; Oliveria *et al.*, 2002). Nurses are a substantial health education resource (Bradford and Winn, 1997; Latter *et al.*, 2000; Runciman *et al.*, 2006). Studies of nurse-led interventions to increase cancer awareness or change behaviour have been successful (e.g. Koinberg *et al.*, 2004; Sharp and Tischelman, 2005). However, most initiatives have not been applied to skin cancer prevention, involve self-examination only (e.g. Oliveria *et al.*, 2002), have a limited theory base and do not evaluate education to reduce risk behaviour (Oliveria *et al.*, 2004).

A systematic review by Saraiya *et al.* (2004) argues for research focused on health outcome, patient behaviour and the 'role of the non-physician provider to help identify if counselling skills to change behaviour might be better suited to providers with the time and skills, such as a nurse' (p. 444); however, there is little evidence of such

studies. Also, resource-efficient models of service delivery are required for primary care. Nurses can effectively increase self-efficacy in targeted patient telephone interventions (Wong *et al.*, 2005) with review evidence finding these safe and acceptable (Bunn *et al.*, 2004).

This section focuses on self-examination for primary disease; however, it also embraces self-examination for metastatic disease. The literature primarily focuses on the former, not the latter. Since primary and secondary prevention are key nursing roles, these are covered in some detail.

Do patients perform self-examination correctly?

Patients' ability to perform self-examination correctly has not been assessed previously. The UK national guidelines (Roberts *et al.*, 2002) do not clearly specify what would constitute a competent SSE. Specific body sites should be examined and there is a need to search for both metastatic disease and other primary melanomas should be.

For competence to be achieved, an individual must possess the appropriate knowledge and skills, be confident to perform the skill safely and trust their own ability to perform the skill without direct supervision. Elements were taken from the definition of competence used by Roach (1992). Whilst it is purported that females in the general population are more knowledgeable about melanoma then men (Bourke *et al.*, 1995; Miller *et al.*, 1996; Melia *et al.*, 2000), the only insight pertaining to the level of knowledge possessed by patients actually diagnosed with melanoma comes from a small retrospective study by Regan *et al.* (1995). Here, patients 'did not clearly know why the examination was being performed or what was being searched for' (p. 13) during self-examination even after regularly submitting to the clinical examination at follow-up. However, if metastases were detected, patients did recognise the importance of their find and reported it: 50% contacted their GP; 28% contacted the hospital; but 22% waited for the next outpatient appointment. Knowledge of skin changes and abnormalities has been found to reduce individuals delay in seeking medical attention for melanoma (Oliveria *et al.*, 1999a). Confidence to carry out SSE for primary skin lesions has been found to be poor (Carli *et al.*, 2002). It is not known how confident individuals diagnosed with melanoma feel to perform self-examination or to detect metastatic disease. The level of trust placed in the hospital health professional and in themselves to perform self-examination is also not known. From the limited literature available on patient's knowledge, confidence and trust, it is impossible to conclude if patients are able to perform self-examination correctly.

Factors which may encourage or inhibit the performance of self-examination

There is little evidence to suggest which factors may encourage individuals to perform self-examination, for metastatic melanoma. A review of the literature on SSE, which is advocated for the detection of primary skin cancer, including melanoma, and the detection of primary melanoma, suggests that many factors may be involved. It is acknowledged that the factors which may encourage or deter an individual from performing self-examination, to detect primary disease, may be different from those involved in the detection of metastatic disease.

Socio-demographic factors

In SSE, several socio-demographic factors such as gender, age, educational attainment, marital status and cohabitation have been investigated. Females are more likely to self-detect their melanoma (Weinstock *et al.*, 1999; Brady *et al.*, 2000) and have been found to perform SSE for primary disease more often than males (Girgis *et al.*, 1991; Hill *et al.*, 1991; Berwick *et al.*, 1996; Miller *et al.*, 1996; Robinson *et al.*, 1998). Similarities in both genders have however also been found (Robinson *et al.*, 2002). Men are more likely to present with melanomas located on the back (Hanrahan *et al.*, 1998). Individuals with melanomas on non-visible areas may incur difficulties in both detecting the primary tumour and performing self-examination. In addition, men are also

less knowledgeable about melanoma and have less favourable attitudes (Brandberg *et al.*, 1996; Miller *et al.*, 1996). The psychological approaches to danger posed by melanoma may be different for men and women (Robinson *et al.*, 2002).

Age and educational attainment have been found to both encourage and discourage the performance of self-examination (Girgis *et al.*, 1991; Friedman *et al.*, 1993; Balanda *et al.*, 1994; Robinson *et al.*, 1998; Oliveria *et al.*, 1999b). Elderly patients have a lower rate of detection compared to younger people and are more likely to be diagnosed with thicker tumours which have a poorer prognosis (Roder *et al.*, 1995). This may result from a failure to identify changes to melanoma more often than younger patients (Hanrahan *et al.*, 1998) or as a result of a less frequent inspection of their skin compared to younger people.

Surprisingly, Miller *et al.* (1996) found that elderly patients are more likely to do self-examinations. In primary disease, patients with a low median educational attainment are more likely to present later, whilst those from more affluent areas generally have thinner melanomas at the time of detection (Bonett *et al.*, 1989; Roder *et al.*, 1995). Patients with melanoma with a lower socioeconomic status are more likely to die of their disease (Vagero and Persson, 1984). Lower socioeconomic status has also been associated with less knowledge and awareness of melanoma. Research by Koh *et al.* (1996) confirms the importance of having a spouse in detecting many primary melanomas. In their study, a spouse was the third most common person (after the index patient and a physician) to detect a melanoma. Having a spouse or partner may provide encouragement or help to carry out the procedure (Brady *et al.*, 2000). This may be especially important when examining inaccessible areas since it has been reported that melanoma arising on more visible body areas are more likely to be diagnosed at an early stage (Hemo *et al.*, 1999). Higher rates of self-examination have been found in those married or cohabitating (Balanda *et al.*, 1994).

Physical factors

A direct plea from a health professional to a patient instructing them to perform self-examination may be a prime motivator (Weinstock *et al.*, 1999). It is suggested that 'by directly informing patients of their risk of the development of melanoma and skin cancer during health care visits, physicians or nurses can promote SSE' (Robinson *et al.*, 1998, p. 755). The literature does not describe which person is best to make this plea or teach self-examination, although both hospital medical and nursing staff may be involved (Poo-Hwu *et al.*, 1999). Persson *et al.* (1995) suggest that this individual should however be trusted by the individual receiving the request. Previously highlighted as important beneficial factors are the following: having heard or read about self-examination (Petro-Nustus and Mikhail, 2002); possessing knowledge (Champion, 1991); (Hajii-Mahmoodi *et al.*, 2002; Jirojwong and MacLennan, 2003) and being motivated (Petro-Nustus and Mikhail, 2002).

The number of visits made to the health professional has been shown to be associated with increased performance of self-examination (Robinson *et al.*, 2002) and attendance at the outpatient clinic has been found to be strongly associated with the practice of SSE for both females and males (Oliveria *et al.*, 1999a). It may provide an opportunity for health professionals to reinforce the importance of self-examination and to promote skin awareness for it is known that behaviours that are reinforced are more likely to be repeated (Redman, 1997). Weinstock *et al.* (1999) reported that one of the reasons given by the general public for not performing self-examination was simply not thinking about it. Having the skin of the body purposely looked at by a health professional, during the physical examination, may be an important factor (Weinstock *et al.*, 1999). It may also act as a reminder.

Knowledge of self-examination and feeling confident are important in encouraging an individual to perform self-examination (Celentano and Holtzman, 1983). Having a high level of confidence in performance was one of the three strongest predictors of SSE, although the measurement used to measure this independent variable was not described (Robinson *et al.*, 2002).

Psychological factors

Earlier in this chapter, the phases of reactions to diagnosis of cancer were highlighted (Perkins, 1993); these psychological effects have relevance to behaviour related to self-examination. During psychosocial Phase 1 (existential crisis), acute anxiety is often experienced due to a poor knowledge of melanoma and 'anticipatory grief'. However, it is argued that some anxiety may cause the individual to act (Redman, 1997) and therefore promote the performance of self-examination. However, extreme anxiety or distress may inhibit patients from 'seeking' professional advice and following through with recommendations (Trask *et al.*, 2001). Perkins (1993) suggests that by recognising key psychosocial phases, health professionals may identify the most 'at risk' patients and provide the appropriate intervention.

Patients who are well informed about melanoma and their risk of metastases, and therefore, 'have a concern for their disease or perceive themselves susceptible to developing cancer may be better able to look after themselves and engage in appropriate self care' (Brown *et al.*, 2000, p. 1148). It has been reported that one of the reasons given by the general public for not performing self-examination was that they did not believe it to be necessary (Weinstock *et al.*, 1999). Patient's perceived risk to developing metastases and understanding of melanoma and the purpose of self-examination, particularly Breslow thickness, is not known. In addition, a belief that self-examination is important may also be required (Rosella, 1994). In Phase 2, referred to as accommodation and mitigation, 'patients feel physically healthy, yet are constantly living with the fear that the disease may return' (Perkins, 1993, p. 162). Self-examination may assist individuals to keep their fears in check. The emotions experienced by individuals before, during and after self-examination are not known. In both breast cancer (Persson *et al.*, 1995) and testicular cancer (Cook, 2000), it is suggested that patients may experience feelings of fear and anxiety when performing self-examination since it involves trying to find something suspicious (Frank and Mai, 1985; Rutledge and Davis, 1988; Persson *et al.*, 1995). Women described that they would be terrified if they found a lump during breast self-examination (Persson *et al.*, 1995). This may discourage its performance. In contrast, it is speculated that the regular practice of self-examination could reassure individuals and therefore reduce anxiety, if no evidence of metastases were found (Best *et al.*, 1996). Thus the performance of self-examination would be encouraged. Whilst as mentioned, Phases 1 and 2 are relevant to those diagnosed with primary disease, in Phase 3 recurrence of the disease occurs. This can be a time of great anxiety for the patient and their family since there are fewer treatment options available. In Phase 4, there is general deterioration and decline as the disease advances. The goal here is the palliation of symptoms.

Teaching of self-examination for metastatic disease

Metastases may become apparent in between hospital visit (Basseres *et al.*, 1995) and may occur many years after the initial diagnosis when follow-up visits at the hospital have ceased (Kelly *et al.*, 1985). Patients can find recurrences (Dickers *et al.*, 1999) and therefore it is advised that they should be taught how to examine their own skin. Whilst many patients who have been taught how to perform self-examination do carry out the health professional's request, often they do not have the necessary knowledge or skills to do so competently as a consequence of current teaching methods (Duncan, 2005). An MDT approach to teaching using innovative aids is suggested (Duncan, 2005). Self-examination should be reinforced at each outpatient appointment and appropriate written materials provided, i.e. 'How to check your lymph nodes' (Wessex Cancer Trust, 2004).

Sun prevention activities

The UK national skin cancer prevention programme *SunSmart* was launched in 2003 and is commissioned by the UK Health Departments and run by Cancer Research UK. SunSmart provides evidence-based information about skin cancer and sun protection and can be accessed at http://info.cancerresearchuk.org/healthyliving/sunsmart (Cancer Research UK, 2009f) (see Box 11.2).

Sunscreens and SPF

Sunscreens can be both chemical absorbers and physical blockers. Chemical absorbers work by absorbing UV radiation and can be further differentiated by the type of radiation they absorb, UVA or UVB, or both. Physical blockers work by reflecting or scattering the UV radiation (DermNet NZ 2009c).

Sun protection factor is a worldwide system, stating how much protection a sunscreen provides, applied to the skin at a thickness of 2 mg/cm^2. The test works out how much UV radiation (mostly UVB) it takes to cause barely detectable sunburn on a given person with and without sunscreen applied. For example, if it takes 10 minutes to burn without a sunscreen and 100 minutes to burn with a sunscreen, then the SPF of that sunscreen is 10 (100/10). There is no recognised international measurement of UVA sun protection factors (DermNet NZ, 2009c). In the UK, a star system is used. Sunscreens can have anywhere from 0 to 5 stars. The number of stars is not an absolute measure and depends on how much UVB protection the sunscreen offers (Cancer Research UK, 2009f). In due course, a new EU symbol is being introduced to convey the UVA and UVB protection offered by some UV protection products.

A sunscreen with an SPF of 15 provides greater than 93% protection against UVB. Protection against UVB is increased to 97% with SPF of 30+. The difference between an SPF 15 and an SPF 30 sunscreen may not have a noticeable difference in actual use as the effectiveness of a sunscreen has more to do with how

Box 11.2   SunSmart – advice on sun protection and prevention of skin cancer

Sunburn can greatly increase the risk of skin cancer. Do not let yourself be caught out – use shade, clothing and sun protection factor15+ (SPF15+) sunscreen to protect you.

Sunburn – Don't let sunburn catch you out. Whether at home or abroad, use shade, clothing and SPF15+ sunscreen to protect your skin.

Clothes and sunglasses – Cover up with a T-shirt, hat and sunglasses.

Sunscreens – Buy sunscreen with SPF of at least 15 'broad-spectrum' sunscreens with a star rating of four stars or more. An SPF 15 is advised as it represents the best balance between protection and price and provides over 90% protection.

Sun beds – Are not a safe alternative to tanning. The more you use a sun bed the greater your risk of skin cancer. Using a sun bed once a month or more can increase your risk of skin cancer by more than half. So when the tan fades, the damage remains.

UV index – Know your skin type and work out your risk of burning. Check the UV Index for the day on the Met Office website (www.metoffice.gov.uk/weather/europe/europe_uv.html). Keep out of the midday sun (12.00–15.00 hrs) and seek the shade.

Vitamin D – Amount of sun needed to make enough vitamin D is always less than the higher amounts that cause tanning or sunburn.

Fake tan – If you really want to change the colour of your skin, it is safer to use a fake tan product on your skin than tan out in the sun or under a sun bed. Fake tan does not protect your skin from the sun.

Protecting children – Young skin is delicate and very easily damaged by the sun. All children, no matter whether they tan easily or not, should be protected from the sun and are at risk.

Working outdoors – Protecting yourself if you work outside during the day. Try to avoid unnecessary midday sun exposure, cover up and use sunscreen.

Source: Adapted from *SunSmart* website (Cancer Research UK, 2009f).

much of it is applied, how often it is applied, whether the person is sweating heavily or being exposed to water. Hence, a sunscreen with SPF15+ should provide adequate protection as long as it is being used correctly. However, most people apply their sunscreen at about one-third the thickness used for testing; they fail to apply it to all exposed areas of skin; and they forget to reapply it every couple of hours. Therefore, the actual protection may be a lot less than the tests indicate. The BBC Weather internet pages provide guidance on the UV Index provided with weather reports and also give updated information on UV Index, offering a basis for guiding to protective behaviour (BBC Weather Centre, 2009).

Conclusion

This chapter has outlined the nature of skin cancer, its epidemiology, clinical presentation, causes and treatment. The different types of pre-malignant, non-melanoma and melanoma cancer have been presented, categorised and examined. Attention has been given to the crucial importance of prevention, patient behaviour, preventative strategies such as self-examination for both primary disease and malignant melanoma. Reference has also been made to reactions to diagnosis and the importance of patient support. The nurse's role in prevention, education and support are of crucial importance and the protective activities that the public can undertake to reduce their risk of UV-related damage have been highlighted.

References

Ajzen, I. (1991). The theory of planned behaviour. *Organisational Behaviour and Human Decision Processes*, **50**: 179–211.

Ajzen, I. (2001). Nature and operation of attitudes. *Annual Review of Psychology*, **52**: 27–58.

All Party Parliamentary Group on Skin (APPGS) (2003). Enquiry into the Treatment, Management and Prevention of Skin Cancer. London: All Party Parliamentary Group on Skin, Portcullis.

All Party Parliamentary Group on Skin (APPGS) (2008). Skin Cancer-Improving Prevention, Treatment and Care. London: APPGS.

American Joint Committee on Cancer. (2002). Melanoma of the Skin. In: Greene, F.L., Page, D.L., Balsh, C.M., Fleming, I.D. and Morrow, M. (eds.) *American Joint Committee on Cancer: Cancer Staging Manual*. (6th edn) New York, Springer Veralog.

Armstrong, B.K. and A. Kricker (2001). The epidemiology of UV induced skin cancer. *Journal of Photochemistry and Photobiology B-Biology*, **63**(1–3): 8–18.

Austoker, J. (1994). Melanoma: Prevention and early diagnosis. *British Medical Journal*, **308**(3944): 1682–1686.

Balanda, K.P., J.B. Lowe *et al.* (1994). Enhancing the early detection of melanoma within current guidelines. *Australian Journal of Public Health*, **18**(4): 420–423.

Balch, C.M., N.R. Pellis *et al.* (1994). Oncology. In: Schwartz, S., Shires, G.T., Spencer, F.C. (Eds), *Principles of Surgery*. New York: McGraw-Hill Incorporated.

Balsh, C.M., S.J. Soong *et al.* (2001). Prognostic factors analysis of 17,600 melanoma patients: Validation of the American Joint Committee on Cancer Melanoma Staging System. *Journal of Clinical Oncology*, **19**(16): 3622–3634.

Bandura, A. (1996). *Social Foundations of Thought and Action: A Social Cognitive Theory*. Englewood Cliffs, NJ: Prentice Hall.

Bandura, A. (1997). *Self-efficacy: The Exercise of Control*. New York: Freeman.

Barnhill, R.L., C. Marhn *et al.* (1993). Neoplasms: Malignant melanoma. In: Fitzpatrick, T.B., Sisen, A.Z., Wolff, K., Freedburg, I.M., Austin, K.F. (Eds), *Dermatology in General Medicine*. New York: McGraw-Hill.

Basseres, N., J. Grob *et al.* (1995). Cost-effectiveness of surveillance of stage 1 melanoma – A retrospective appraisal based on a 10 year experience in a dermatology department in France. *Dermatology*, **191**(3): 199–203.

Bath-Hextall, F. and W. Perkins (2008). Basal cell carcinoma. In: Williams, H.C., Bigby, M., Diepgen, T. *et al.* (Eds), *Evidence-based Dermatology*. Oxford: Blackwell Publishing/ BMJ Books.

BBC Weather Centre (2009). The Sun – how the index works. *BBC Weather*. Retrieved 8 May 2009, from http://www.bbc.co.uk/weather/ world/features/sun_index.shtml.

Berwick, M., C. Begg *et al.* (1996). Screening for cutaneous melanoma by skin self-examination. *Journal National Canadian Institute*, **88**(1): 17–23.

Berwick, M., S. Oilveria *et al.* (2000). A pilot study using nurse education as an intervention to increase skin self-examination for melanoma. *Journal of Cancer Education*, **15**(1): 38–40.

Best, D., S. Davis *et al.* (1996). Testicular cancer education: A comparison of teaching methods. *American Journal of Health Behaviour*, **20**(4): 229–241.

Bonett, A., D. Roder *et al.* (1989). Epidemiological features of melanoma in South Australia: Implications for cancer control. *Medical Journal Australia*, **15**(9): 502–504, 506–509.

Bonevski, B., R.P.H. Sanson-Fisher *et al.* (1999). Assessing the perceived needs of patients attending an outpatient melanoma clinic. *Journal of Psychosocial Oncology*, **17**(3/4): 101-118.

Bourke, J., M. Healsmith *et al.* (1995). Melanoma awareness and sun exposure in Leicester. *British Journal of Dermatology*, **132**(2): 251–256.

Bradford, S. and M. Winn (1997). Practice nursing and health promotion: A case study. In: Siddell, M., Jones, L., Katz, J., Perberdy, A.I. (Eds), *Debates and Dilemmas in Promoting Health. A. Reader*. Basingstoke: Macmillan and Open University Press.

Brady, M.S., S.A. Oliveria *et al.* (2000). Patterns of detection in patients with cutaneous melanoma. *Cancer*, **89**(2): 342–347.

Brandberg, Y., M. Bergenmar *et al.* (1996). Six-month follow-up effects of an information programme for patients with malignant melanoma. *Patient Education and Counselling*, **28**(2): 201–208.

British Association of Dermatologists (BAD) (2009). Skin cancer. *Patient Information and Leaflets*, 3 May 2009, from http://www.bad.org.uk//site/574/default.aspx.

Brown, J., P. Butow *et al.* (2000). Psychological predictors of outcome: Time to relapse and survival in patients with early stage melanoma. *British Journal of Cancer*, **83**(11): 1448–1453.

Buchanan, P. and M. Courtenay (2006). *Prescribing in Dermatology*. Cambridge: Cambridge University Press.

Buckman, R. (1996). Talking to patients about cancer. *British Medical Journal*, **313**(7059): 699–700.

Bunn, F., G. Byrne *et al.* (2004). Telephone consultation and triage: Effects on health care use and patient satisfaction. *Cochrane Database of Systematic Reviews*, **18**(4): CD004180.

Burns, T., S. Breathnagh *et al.* (2004). *Rook's Textbook of Dermatology*. Oxford: Blackwell Publishing Ltd.

Cancer Research UK (2004). Brief sheets: Skin Cancer. CRUK.

Cancer Research UK (2009a). Malignant Melanoma – Cancerstats, from http://info.cancerresearchuk.org/cancerstats/types/skin/incidence/.

Cancer Research UK (2009b). UK Skin Cancer Incidence Statistics, from http://www.cancerhelp.org.uk/help/default.asp?page=3010.

Cancer Research UK (2009c). Malignant Melanoma Mortality by Age and Sex, from http://www.cancerresearchuk.org/cancerstats/types/skin/mortality/?a=5441 and http://www.cancerresearchuk.org/cancerstats/type/skin/in/#age.

Cancer Research UK (2009d). The National Awareness and Early Diagnosis Initiative (NAEDI). Retrieved 3 May 2009, from http://info.cancerresearchuk.org/publicpolicy/naedi/?a=5441.

Cancer Research UK (2009e). Cancer Help. Retrieved 3 May 2009, from http://www.cancerhelp.org.uk/.

Cancer Research UK (2009f). SunSmart. Retrieved 3 May 2009, from http://info.cancerresearchuk.org/healthyliving/sunsmart/.

Carli, P., V.D. Giorgi *et al.* (2002). Melanoma detection rate and concordance between self-skin examination and clinical evaluation in patients attending a pigmented lesion clinic in Italy. *British Journal of Dermatology*, **146**(2): 261–266.

Celentano, D. and D. Holtzman (1983). Breast self examination: An analysis of self reported practice and associated characteristics. *American Journal Public Health*, **73**(11): 1321–1323.

Champion, V.L. (1991). The relationship of selected variables to breast cancer detection behaviours in women 35 and older. *Oncology Nursing Forum*, **18**(4): 733–739.

Clark, J. and N. Dodge (1999). Exploring self-efficacy as a predictor of disease management. *Health Education and Behaviour*, **26**: 72–89.

Cokkinides, V.E., M.A. Weinstock, M.C. O'Connell and M.J. Thun (2002). Use of indoor tanning sunlamps by US youth, ages 11–18 years, and by their parent or guardian caregivers: Prevalence and correlates. *Pediatrics*, **109**(6): 1124–1130.

Connor, M. and P. Sparks (2005). Theory of planned behaviour and health behaviour. In: Connor, M., Sparks, P. (Eds), *Predicting Health Behaviour: Health and Practice with Social Cognition Models*. Maidenhead: Open University.

Cook, N. (2000). Teaching and promoting testicular self examination. *Nursing Standard*, **14**(24): 48–51.

de Berker, D., J. McGregor *et al.* (2007). Guidelines for the management of actinic keratosis. *British Journal of Dermatology*, **156**(2): 222–230.

Department of Health (1999). *Saving Lives: Our Healthier Nation*. London: The Stationery Office.

Department of Health (2000). The NHS Cancer Plan: A Plan for Investment, a Plan for Reform. London: The Stationery Office.

Department of Health (2006). Cancer Waiting Targets – A guide Version 5. Retrieved 6 May 2009, from http://www.performance.doh.gov.uk/cancerwaits.

Department of Health (2007). What the Cancer Reform Strategy means to Patients. London: Crown.

DermNet NZ (2009a). Basal cell carcinoma. Retrieved 20 April 2009, from http://www.dermnetnz.org/lesions/basal-cell-carcinoma.html.

DermNet NZ (2009b). Cutaneous T-cell lymphoma. Retrieved 27 April 2009, from http://www.dermnetnz.org/dermal-infiltrative/cutaneous-t-cell-lymphoma.html.

DermNet NZ (2009c). Sunscreens. Retrieved 27 April 2009, from http://www.dermnetnz.org/treatments/sunscreens.html.

Dickers, T.J., G.M. Kavanagh *et al.* (1999). A rational approach to melanoma follow-up in patients with primary cutaneous melanoma. *British Journal of Dermatology*, **140**(2): 249–254.

Duncan, R. (2005). A Survey of the Factors which Influence Patients Diagnosed with Cutaneous Melanoma to Perform Self-Examination for Metastatic Disease. Birmingham, Birmingham, UK.

Electronic Medicines Compendium (2009). Summary of product characteristics (SPC) for Imiquimod cream.

Essner, R. (2001). Is it worthwhile to detect and resect metastases early? *Melanoma Research*, **11**(Suppl 1): S2.

Evans, A.V., F.J. Child and R. Russell-Jones (2003). Zosteriform metastasis from melanoma. *British Medical Journal*, **326**: 1025–1026.

Fawzy, F.I., N. Cousins *et al.* (1990). A structured psychiatric intervention for cancer patients. 1. Changes over time in methods of coping and affective disturbance. *Archives General Psychiatry*, **47**(8): 720–725.

Fawzy, F.I., A.L. Canada *et al.* (2003). Malignant melanoma: Effects of a brief structured psychiatric intervention on survival and recurrence at 10 year follow-up. *Archives of General Psychiatry*, **60**(1): 100–103.

Forman, D., D. Stockton *et al.* (2003). Cancer prevalence in the UK: Results from the EUROPREVAL study. *Annals of Oncology*, **14**(4): 648–654.

Frank, J. and Mai, V. (1985). Breast Self Examination in Young Women: More Harm Than Good? *The Lancet* **2**(8456): 645–7.

Friedman, L.C., S. Bruce *et al.* (1993). Skin self-examination in a population at increased risk for skin cancer. *American Journal of Preventative Medicine*, **9**(6): 359–364.

Girgis, A., E.M. Campbell *et al.* (1991). Screening for melanoma: A community survey of prevalence and predictors. *Medical Journal of Australia*, **154**(5): 338–343.

Hajii-Mahmoodi, M., A. Montazeri *et al.* (2002). Breast self examination, knowledge, attitudes and practices among female health care workers in Tehran." *Breast Journal*, **8**(4): 222–225.

Hanrahan, P.F., P. Hersey *et al.* (1998). Factors involved in presentation of older people with thick melanoma. *Medical Journal Australia*, **169**(8): 410–414.

Havas, S., K. Treimen *et al.* (1998). Factors associated with fruit and vegetable consumption among women participating in WIC. *Journal of American Dietetic Association*, **98**: 1141–1148.

Health Development Agency (2002). *Cancer Prevention: A Resource to Support Local Action in Delivering The NHS Cancer Plan*. London: Health Development Agency.

Hemo, Y., M. Gutman *et al.* (1999). Anatomical site of primary melanoma is associated with depth of invasion. *Archives of Surgery*, **134**(2): 148–150.

Hill, D., V. White *et al.* (1991). Cancer related beliefs and behaviours in Australia. *Australian Journal Public Health*, **15**: 14–23.

International Cancer Research Funding Organisations. (2008). International Cancer

Research Portfolio, from http://www.cancerportfolio.org/index.jsp.

Jirojwong, S. and R. MacLennan (2003). Health beliefs, perceived self efficacy and breast self-examination among Thai migrants in Brisbane. *Journal of Advanced Nursing*, 41(3): 241–249.

Karim-Kos, H.E., E. de Vries *et al.* (2008). Recent trends of cancer in Europe: A combined approach of incidence, survival and mortality for 17 cancer sites since the 1990's. *European Journal Cancer*, 44: 1345–1389.

Kelly, J., M. Blois and R.W. Sagebiel (1985). Frequency and duration of patient follow up after treatment of a primary malignant melanoma. *Journal of the American Academy of Dermatology*, 13(5): 756–760.

Kersey, P., N. Iscoe *et al.* (1995). The value of staging and serial follow-up investigations in patients with completely resected primary cutaneous melanoma. *British Journal of Surgery*, 72(8): 614–617.

Kim, C.J., D.S. Reintgen *et al.* (2002). The new melanoma staging system. *Cancer Control*, 9(1): 9–15.

Koh, H., A. Geller *et al.* (1996). Detection and early prevention strategies for melanoma and skin cancer: Current status. *Archives of Dermatology*, 132(4): 436–442.

Koinberg, I.L., B. Fridlund *et al.* (2004). Nurse-led follow-up on demand or by a physician after breast cancer surgery: A randomised study. *European Journal of Oncology Nursing*, 8: 109–117.

Latter, S., P. Yerrell *et al.* (2000). Nursing, medication education and the new policy agenda: The evidence base. *International Journal of Nursing Studies*, 37(6): 469–479.

Levi, F., L. Randimbison *et al.* (2005). High constant incidence rates of second cutaneous melanomas. *International Journal of Cancer*, 117(5): 877–879.

Lookingbill, D., N. Spangler *et al.* (1993). Cutaneous metastases in patients with metastatic carcinoma: A retrospective study of 4020 patients. *Journal of the American Academy of Dermatology*, 29(2 Pt 1): 228–236.

Luke, C., B. Coventry *et al.* (2003). Are cutaneous melanomas of a specified thickness showing deeper levels of invasion? *Asian Pacific Journal of Cancer*, 4(4): 307–311.

Mackie, R.M. (2000). *Primary Cutaneous Malignant Melanoma: A Guide to Clinical, Differential Diagnosis and Current Management*. Edinburgh: Lothian Print.

Mackie, R.M. (2003). *Cancer Scenarios: An Aid to Planning Cancer Services in Scotland in the Next Decade. 06 Malignant Melanoma of the Skin*. Edinburgh: Scottish Executive Publications.

Macmillan Cancer Support (2009). Cancerbacup. Retrieved 3 May 2009, from www.cancerbackup.org.uk/.

McCarthy, W., H. Shaw *et al.* (1988). Time and frequency of recurrence of cutaneous stage 1 malignant melanoma with guidelines for follow-up study. *Surgery Gynecology and Obstetrics*, 166(6): 497–502.

Melia, J., L. Pendrey *et al.* (2000). Evaluation of primary prevention initiatives for skin cancer: a review from a UK perspective. *British Journal of Dermatology*, 143: 701–708.

Miles, A., J. Waller *et al.* (2005). SunSmart? Skin cancer knowledge and preventative behaviour in a British population representative sample. *Health Education Research*, 20(5): 579–585.

Miller, D., A. Geller *et al.* (1996). Melanoma awareness and self examination practices: Results of a United States survey. *Journal of the American Academy of Dermatology*, 34: 962–970.

Motley, R., P. Kersey *et al.* (2002). Multiprofessional guidelines for the management of the patient with primary cutaneous cell carcinoma. *British Journal of Dermatology*, 146: 18–25.

National Cancer Research Institute (2005). *Strategic Plan 2005–2008*. London: NCRI.

National Institute for Health and Clinical Excellence (2006a). *Guidance on Cancer Services: Improving Outcomes for People with Skin Tumours including Melanoma: The Manual*. London, NICE.

National Institute for Health and Clinical Excellence (NICE) (2006b). Photodynamic therapy for non-melanoma skin tumours (including premalignant and primary non-metastatic skin lesions). Retrieved 23 April 2009, from http://www.nice.org.uk/nicemedia/pdf/ip/IPG155guidance.pdf.

National Institute for Health and Clinical Excellence (2007). *The Most Appropriate Means of Generic and Specific Interventions to Support Attitude and Behaviour Change at Population and Community Levels*. London: NICE.

Norton, E.A. (2008). *A Grounded Theory of Female Adolescent Behaviour in the Sun: Comfort Matters*. Bournemouth: Bournemouth University.

Office of National Statistics (2009). Cancer. *National Statistics*. Retrieved 19 April 2009, from http://www.statistics.gov.uk/CCI/nugget.asp?ID=915&Pos=2&ColRank=1&Rank=310.

Oliveria, S.A., P.J. Christos, A.C. Halpern, J.A. Fine, R.L. Barnhill and M. Berwick (1999a). Patient knowledge, awareness, and delay in seeking medical attention for malignant melanoma. *Journal Clinical Epidemiology*, **52**(11): 1111–1116.

Oliveria, S.A., P.J. Christos *et al.* (1999b). Evaluation of factors associated with skin self-examination. *Cancer Epidemiology Biomarkers and Prevention*, **8**(11): 971–978.

Oliveria, S.A., J.F. Altman *et al.* (2002). Use of nonphysician health care providers for skin cancer screening in the primary care setting. *Preventive Medicine*, **34**(3): 374–379.

Oliveria, S.A., S.W. Dusza *et al.* (2004). Patient adherence to skin self-examination – Effect of nurse intervention with photographs. *American Journal of Preventive Medicine*, **26**(2): 152–155.

Perkins, P.J. (1993). Psychosocial support and malignant melanoma. *European Journal of Cancer Care*, **2**(4): 161–164.

Persson, K., I. Johansson *et al.* (1995). Breast self examination. A survey of frequency, knowledge and attitudes. *Journal of Canadian Education*, **10**(3): 163–167.

Petro-Nustus, W. and B. Mikhail (2002). Factors associated with breast self examination among Jordanian women. *Public Health Nursing*, **19**(4): 263–271.

Poo-Hwu, W., S. Ariyan *et al.* (1999). Follow-up recommendations for patients with American Joint Committee on Cancer Stages I–III. Malignant melanoma. *Cancer Control*, **86**(11): 2252–2258.

Preston, D.S. (1992). Non-melanoma cancers of the skin. *New England Journal of Medicine*, **327**: 1649–1662.

Redman, B. (1997). *The Practice of Patient Education*. St Louis: Mosby.

Regan, M., C. Reid *et al.* (1995). Malignant melanoma, evaluation of clinical follow-up by questionnaire survey. *British Journal of Plastic Surgery*, **38**: 11–14.

Roach, S. (1992). *Human Act of Caring: A Blueprint for the Healthcare Professional* (Revised edition). Ottawa: Canadian Health Association Press.

Roberts, D. and T. Crosby (2008). Cutaneous melanoma. In: Williams, H.C., Bigby, M., Diepgen, T. *et al.* (Eds), *Evidence-based Dermatology*. Oxford: Blackwell Publishing/BMJ Books.

Roberts, D.L.L., A.V. Anstey *et al.* (2002). U.K. guidelines for the management of cutaneous melanoma. *British Journal of Dermatology*, **146**(1): 7–17.

Robinson, J., D. Rigel *et al.* (1998). What promotes skin self-examination? *Journal of the American Academy of Dermatology*, **39**(5): 752–757.

Robinson, J.K., S.G. Fisher *et al.* (2002). Predictors of skin self-examination performance. *Cancer*, **95**(10): 135–146.

Roder, D.M., C.G. Luke *et al.* (1995). Trends in prognostic factors of melanoma in South Australia 1981–1992: Implications for health promotion. *Medical Journal Australia*, **162**(1): 25–29.

Rosal, M.C., J.K. Ockene *et al.* (1998). Coronary Artery Smoking Intervention Study (CASIS): 5 year follow up. *Health Psychology*, **1**(7): 476–478.

Rosella, J.D. (1994). Testicular cancer health education: An integrative review. *Journal Advanced Nursing*, **20**(4): 666–671.

Royal College of Physicians (2007). *The Prevention, Diagnosis, Referral and Management of Melanoma of the Skin: Concise Guidance to Good Practice. Number 7 Clinical Standards: Royal College of Physicians and British Association of Dermatologists.* London: Royal College of Physicians.

Runciman, P., H. Watson *et al.* (2006). Community nurses' health promotion work with older people. *Journal of Advanced Nursing,* 55(1): 46–57.

Rutledge, D. and Davis, G. (1988). Breast Self Examination Compliance and the Health Belief Model. *Oncology Nursing Forum* 15(2): 175–9.

Saraiya, M., K. Glanz *et al.* (2004). Interventions to prevent skin cancer by reducing exposure to ultraviolet radiation: A systematic review. *American Journal of Preventive Medicine,* 27(5): 422–466.

Schofield, P.E., L.J. Beeney *et al.* (2001). Hearing the bad news of a cancer diagnosis: The Australian melanoma patient's perspective. *Annals of Oncology,* 12: 365–371.

Scottish Intercollegiate Guidelines Network (SIGN) (2003). Cutaneous melanoma: A National Clinical Guideline. Section 10 Information for Patients, from www.sign.ac.uk/guidelines/fulltext/72/section10.html.

Scottish Intercollegiate Guidelines Network (SIGN) (2009). Cutaneous melanoma: A National Clinical Guideline, from http://www.sign.ac.uk/pdf/sign72.pdf.

Sharp, L. and C. Tischelman (2005). Smoking cessation for patients with head and neck cancer. *Cancer Nursing,* 28(3): 226–235.

Shumate, C.R., M.M. Urist *et al.* (1995). Melanoma recurrence surveillance, patient or physician based? *Annals of Surgery,* 221(5): 566–571.

Sober, A.J., T.Y. Chuang *et al.* (2001). Guidelines for care for primary cutaneous melanoma. *Journal of the American Academy of Dermatology,* 45(4): 579–586.

Strohl, R.A. (1998). Cutaneous manifestations of malignant disease. *Dermatology Nursing,* 10(1): 23–25.

Taylor, P. and D. Roberts (1997). Skin cancer prevention. *Nursing Standard,* 11(50): 42–45.

Telfer, N., G. Colver *et al.* (2008). Guidelines for the management of basal cell carcinoma. *British Journal of Dermatology,* 159: 35–48.

Thompson, A. (2009). Psychosocial impact of skin conditions. *Dermatological Nursing,* 81(1): 43–47.

Tortora, G.J. and B.H. Derrickson (2005). *Principles of Anatomy and Physiology.* New Jersey: John Wiley & Sons.

Trask, P., A. Paterson *et al.* (2001). Psychological characteristics of individuals with non-stage iv melanoma. *Journal of Clinical Oncology,* 19(1): 1844–1850.

Vagero, D. and G. Persson (1984). Risks, survival and trends of malignant melanoma among white and blue collar workers in Sweden. *Social Science and Medicine,* 19(4): 475–478.

Van der Molen, B. (1999). Relating information needs to the cancer experience: 1. Information as a key coping strategy. *European Journal of Cancer Care,* 8(4): 238–244.

Weinstock, M.A., R. Martin *et al.* (1999). Thorough skin examination for the early detection of melanoma. *American Journal of Preventative Medicine,* 17(3): 169–175.

Wessex Cancer Trust (2004). *How to Check Your Lymph Nodes.* Southampton: Wessex Cancer Trust.

Wong, K., F.K. Wong *et al.* (2005). Effects of nurse-initiated telephone follow-up on self-efficacy among patients with chronic obstructive pulmonary disease. *Journal of Advanced Nursing,* 49(2): 210–222.

Wright, S., Becker, S., Smith, J. & South West Cancer Intelligence Service Skin Cancer Tumour Panel (2004). *Use of focus groups to inform the development of skin cancer patient information.* Bristol. South West Cancer Intelligence Service.

Infective skin conditions and infestations

12

Jean Robinson

Introduction

Healthy skin provides a tough barrier to keep out allergens and pathogens but if this barrier function breaks down or is penetrated, infections and infestations can cause disease (Gawkrodger, 2003). Skin infections and infestations are common problems and nurses need to be confident in their assessment and management. This includes not only treating the physical problem and ensuring patients and their families understand how to use the treatments correctly, in order to be effective, but also addressing practical considerations and reducing potential for recurrence if possible. This chapter will look at bacterial, viral and fungal skin infections and infestations. Risk factors such as age and concomitant conditions, treatment and, where possible, prevention will be considered for each subgroup.

Infections and infestations are common and many are treated by the primary care team. It is therefore important to understand the fundamentals of diagnosing these common skin conditions. Children, parents and patients who miss school or work while waiting for proper diagnosis contribute to the financial burden of these common conditions which are usually very easily treated. Infections such as impetigo and tinea are highly visible and can lead to stigmatisation and create difficulties for children at school (Popovich and McAlhany, 2007). Impetigo is also very contagious and therefore easily spread.

Early access to appropriate diagnosis and treatment can alleviate these aspects. Nurse prescribers in the community have much to contribute to the improvement of health care provision for dermatology patients (Courtenay *et al.*, 2007), but this does mean that there is a continuing need for nurses to receive additional educational support to be 'upskilled' and confident in the assessment and management of such problems. There have long been calls for nurses with experience in dermatology nursing to be available in every primary care setting so that patients with skin conditions can all have access to quality dermatological care from appropriately informed nurses. An increase in the number of such nurse-clinicians would allow for greater support and advice for people with skin conditions and those that are affected. In addition and very importantly, it would lead to an improvement in the dissemination of accurate information and treatments and encourage greater adherence to therapies (APPGS, 2008).

While Watson and de Bruin's (2007) work focuses on the experiences of patients with psoriasis, it clearly demonstrates how influential the doctor/patient relationship is to the patient's self-concept: the participants all agreed that they would have felt more empowered by their doctors had they empathised with their suffering, given good explanations about the disease and treatment and been alert to their related underlying emotional struggles. Such findings can be transferred across the spectrum of dermatological disease and for patients it cannot be overemphasised that a caring, empathetic nurse is therefore important for holding and addressing the patients' physical and psychological well-being.

Skin infections (bacterial, viral and fungal) and infestations (parasites or mites which can be direct as in scabies or lice or indirect, e.g. bedbugs or fleas) cover a huge spectrum. They may range from minor conditions which neverthe-less can be embarrassing and uncomfortable to life-threatening infection where patients are systemically unwell. Dermatology is a very visual and practical field where touch is also important and nurses need an ability to recognise the changes which infection may make in the appearance and feel of skin along with an ability to accurately describe what they observe and feel. With this need to touch skin must also come education of the patient and public in infection control measures, i.e. hand washing to promote best practice in preventing transmission (Docherty, 2001).

In this chapter, the most commonly seen bacterial, viral and fungal infections are considered.

Bacterial skin infections

Impetigo

Impetigo is a highly infectious superficial bacterial skin infection which is most frequently seen in children (Figure 12.1). It is more common in the summer (Loffeld *et al.*, 2005). Both *Staphylococcus aureus* (*S. aureus*) and

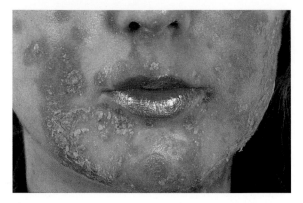

Figure 12.1 Impetigo. (Source: Graham-Brown and Burns, 2006.)

Streptococcus pyogenes (group A – haemolytic streptococcus, GABHS) can cause this type of superficial pyoderma or purulent skin disease. In British general practice, 2.8% of children aged 0–4 years and 1.6% of children 5–15 years consult their GP about impetigo each year (McCormick *et al.*, 1995). It is the most common form of bacterial infection in individuals with human immunodeficiency virus (HIV).

Primary impetigo is direct bacterial invasion of skin which was previously normal whereas secondary impetigo occurs in skin where there is some underlying skin disease, for example atopic eczema or scabies, disrupting the skin barrier. Impetigo is characterised by inflammation and infection localised in the epidermis. Impetigo is also classified as non-bullous or bullous. Non-bullous impetigo is sometimes also termed impetigo contagiosa, although this terminology may be used at times synonymously as any impetigo.

Non-bullous impetigo is the most common type and accounts for more than 70% of cases (Burr, 2003). It is more common in children over the age of 2 years. Initial lesions are thin walled vesicles on skin which has previously been normal. Subsequently any areas where the skin barrier has been disrupted, for example minor abrasions, insect bites or atopic eczema, may be infected. The initial lesions rupture leaving erosions which are covered by the yellowish brown or honey-coloured crusts which are very characteristic of the condition. Individual lesions enlarge to 1–2 cm and satellite lesions appear. These can coalesce resulting in larger areas of crusted involvement. The infection can occur on any part of the body but the face, especially around the mouth and nostrils, extremities and buttocks are common. The problem usually remains localised. Widespread impetigo is most common in secondarily infected or impetiginised eczema. Diagnosis is not usually difficult. The most important point to remember is that any underlying skin disease, for example shingles, cold sores, fungal skin infections and eczema, needs recognition and must also be treated (Resnick, 2000). Although not painful, impetigo can be itchy and sore.

Bullous impetigo is less common and characterised by vesicles and bullae which rupture less easily and can persist for several days (Koning *et al.*, 2003). There are usually fewer lesions and it can affect the trunk more commonly than in non-bullous impetigo. It is more common in infants and children under 2 years of age. Neonatal bullous impetigo tends to occur in the inguinal area and on the buttocks. The lesions appear to develop on intact skin as a result of localised toxin production by *S. aureus*. It can be confused with thermal burns, blistering disorders (e.g. bullous pemphigoid), herpes infections and Stevens–Johnson syndrome (Koning *et al.*, 2003).

Causes

Bullous impetigo is always caused by *S. aureus*. Non-bullous impetigo can be caused by staphylococci or streptococci; it is possible to culture both organisms from lesions in many cases (Resnick, 2000). Historically in Britain *S. aureus* was the main cause of impetigo in the 1940s and 1950s after which *S. pyogenes* was the main causative agent for about 30 years. Currently *S. aureus* is the dominant cause again (Koning *et al.*, 2003) with 10% of impetigo cases in Britain due to *S. pyogenes*.

Prognosis

The prognosis is generally good. Impetigo can be self-limiting but will usually persist and spread if untreated and be a source of infection for others. Local and systemic spread can rarely result in cellulitis, lymphangitis or septicaemia (Koning *et al.*, 2003). Severe progression such as septic arthritis, pneumonia and osteomyelitis are very rare and usually limited to those with acquired in inherited immune deficiencies (Resnick, 2000). Post-streptococcal glomerular nephritis is a serious but rare complication while guttate psoriasis can also occur but probably only in those already genetically predisposed.

Management

Koning *et al.*'s (2003) review of 36 treatments for impetigo highlight that there is no standard therapy for impetigo. Trials show that Penicillin is not effective for impetigo and there is little evidence supporting the value of disinfecting measures. Knowledge of local resistance patterns on the basis of surveillance of specimens should be incorporated into any regional guidelines.

(1) Consider taking a swab for microscopy, culture and sensitivity of in non-bullous impetigo of purulent material or bullae fluid in bullous impetigo especially if MRSA is a possibility (Box 12.1). If the child or adult is systemically unwell, consider taking blood for blood cultures.
(2) *Hygiene measures to reduce the spread to others*: Careful hand washing, use of individual towels and bedding, avoidance of skin-to-skin contact with the child or adult until lesions have been treated.
(3) Children should stay away from nursery or school until the lesions have stopped

---

Box 12.1 Bacterial swab

Moisten the tip of the swab;
Apply to the affected skin;
Rotate the swab between the fingers to pick up debris;
Put into transport medium.

Source: RCN/BDNG (2008).

blistering or crusting or they have had 48 hours of antibiotics.

(4) In limited disease topical antibiotics, for example fusidic acid, may be sufficient (other topical antibiotics seem less effective) (Koning *et al.*, 2003).

(5) Oral Flucloxacillin or Erythromycin, although there is insufficient evidence that they are better than topical (Koning *et al.*, 2003).

(6) If culture reveals both staphylococcus and streptococcus, both pathogens must be treated with appropriate antibiotics.

(7) Most importantly any underlying skin condition must also be treated, e.g. impetiginised atopic eczema should be treated concurrently with appropriate topical corticosteroids and emollients (Charman and Lawton, 2006).

Folliculitis and related conditions

Folliculitis is an acute pustular infection of multiple hair follicles. A furuncle or boil is a localised acute abscess formed in hair follicles next to each other and a carbuncle is a deep abscess of the skin and subcutaneous tissue formed in a group of follicles which is painful. Anything which tends to increase the numbers of skin surface bacteria may lead to the development of folliculitis (Resnick, 2000) and this can include occlusion, overhydration and maceration. Folliculitis is more common in tropical climates and in those who live in overcrowded conditions or practice poor hygiene. It is also more common in patients who are obese, have diabetes mellitus or wear tight occlusive clothing.

Follicular pustules occur in hair bearing areas such as the legs, face, buttocks and groin. In women it can happen after hair removal by shaving or waxing and in men it can affect the beard area. It is usually, but not always, caused by *S. aureus*. Boils appear as tender, red pustules which grow over a few days into a large red lump under the skin surface. It may burst through the skin releasing pus or may gradually settle without bursting. They often occur on the face, neck, scalp, axillae and perineum as the bacteria survives best in moist areas. They can recur. Large boils or carbuncles can result in systemic illness.

Furuncles, carbuncles and other abscesses appear to be the most frequently reported clinical manifestations of MRSA (Nathwani *et al.*, 2008).

Management

(1) Swabs should be taken for bacterial culture from the lesion only if: furuncles or boils are recurrent, there is a history of spread in the family or close contacts, the infection is severe or MRSA is suspected (Nathwani *et al.*, 2008).

(2) Acute staphylococcal infections should be treated with antibiotics in either topical or systemic forms.

(3) Furuncles and carbuncles can be treated surgically by lancing or incision and drainage if they are <5 cm in diameter (Gould *et al.*, 2009), and if cellulitis is not present antibiotics may not be required.

(4) Recurrent and chronic cases are more difficult to treat and measures to help break the cycle of infection are needed (BAD, 2007). Antiseptic washes, for example iodine or chlorhexidine, can be used. Nasal carriage of staphylococcus should be treated with topical antibiotic, e.g. Mupirocin.

(5) Other family members should be swabbed and if carriers should also be treated.

(6) Hands and finger nails should be kept clean and short and clothing washed frequently using a hot wash.

(7) Obese patients should be advised about the need to lose weight to reduce the survival of bacteria in the skin folds.

Staphylococcal scalded skin syndrome

This is an acute toxic illness usually seen in infants but can affect adults with renal failure or immunodeficiency (BAD, 2006). It is caused by *S. aureus* which produces a toxin leading to damage of a key protein called desmoglein which binds skin together. The resulting shedding of sheets of superficial parts of the epidermis resembles a scald, giving rise to the name of the condition (Gawkrodger, 2003).

The original infection can be minor, for example a graze or sticky eye, after which a patchy red rash will develop and quickly spread and increase in size. There is often redness around the mouth but there is no mucosal involvement of the lips or eyes which differentiates this from the more serious toxic epidermal necrolysis (TEN). TEN is a similar looking condition but rare in children and nearly always caused by a drug reaction. The baby or child is usually miserable and feverish and the condition is painful. A thin layer of skin will loosen, with fluid-filled blisters or just with sheets of skin sliding off the underlying areas (BAD, 2006). If large areas of denuded erythematous areas occur, there will be exudate with possible electrolyte imbalance and the risk of septicaemia.

Management

(1) Swab surface fluid or pus for bacterial culture.
(2) *Give systemic antibiotics*: including Flucloxacillin or Erythromycin which may need to be given intravenously.
(3) Clean skin gently and apply emollient, e.g. Liquid and White Soft Paraffin, NPF ointment (WSP:LP 50:50).

Cellulitis and erysipelas

Cellulitis is a relatively common infection of the dermis and subcutaneous tissues, often due to streptococci (Figure 12.2). Erysipelas is an infection of the dermis only with a well-defined, raised edge which usually affects the face or lower leg or areas where there is less subcutaneous tissue. It can be hard to distinguish between the two and in practice the terms may be used interchangeably (Kilburn *et al.*, 2003). Important precipitants include tinea pedis, lymphoedema venous insufficiency and being overweight as they all lead to skin barrier breakdown and the consequent entry points for infection (DTB, 2003). Cellulitis

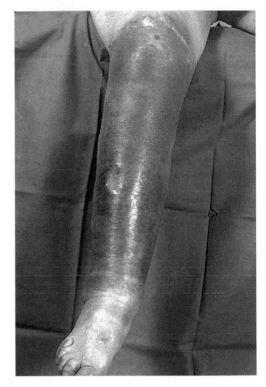

Figure 12.2   Cellulitis. (Source: Graham-Brown and Burns, 2006.)

presents with an acute onset of red, painful, hot, swollen, smooth, shiny and tender skin, sometimes with bullae. There may also be systemic upset with nausea, shivering, malaise, fevers and rigors. It usually affects one limb only, nearly always a leg. Some cases arise through a break in the skin, e.g. bites, burns and scalds and cuts, eczema or ulcers.

It is important to distinguish between cellulitis of the leg and varicose eczema as the two are often confused due to the erythematous inflammation found in both conditions (Quartey-Papafio, 1999). However, there are other clinical features by which to differentiate the two conditions. Crusting or scaling is the most important sign in varicose eczema and not present in cellulitis where the skin is smooth and shiny. Small vesicles are common in varicose eczema. These break down with the release of serous fluid which dries to form crusts which coalesce. Such blister formation is rare in cellulitis. Itching is present in varicose eczema but not cellulitis and the patient may have a history of varicose veins or deep vein thrombosis.

Varicose eczema should always be considered in the differential diagnosis of cellulitis of the leg. In varicose eczema, intravenous antibiotics are unnecessary. Treatment will be needed with 1:10,000 potassium permanganate solution and topical steroid and emollients (Quartey-Papafio, 1999).

Management

(1) There are no published UK guidelines or consensus for treating cellulitis.
(2) Hospital admission is advisable for neonates, the immunocompromised or those unwell with co-existing disease, those with severe cellulitis or with periorbital cellulitis and those who lack support at home or are not improving on treatment (DTB, 2003).
(3) Treatment with phenoxymethylpenicillin or benzylpenicillin can be started 'blind' for mild uncomplicated cellulitis, as unless there is a likely portal of entry or secondary blistering, it is usually difficult to identify a specific bacteriological cause (DTB, 2003).
(4) Drawing around the extent of the infection with a permanent marker pen can help to track for future comparison.
(5) Flucloxacillin may be given in addition and this is common practice in more severe cases. Whether these are given orally or intravenously will depend on the patient's condition.
(6) Co-existing disease such as leg ulcers, toe-web intertrigo, lymphoedema, venous insufficiency, leg oedema and obesity should also be addressed.
(7) Recurrence is common (up to 30%) (DTB, 2003). There is a strong association with oedema and multiple episodes of cellulitis (Cox, 2006) where the vicious cycle of oedema predisposing to cellulitis and cellulitis being a cause of persistent oedema must be appreciated. Cox suggests that interventions such as the reduction of oedema or more prolonged antibiotic therapy may reduce the risk of recurrent infection.

Viral infections

Herpes simplex

Herpes simplex virus (HSV) is a very common acute, self-limiting vesicular eruption. Humans are the only natural host of HSV and the virus does not survive for long in the external environment (Goodyear, 2000). It is highly contagious and spreads by direct contact with infected individuals when the virus comes into contact with mucosal surfaces or broken skin. In primary infection, a non-immune person is exposed to contaminated saliva or secretions from the pharynx, genitalia or eyes at close contact. The virus penetrates the epidermis and replicates in the epithelial cells at the site of the infection (Gawkrodger, 2003) in the primary infection. The latent non-replicating virus then travels down to the dorsal root ganglion where it can lie dormant. At some later date, following exposure to a trigger it can reactivate and travel back down the sensory nerve and reinfect the epithelial cells at the nerve ending. This ability to recur is a hallmark of HSV infection. It usually happens at the same site, e.g. cold sore. Common triggers are colds, strong sunlight, stress and menstruation (Docherty, 2001). HSV is preceded by tingling or burning in the affected area – the prodromal phase. The highest rate of HSV infections is in the first 5 years of life and then after the onset of sexual maturity (Goodyear, 2000). It is rare under 6 months of age due to passive transfer of maternal antibodies.

There are two types of HSV. Type 1 is usually facial or non-genital and Type 2 is genital due to sexual contact but crossover is seen.

Primary infection usually occurs in children which may often go unrecognised as they are sub-clinical. In those with symptoms, acute inflammation of the gums and mouth (gingivostomatitis) is common. The children have vesicles on their lips and mucous membranes which rapidly erode and are painful. Clusters of vesicles arise on a background of erythema and over about 10–12 days erode to become crusted lesions. Children are miserable, may be pyrexial and can have problems eating and drinking. In severe cases, intravenous fluids may be needed. Some children may also have corneal involvement. There may be local lymphadenopathy. This can last for about 2 weeks.

Herpetic whitlow

This is a local painful presentation where a painful vesicle or pustule is found on a finger.

Type 2 HSV occurs as a primary infection due to sexual contact in young adults as acute vulvovaginitis, penile or perianal lesions sometimes with associated dysuria, difficulties in passing urine, fever, headache and muscle pains.

Differential diagnosis

HSV may be confused with impetigo. The virus can be cultured or identified by immunofluorescence from a swab (Box 12. 2).

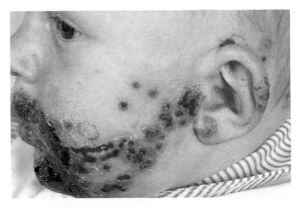

Figure 12.3 Eczema herpeticum. (Source: Graham-Brown and Burns, 2006.)

> ## Box 12.2   Viral swab
>
> Use the appropriate medium;
> Pierce the roof of the blister and place swab in the fluid and rotate.
>
> *Source*: RCN/BDNG (2008).

Complications

Complications are rare but serious (Gawkrodger, 2003). Secondary bacterial infection is usually due to *S. aureus*. Eczema herpeticum where eczema becomes infected with herpes simplex is a serious potentially fatal complication (Figure 12.3). Disseminated herpes simplex can occur in neonates or immunosuppressed patients. Chronic and atypical lesions can occur in patients with HIV. Herpes encephalitis is a serious complication. Lastly, infection with HSV is the most common cause of recurrent erythema multiforme (Gawkrodger, 2003).

Management

(1) Mild HSV may not require any treatment. Those with more severe disease will require symptomatic treatment with oral fluids and paracetamol.
(2) Recurrent or mild facial or genital HSV can be treated with aciclovir topically five times daily for 5 days. This helps to reduce the length of the attack and the duration of viral shedding if given early. Viral shedding occurs when the virus is active and transmittable. More severe episodes require oral aciclovir. Those with recurrent attacks may require prophylactic treatment with aciclovir.
(3) Intravenous aciclovir may be needed for severe attacks in the immunosuppressed and those with eczema herpeticum.
(4) Genital herpes can be treated with valaciclovir or famciclovir. Barrier contraception methods are advised during intercourse which ideally should be avoided while the patient is symptomatic.

Varicella zoster (chickenpox)

Varicella is an acute, highly infectious disease caused by the varicella zoster virus (VZV) which also causes shingles. It is typically a disease of childhood (Macartney and McIntyre, 2008) with an incubation period of 7–21 days.

It is communicable from 5 days before a rash develops until 6 days after. The disease is characterised by a widespread maculopapular rash which often starts on the trunk and then moves to the limbs. Lesions are often seen at all stages at once: vesicles, papules and crusted lesions. Fever and general malaise are also present.

Management

(1) Treatment is supportive.

(2) Paracetamol may be given for pyrexia.

(3) Traditionally lotions, for example calamine lotion, are used. The effect of calamine lotion on pruritis has not been evaluated but it has a good safety profile and Tebruegge *et al.* (2006) report some symptomatic relief. They found limited evidence to support the use of systemic antihistamines in this context.

(4) Lukewarm baths may provide some relief and light cotton clothing is probably more comfortable (Shuru, 2003).

(5) Scabs should not be picked but allowed to fall off spontaneously.

(6) Children with sores in their mouths may be reluctant to eat or drink, so small amounts of clear liquids should be encouraged frequently.

(7) Aciclovir can reduce the number of days with fever in otherwise healthy children but its effect on soreness and itching is not certain (Klassen *et al.*, 2005).

(8) Live attenuated varicella vaccines are now licensed for use in some countries (not the UK) and are a potential strategy for the prevention of morbidity from varicella infection. Macartney and McIntyre's 2008 review of the efficacy and safety of vaccines for the post-exposure prophylaxis against varicella shows that varicella vaccine administered within 3 days to children following household contact with a varicella case reduced infection rates and severity of cases but did not adequately address safety aspects.

(9) Neonates with chickenpox should be treated with parenteral aciclovir regardless of immune function to reduce the risk of severe disease.

(10) Neonates and children and adults who are immunocompromised and have been exposed to the virus may require prophylaxis with varicella-zoster immunoglobulin (VZIG).

Complications

In healthy children, the disease is mostly self-limiting. The most common complication is secondary bacterial infection (Macartney and McIntyre, 2008). However, there are the more serious well-recognised complications of pneumonia and encephalitis, dehydration, hepatitis and ataxia and these usually lead to hospitalisation. Women who contract varicella in the first 20 weeks of pregnancy have a 2% risk of the foetus developing congenital varicella syndrome with women who contract varicella in the last trimester being at increased risk of pneumonia. The onset of varicella in pregnant women from 5 days prior to delivery to 2 days after can result in neonatal varicella in 17–30% (Macartney and McIntyre, 2008).

VZV also remains dormant in the dorsal ganglia of individuals and can reactivate to cause herpes zoster. Primary infection usually provides lifetime immunity but secondary infections do occur.

Immunocompromised patients are at particular risk from primary VZV infection or reactivation.

Herpes zoster (shingles)

Herpes zoster or shingles is an acute self-limiting vesicular eruption occurring in a dermatomal (localised area of skin that has its sensation via a single nerve from a single nerve root) distribution. It is caused by a reactivation of VZV. It is not known what causes this but is more likely in the elderly, those who are under stress or immunosuppressed.

It always occurs in people who have previously had varicella (chickenpox). The virus lies dormant in the sensory root ganglion of the spinal cord and when reactivated, the virus replicates and travels down the nerve to the skin to induce the cutaneous lesions of shingles. Viraemia (the presence of virus in the bloodstream) is frequent and involvement may be disseminated (Gawkrodger, 2003). The thoracic dermatomes are involved in 50% of cases. Involvement of the ophthalmic division of the trigeminal nerve is particularly common in the elderly.

Presentation

Pain, tenderness and paraesthesia in the dermatome may precede the eruption by 3–5 days. These are followed by erythema and groups of vesicles scattered in the dermatomal area. The vesicles become pustular and then form crusts (Figure 12.4). Secondary infection can occur. These separate after 2–3 weeks and leave scarring. Herpes zoster is usually unilateral and can involve adjacent dermatomes. Local lymphadenopathy is common. Shingles recurs in about 5% of cases.

Complications

Serious complications can occur depending on which nerve is involved (Gawkrodger, 2003).

> *Opthalmic disease*: If the first trigeminal division is affected, corneal ulcers and scarring can result.
>
> *Motor palsy: The viral involvement may spread fr*om the posterior horn of the spinal cord to the anterior horn which results in a motor disorder. Cranial nerve palsy or paralysis of the diaphragm or other muscle groups can happen.
>
> *Disseminated herpes zoster*: Immunosuppressed patients can develop confluent haemorrhagic involvement which spreads and can become necrotic or gangrenous.
>
> *Postherpetic neuralgia*: The pain of shingles may go on long after the rash has disappeared. Neuralgia is rare in patients under 40 years of age but affects a third of those over the age of 60 years and usually subsides within 6 months but may go on for more than a year.

Management

(1) The goals of treatment are to shorten the attack, reduce pain, deal with complications and prevent postherpetic neuralgia if possible and to treat pain should it occur (BAD, 2004).

(2) In mild disease, treatment is symptomatic with rest and analgesia. Basic hygiene should be maintained (Docherty, 2001) and the principles of care for chickenpox applied.

(3) Any secondary bacterial infection may make the neuralgia worse and should be treated with antibiotics.

(4) Patients should stay away from young babies and the immunocompromised and may need to stay off work for 2–3 weeks (BAD, 2004).

(5) More severe cases may be treated if seen within 72 hours of onset with aciclovir or famciclovir to reduce the length of the attack and reduce viral shedding. Immunosuppressed patients will need intravenous aciclovir.

(6) Except in the immunosuppressed, oral prednisolone can reduce the incidence of postherpetic neuralgia. There is evidence to show that gabapentin which was originally developed to treat epilepsy, but is now widely used to relieve neuropathic pain, may be effective but ineffective in acute pain (Wiffen *et al.*, 2005). In severe cases, referral to pain clinics may be needed.

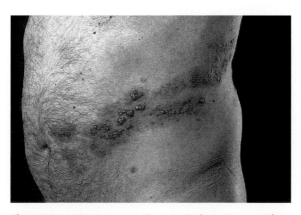

Figure 12.4 Herpes zoster. (Source: Graham-Brown and Burns, 2006.)

Molluscum contagiosum

Molluscum contagiosum is a viral skin infection seen most often in normal immunocompetent children. They usually present as single or multiple (usually no more than 20), discrete, smooth, pearly papules with a classic dimple (van der Wouden *et al.*, 2006) (Figure 12.5). The infection is caused by a pox virus and follows contact with infected people or contaminated objects. They occur worldwide but are more common in areas with warm climates with an association with swimming pool use, age, living in close proximity and skin-to-skin contact while gender, seasonality and hygiene show no association (Braue *et al.*, 2005). Infection is rare under the age of 1 year and most common in the 2- to 5-year age group. Affected people and the parents of affected children frequently seek help for social reasons; for children name calling and bullying are not uncommon. A large proportion of the parents interviewed by Braue *et al.* (2005) reported that they were moderately or greatly concerned and these concerns focused on physical issues such as scarring, itching and the chance of spread to peers, pain and the effects of treatments.

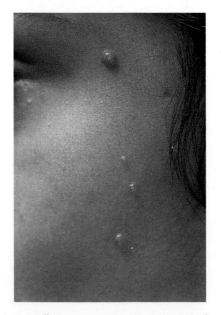

Figure 12.5 Molluscum contagiosum. (Source: Graham-Brown and Burns, 2006.)

The estimated incubation period varies from 14 days to 6 months. The lesions grow slowly and can reach a diameter of 5–10 mm in 6–12 weeks. They usually resolve spontaneously within 6–9 months without leaving scars but the duration of individual lesions and the entire episode can be very variable with some lasting for 3–4 years (van der Wouden *et al.*, 2006) and the virus may spread to other areas of skin. Trauma such as scratching may result in pus, crusting and the destruction of the lesion.

It should be noted that there is also a sexually transmitted variant which occurs in genital, perineal, pubic and surrounding skin. Molluscum contagiosum has also been observed with other diseases in people with a damaged immune system and people with HIV infection are particularly prone (van der Wouden *et al.*, 2006). As immunodeficiency progresses in HIV-infected individuals, they become more common and resistant to treatment. Multiple lesions on atypical areas such as the face and neck are often seen. There is limited data on the disease course in this group.

Management

(1) The option of no treatment is reasonable especially in young children (van der Wouden *et al.*, 2006).
(2) Cryotherapy can be very effective but is painful and not usually tolerated by children.
(3) Topical therapies include salicylic acid or podophyllotoxin cream. Crystacide cream can be used off license and 5% Imiquimod cream can be used in difficult cases.
(4) A recent review of treatments could find no reliable evidence for any of the treatments currently used (van der Wouden *et al.*, 2006) and recommends that until better evidence on treatment options is found, lesions should be left to heal naturally.

Viral warts

Warts (verrucae) are common cutaneous tumours due to infection via direct inoculation

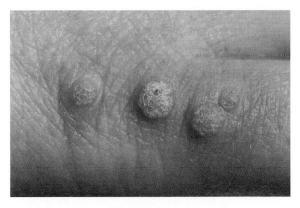

Figure 12.6 Viral warts. (Source: Graham-Brown and Burns, 2006.)

of epidermal cells with human papilloma virus (HPV) and most people will experience them at some time in their life (Figure 12.6). They are spread by touch, sexual contact or indirectly via fomites or inanimate objects or substances capable of carrying infectious organisms. They are common in children and the immunosuppressed are particularly susceptible. Approximately 50% of renal transplant patients develop warts within 5 years of transplantation. The epidermis becomes thickened and hyperkeratotic due to vacuolation of keratinocytes infected by the wart virus whereby the keratinocytes become filled with fluid-filled vesicles bounded by a membrane within the cytoplasm. Up to half of common warts disappear spontaneously in children within 6 months. Benign warts almost never undergo malignant transformation in immunocompetent individuals. Sterling *et al.* (2001) advise that periungual warts in combination with genital HPV disease warrant careful attention. In immunosuppressed patients, dysplastic change is quite common and there is often a poor correlation between clinical and histological appearance.

Common warts

These are dome-shaped papules or nodules with papilliferous surfaces. They are rough, scaly, pink or skin-coloured and usually multiple. They are most common on hands or feet in children but may also be found on faces or genitalia. Their surfaces interrupt skin lines. Some facial warts can resemble a thread or filament (filiform appearance).

Plane warts

These are smooth, flat-topped papules which are often light brown in colour. They are most common on the face and dorsum of hands and usually multiple and painless. They are hard to treat and eventually resolve spontaneously. They can Koebnerise, i.e. appear in areas where the skin is injured.

Plantar warts

These are common in children and adolescents and can be solitary or multiple. They usually have a rough surface and affect the soles of feet, are painful and covered by callus. They grow into the dermis due to pressure.

Genital warts

In females they are found on the vulva, perineum and vagina. In males they are found on the penis. The perianal area can be affected in those who have anal sex. They may be small but can grow into large cauliflower-like lesions (Gawkrodger, 2003).

Management

(1) No treatment is a valid option but pain, interference with function, cosmetic embarrassment and risk of malignancy are indications for treatment (Sterling *et al.*, 2001). An immune response is needed for clearance, so immunocompromised patients may never show clearance.
(2) The majority can be treated in primary care. There is no treatment which is 100% effective and different types of treatment may need to be combined. Gibbs and Harvey (2006) found a considerable lack of evidence on which to base the rationale of topical treatments for warts, although they found evidence to support the use of simple topical treatments containing salicylic acid. There was less evidence for the efficacy of liquid nitrogen.

(3) In hand and foot warts, the hyperkeratotic areas can be pared down with a pumice stone and allows for topical treatment. There are many wart paints now available, most of which contain salicylic acid. This is a keratolytic which slowly destroys the virus-infected epidermis. They should be applied after bathing which will help to moisten the warts. Treatment needs to be continued for at least 3 months. Wart paints are not suitable for the management of facial and anogenital warts or warts on or near areas of atopic eczema.

(4) Topical treatments should always be tried before cryotherapy. Cryotherapy with liquid nitrogen is painful and should not be carried out on small children. It should be applied every 2–3 weeks and can be carried out on hand, foot and genital warts. It can cause blistering, scarring and damage to nail growth. Hypo- and hyperpigmentation can occur in skin types 5 and 6.

(5) Surgical removal by curettage or blunt dissection followed by cautery may be useful for filiform warts on the face and limbs but can result in scarring.

(6) Patients with anogenital warts should be managed by genito-urinary physicians to exclude the possibility of other sexually transmitted infections (Sterling *et al.*, 2001).

(7) While many children under 3 years of age have vertical transmission of anogenital warts, sexual transmission (and therefore sexual abuse) should always be considered, especially in older children with no warts elsewhere. This emphasises the need for careful physical examination and history-taking as well as thorough assessment of the social and family dynamics (Wyatt, 2008).

Hand, foot and mouth disease

This occurs as epidemics in young children and is due to coxsackie A16 virus. Children present with oral blisters or ulcers, red-edged vesicles on the hands and feet and mild fever. It usually fades within a week.

Management

(1) Supportive measures only are needed, e.g. paracetamol, encouragement with oral fluids.

Kawasaki disease

This is an acute systemic vasculitis involving small and medium arteries with a predilection for coronary arteries. Peak occurrence in the winter and spring has been reported with peak incidence in children aged 9–11 months with a range of 6 months to 5 years. It is the second commonest vasculitic illness of childhood and associated with the development of systemic vasculitis complicated by coronary and peripheral arterial aneurysms and is the commonest cause of acquired heart disease in children in the UK (Brogan *et al.*, 2002). The causative agent is unknown but clinical and epidemiological features are strongly suggestive of an infectious trigger, although there is no correlation with any specific viruses (Brogan *et al.*, 2002; Harnden *et al.*, 2009).

There is no diagnostic test for this illness seen in young children, so diagnosis is based on clinical criteria which are:

Fever of 5 days duration plus four of the following:

(1) Conjunctivitis which is bilateral, bulbar and non-suppurative;
(2) Lymphadenopathy which is cervical and |>1.5 cm;
(3) Polymorphic rash with no vesicles or crusts;
(4) Changed lip or oral mucosa with red cracked lips, 'strawberry' tongue or diffuse erythema of the oropharynx;
(5) Changes of the extremities initially with erythema and oedema of palms and soles. At the convalescent stage, peeling of skin from the fingertips is seen.

It can be diagnosed with less than four of these features if coronary artery aneurysms are detected (Brogan *et al.*, 2002).

Management

(1) This aims to reduce inflammation and prevent the occurrence of coronary arterial aneurysms (CAA) and arterial thrombosis.
(2) Early treatment with aspirin and intravenous immunoglobulin has been shown to reduce the occurrence of CAA.

Fungal infections

Superficial fungal skin infections are very common in people of all ages (Penzer, 2005). They are usually considered mild but can be unpleasant and difficult to eradicate; this underlines the need for accurate assessment and treatment. They can be more serious in immunosuppressed people. They can also lead to compromised skin barrier function which can predispose to bacterial infections such as cellulitis. They can be due to two groups of fungi:

(1) Dermatophytes (ringworm): multicellular filaments or hyphae;
(2) Yeasts: unicellular forms which replicate by budding (Gawkrodger, 2003).

Dermatophyte (ringworm) infections

These fungi reproduce by spore formation. They invade and colonise the stratum corneum of the skin and keratinised tissues, e.g. hair and nails (Clayton, 2000) and induce inflammation by delayed hypersensitivity or by metabolic effects. They are classified by associating the Latin word for the body part they affect with the word tinea: thus *tinea capitis* (scalp ringworm), *tinea corporis* (ringworm on the body), *tinea pedis* (ringworm of the foot) and *tinea cruris* (ringworm of the groin and upper thighs), *tinea unguium* (ringworm of nail plate).

They are caused by three groups of fungal organisms: *Trichophyton*, *Microsporum* and *Epidermophyton*. These organisms can also be distinguished as anthrophilic if they prefer 'living on' human bodies or zoophilic if associated with animals. Zoophilic organisms will also live on humans (Clayton, 2000).

Tinea capitis

This is usually seen in pre-adolescent children. Adult cases are rare. The key symptoms are scalp hair loss and scaling. Sometimes there is a black-dot pattern (studded with broken-off hairs) (Figure 12.7). Acute inflammation with erythema and pustule formation may also occur. Infection may also be associated with painful regional lymphadenopathy. In some cases, kerions or boggy tumours studded with pustules may develop which may be misdiagnosed as bacterial abscesses. A generalised eruption of small itchy papules particularly around the outer helix of the ear, although it can occur anywhere, can occur as a reactive phenomenon or 'id' response (Higgins *et al.*, 2000; González *et al.*, 2007).

Fungus can either penetrate the hair shaft (endothrix infection) or penetrate the hair shaft and grow over the outside of the hair shaft at the same time (exothrix infection). Some other conditions can be confused with *tinea capitis* (Health Protection Agency, 2007). In alopecia areata, there is rarely inflammation in the area of alopecia and no scaling or itching. Seborrhoeic dermatitis occurs in children of all ages but the scaling is diffuse and there is seldom associated hair loss. Scalp psoriasis produces more scaling.

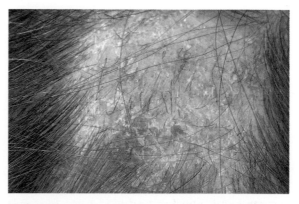

Figure 12.7 Tinea capitis. *Source*: Graham-Brown and Burns, 2006.

The pattern of *tinea capitis* has changed in the UK over the past 10 years (Health Protection Agency, 2007) with a significant rise in the incidence and prevalence of causes of infection due to the anthrophilic organism, *Trichophyton tonsurans* (*T. tonsurans*), which causes endothrix infection. The main focus of the infection has historically been linked to Afro Caribbean communities and therefore cities where there are long standing or recently established black communities but the Health Protection Agency (2007) makes it clear that infection can occur in any child irrespective of their ethnic origin. Indeed Higgins *et al*. (2000) recommend that as it is now so widespread it should be considered in the diagnosis of any child over 3 months with a scaly scalp.

Laboratory diagnosis

Specimens should be taken whenever possible to confirm the diagnosis as systemic therapy will be required. Skin scrapings (Box 12.3) or brushings which include hair and hair fragments (Box 12.4) should be used and sent for mycology. Cut hair is not helpful because of the endothrix nature of the infection; hairs should be plucked. Culturing of the scrapings allows for accurate identification of the organism. These should be repeated after treatment to determine whether the treatment has been effective or not. The use of Wood's light examination is not usually helpful as *T. tonsurans* is an endothrix infection so does not fluoresce.

Box 12.3   **Skin scraping sample**

Hold a blunt blade at an angle of 45 degrees;
Scrape along the active scaly edge of the lesion without cutting the patient;
Wipe the blade edge or catch the keratin scale onto the black filter paper container.

Source: RCN/BDNG (2008).

Box 12.4   **Hair debris**

Identify affected hair follicles and remove skin, hair and/or debris for collection suing a firm toothbrush.
Fold inside the black filter paper container.

Source: RCN/BDNG (2008).

Management

(1) Treatment must be systemic. Most superficial fungal infections can be treated topically. However tinea capitis (like fungal nail infections) always requires systemic medication (González, 2007) as the infection is found at the root of the hair follicle which cannot be reached by topical agents.
(2) Incision and drainage of kerions is not helpful and must be avoided.
(3) Removal of surface crusts from a kerion is often helpful as it relieves itching and secondary infection. It can be painful but can be done gently after soaking the kerion with lukewarm water or saline (Health Protection Agency, 2007).
(4) Griseofulvin remains the only licensed treatment for scalp ringworm in the UK. Absorption is improved if taken with fatty foods. The dose is at least 10 mg/kg per day for 6–8 weeks but up to 20 mg/kg may be required (Higgins *et al*., 2000).
(5) Terbinafine is now well documented for treatment at doses based on weight: <20 kg, 62.5 mg/day; 20–40 kg, 125 mg/day and 40 kg, 250 mg/day for 4 weeks. Terbinafine tablets only are available. The newer treatments (Terbenafine, Itraconazole) are similar to Griseofulvin and may be preferred because the treatment durations are shorter and all have reasonable safety profiles (González *et al*., 2007). However, they are not licensed

for use in the UK and are not all available in paediatric suspensions (Health Protection Agency, 2007).

(6) The use of a topical treatment, for example selenium sulphide or ketaconazole shampoo, or another topically active antifungal, for example Terbenafine cream, is recommended for the first 2 weeks of therapy as this may allow the scalp to heal and prevent formation of crusts where there are kerions (Health Protection Agency, 2007). Carriers should also be given a topical preparation.

(7) Hairbrushes and combs should be cleaned with simple bleach or Milton (Higgins *et al.*, 2000).

Parents are often horrified that their child has a fungal infection and need reassurance that this is not due to a worm (Broomhead, 2007). Children do not need to be kept off school (Health Protection Agency, 2007) as although theoretically there is a potential risk to non-infected children; the method of spread is not clear and the infected child is likely to have been at school for sometime before detection of the infection. Exclusion is probably too late to prevent spread and in addition only reinforces a child's isolation.

Other children in the household should also be examined. Adults in contact with tinea capitis can very rarely develop tinea corporis.

Tinea corporis

This term covers infections of the trunk and limbs with characteristic annular or ring-like lesions which are usually unilateral. They appear as pink scaly plaques or papules which extend outwards and heal form the centre (Figure 12.8). The degree of inflammation depends on whether the infection is anthrophilic, for example *T. rubrum* or *tonsurans* when the lesions are usually less erythematous, or zoophilic, for example *M. canis*, which produces erythematous scaly lesions (Clayton, 2000). It is common in children of all ages and adults but rare cases have been seen in the newborn.

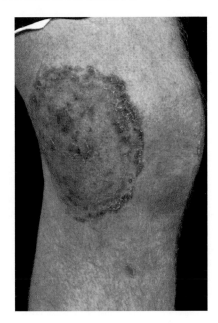

Figure 12.8 Tinea corporis. (Source: Graham-Brown and Burns, 2006.)

Tinea cruris

This is rare before puberty but is frequently seen in adolescent males and adults. Erythematous and scaly lesions extend symmetrically from the groin down the inner thigh and may contain pustules at the edges. Lesions are often very itchy. The causative fungi are either *T. rubrum*, *T. interdigitale* or *E. floccosum*. The last is always the cause of outbreaks in groups of sportspeople or those living in close communities with shared bathing facilities, for example boarding schools (Crawford and Hollis, 2007).

Tinea pedis or athlete's foot

This is the most common form of tinea in temperate climates (Clayton, 2000). It occurs more often in males than females but rarely before puberty. The responsible fungi are all anthrophilic with *T. rubrum* the commonest species. It usually starts in the toe spaces, often between the 4th and 5th toe with peeling, white skin and fissures which are usually itchy. It can spread to the toes and soles of the feet. *T. rubrum* usually results in fine dry scaling on the toes which can become more widespread and chronic. *T. interdigitales* results in small clear vesicles which can spread onto the dorsum of the foot before they rupture and dry with a scaly edge.

Diagnosis

Scrapings can be taken for microscopy.

Management

(1) These lesions respond well to topical antifungals, for example imidazole creams, Clotrimazole twice daily for 2–4 weeks or Terbinafine twice daily for 7–10 days, which is said to be most effective (Crawford and Hollis, 2007).

(2) Particularly in tinea pedis, patients should be educated about the importance of good foot hygiene and careful drying, especially between the toes because moisture encourages fungal growth. Patients should also be advised to change socks and shoes frequently if they become moist with cotton socks and natural fibre shoes providing better ventilation. The wearing of flip flops in communal showering facilities or locker rooms should also be advised.

(3) It is particularly important to treat tinea pedis in those who are prone to cellulitis.

Tinea unguium

Onychomycosis or invasion of the nail plates by species of dermatophytes (mostly *Trichophyton rubrum*) is one of the most common dermatological conditions (Figure 12.9). It is very rare in children but increases with age with toenails more commonly affected than finger nails. It is often associated with existing fungal skin infections, e.g. *tinea pedis*. Although sometimes considered to be a trivial cosmetic problem, it is relentlessly progressive and in the elderly can give rise to complications such as cellulitis and in those with diabetes or peripheral vascular disease can further compromise the limb. It can affect choice of footwear and mobility. It is therefore not surprising that it gives rise to many medical consultations and absence from work (Roberts *et al.*, 2003).

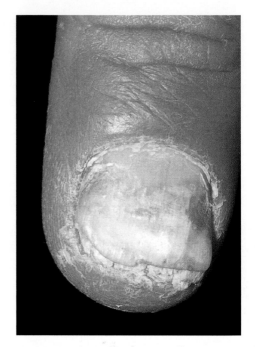

Figure 12.9   Fungal toenail. (Source: Graham-Brown and Burns, 2006.)

It is clinically classified as (Hay and Moore, 2004):

(1) *Distal and lateral subungual onychomycosis (DLSO)*: This is the most common and nearly always due to dermatophyte infection. It often starts with a streak or patch of discoloration, white or yellow at the free edge of the nail plate, often near the lateral nail fold. It then spreads to the base of the nail and may become darker brown or black. The nail plate then thickens and lifts from the nail bed (onycholysis). Surrounding skin nearly always shows signs of tinea pedis. It commonly starts as one affected nail with other digits invaded later. There may be a marked variation in the degree of damage.

(2) *Superficial white onychomycosis (SWO)*: So called due to the 'creamy' white discolouration, distally this is less common than DLSO and affects the surface of the nail plate rather than the nail bed. The dorsal surface of the nail plate is eroded in well-circumscribed powdery white patches where the

white material can be easily scraped away. Toenails are usually affected. Onycholysis is unusual.

(3) *Endonyx onychomycosis*: The organism invades the nail plate from the top surface penetrating deep into the nail plate. There is white creamy discolouration. The nail plate is scarred with pits and lamellar splits. It is usually caused by dermatophytes which cause endothrix scalp infections, notably *T. soudanense*.

(4) *Proximal subungual onychomycosis (PSO)*: Fungi invade the nail bed and plate via the cuticle. The lanula (half moon) of the nail appear as patches of white or yellow discolouration. This is a rare variety of dermatophyte infection which is now more common particularly associated with immunosuppressed patients or those with diabetes or peripheral vascular disease. It is therefore important to think about intercurrent disease, especially HIV in these cases.

Differential diagnosis

The changes of the nail plate and bed can be mimicked by psoriasis, although fine pitting of the nail plate is never seen in fungal infections. Irregular buckling of the nail can be seen in eczema and in lichen planus there may be a ridged or dysplastic nail. Candida can cause paronychia of the nail where there is a tender area of infection where the nail and skin meet at the side or the base of a finger or toenail. However, this usually affects the nail plate proximally and laterally while the free edge is often spared initially. Ringworm of the finger nails is rarely symmetrical and it is common to find the nails of only one hand affected.

Management

This is not a trivial problem and affects many patients' quality of life, functional activity and general well-being. On the grounds of complications, there is a real need to treat. Toenails can take 12 months to grow out and 70–80% cure rates can be expected with fingernails taking 6 months with a cure rate of 80–90% (Roberts *et al.*, 2003). It is therefore vital that patients

understand the nature of the disease and how it is spread along with an acceptance of the long-term nature and slow clinical improvement of antifungal treatments.

(1) Careful clinical examination of the skin of the feet and of the palms is essential.

(2) Treatment should not be started on clinical grounds alone because although 50% of nail dystrophies are due to fungal infection it is not always possible to identify these. A nail sample and clippings should be sent for mycological examination (Box 12.5). The sample needs to be from nail tissue where active disease is present which may mean paring down the nail with a scalpel and clippers to access the nail bed and debris in the middle of the suspected area of infection (Buchanan, 2006). Sampling white superficial nail infection involves scraping the upper surfaces of the nails with a curette or scalpel.

(3) Evidence for the effective use of topical therapies to treat dermatophyte nail infections is limited (Crawford and Hollis, 2007) and systemic treatments are usually used. These include Terbinafine, Itraconazole, Griseofulvin.

(4) Proper early treatment of tinea pedis and tinea manum (ringworm of the hand) would almost certainly reduce the prevalence of tine unguium (Hay and Moore, 2004). Candida species can be treated topically with an imidazole lotion or cream twice daily to the nail fold or oral Itraconazole for 14 days.

Box 12.5 Nail clipping sample

Identify the active edge of the nail;
Clip carefully and catch the keratin pieces in the black filter paper container.

Source: RCN/BDNG (2008).

(5) Early diagnosis and treatment is the most effective way to manage onychomycosis (Buchanan, 2006), so patient and carer education is fundamental.

(6) Effective treatment of concomitant tinea infections of the skin, e.g. tinea pedis, to try and prevent ongoing nail involvement and infection is very important.

(7) Patients also need practical advice on foot and nail care especially if they are high risk, e.g. elderly, those with psoriasis, diabetes, peripheral vascular disease or immunocompromised.

(8) Advice should cover a good foot care regime encompassing:

- Daily washing with warm (not hot) water and mild soap or soap substitute;
- Careful drying, especially between toe webs;
- Moisturising of dry, scaly skin on feet and heels with emollient, although this should be avoided between toes;
- Avoiding the use of dusting powder between toes;
- Socks, tights and shoes should fit well and socks and tights should be changed every day;
- Daily checking for any redness, itching or swelling of skin between and around toes and any changes in colour, shape, thickness or smoothness of nails;
- Cutting toe nails straight across in line with toe shape and avoiding cutting close to corners of nails;
- Seeking advice for treatment of corns and calluses;
- Prompt advice if fungal infection is suspected;
- Possible referral to a podiatrist.

Buchanan (2006).

Tinea incognito

This is not a specific type of lesion but describes an infection where the usual clinical signs of tinea have been modified by the application of topical corticosteroids. The rash may have become more widespread and the active margins may be lost.

Yeast infections

These infections are common (Crawford and Hollis, 2007) and generally caused by commensal organisms; organisms which normally live on the skin (particularly of the oral cavity and genital tracts) in symbiosis with their human hosts. This non-parasitic relationship becomes pathogenic when opportunistic situations which favour its multiplication arise. This is common while patients are taking oral antibiotics or oral contraceptives or in patients who are immuno-suppressed.

Candida albicans is a commensal of the mouth and gastrointestinal tract which can result in opportunistic infection (Gawkrodger, 2003). There are predisposing factors which good nursing advice may help patients to address:

(1) *Moist and opposing skin folds*: advise patients to dry the skin well after washing especially in skin folds with the use of individual towels;
(2) Obesity patients require advice about weight reduction strategies;
(3) Immunosuppressed patients require education about such opportunistic infections in order to recognise them and seek advice early;
(4) Pregnancy
(5) *Poor hygiene*: patients need advice about good skin hygiene and careful drying;
(6) *Humid environments*: patients should be advised to avoid skin occlusion in order to aid healing and prevent recurrence;
(7) *Wet work occupations*: offer advice about careful hand drying and hand protection during wet work, e.g. gloves;
(8) Use of broad-spectrum antibiotics should be avoided unless necessary.

Presentation

Yeast infections may present in a number of different ways.

Genital thrush commonly presents as an itchy, sore vulvovaginitis. Mucous membranes are inflamed and white plaques adhere to these. There may be a white vaginal discharge or penile discharge. Thrush can be spread by sexual intercourse.

Intertrigo

There is a moist macerated appearance to this super-infection with *Candida albicans* in the sub mammary, axillary or inguinal folds and in the interdigital clefts. Red macerated skin with satellite lesions just ahead of the advancing edge is very distinctive of candida.

Oral

White plaques stick to the buccal mucosa (Figure 12.10). Unlike leukoplakia (white plaques on the mucous membranes), these can be scraped off and leave small bleeding points underneath. Broad-spectrum antibiotics, false teeth, poor oral hygiene and poorly sterilised feeding equipment in babies can predispose to this.

Systemic

Systemic candidiasis can occur in immunosuppressed patients. Red nodules or pustules are seen in the skin.

Management

(1) There is little evidence on the optimal treatment of candidal skin infections.
(2) It is generally agreed that general measures such as good hygiene and careful drying should be improved and other predisposing factors addressed.
(3) Topical imidazoles, for example clotrimazole, ketaconazole, are recommended for first-line treatment.

(4) Oral treatment is required for people with severe or extensive disease or when topical treatment has failed.
(5) Oral Fluconazole is recommended as the first-line treatment if systemic treatment is needed.
(6) In children under the age of 12 years specialist advice should be sought.

Pityriasis versicolor

This is a chronic yeast infection which is often asymptomatic. It is seen in adolescents and adults but not younger children. It is characterised by pigmentary changes, often on the trunk and proximal parts of the limbs. Brown or pinkish oval or round scaly patches are seen (Gawkrodger, 2003) (Figure 12.11). In tanned or pigmented skin, the lesions may be hypopigmented. It is caused by overgrowth of a yeast called *Pityrosporum orbiculare*. It is common in young adults.

Management

(1) Topical imidazole antifungal, e.g. Canesten or Daktarin, or alternatively selenium sulphide shampoo (Selsun) or ketaconazole shampoo should be applied and showered off after 5–10 minutes three times a week for 2 weeks. The best way to do this may be to lather the shampoo on the scalp and then allow the lather to sit on the skin.

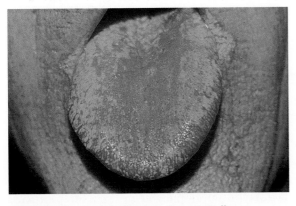

Figure 12.10 Candida albicans. (Source: Weller *et al.*, 2008.)

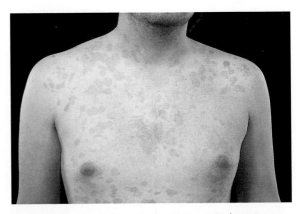

Figure 12.11 Pityriasis versicolor. (Source: Graham-Brown and Burns, 2006.)

While redness and scaling rapidly improves, colour disturbances can take months to recover.

(2) Recurrence is common, so patients need to be made aware of the difference between prolonged repigmentation and recurrence of the active condition.

(3) For resistant cases, Itraconazole 200 mg daily for 7 days may be given.

Infestations

Infestations are defined as the harbouring of insect or worm parasites in or on the body (Gawkrodger, 2003) and these are also common presenting problems in primary care.

Scabies

Scabies is a contagious parasitic infection of the skin endemic throughout the world with a global prevalence of 300 million but particularly problematic in areas of poor sanitation, overcrowding and social disruption (Strong and Johnstone, 2007). Despite its incidence, it is often missed or misdiagnosed. It can affect people of any age but is mostly seen in children, young adults, elderly people especially those in institutions and those who are immunocompromised. It is more common in overcrowded situations and in urban areas. It is a huge source of embarrassment and misery from severe itching and sleepless nights. Disease control is often hampered by inappropriate or delayed diagnosis and poor treatment compliance (Heukelbach and Feldmeier, 2006).

It is caused by the *Sarcoptes scabeii* mite and spreads from person to person by direct skin contact which includes sexual, though transfer via clothing or furnishings is possible. The pregnant female lays eggs in burrows in the stratum corneum; 50–72 hours later, the larvae appear and make new burrows. They mature, mate and repeat this 10- to 17-day cycle. Physical findings include burrows (Figure 12.12), erythematous

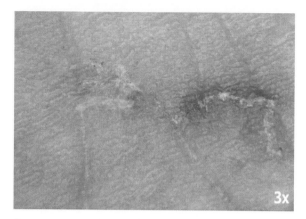

Figure 12.12 Scabies burrow. (Source: Graham-Brown and Burns, 2006.)

papules, excoriations, nodules, vesico-pustular or bullous lesions and secondary bacterial infection. The classic sites of infection are between the fingers, the wrists, axillary areas, female breasts (particularly the skin of the nipples), peri-umbilical area, penis, scrotum and buttocks (Strong and Johnstone, 2007). Infants are usually affected on the face, scalp, palms and soles. There are more pustules in younger children. The condition is very itchy which is often worse at night. The host immune reaction to the presence of mites and their products in the epidermis (Heukelbach and Feldmeier, 2006) is the source of much of the itching and can appear about a month after initial infection and persist for up to 6 weeks after treatment.

Crusted (Norwegian) scabies is much more severe and is associated with extreme incapacity and immunosuppression such as in HIV infection. This form of scabies presents with a hyperkeratotic dermatosis which can resemble psoriasis and lymphadenopathy and eosinophilia may also be present. Itching may be surprisingly mild. These patients are highly infectious and may harbour millions of mites which may also be on the scalp (Strong and Johnstone, 2007). Complications are few but secondary bacterial infection with *S. aureus* or *Group A Streptococcus* can occur. Scabies is a risk factor for developing acute post-streptococcal glomerulonephritis (Heukelbach and Feldmeier,

2006). In crusted scabies, a generalised lymphadenopathy is common and secondary sepsis can lead to death.

Diagnosis

This is usually made on clinical grounds and good history-taking. Other family members may be infected and although they may be asymptomatic, more classically itching which starts at the same time amongst family members or those living in an institution, indicates scabies. Differential diagnosis includes atopic eczema, allergic contact dermatitis, insect bites, papular urticaria and impetigo.

Microscopic identification of the mite can be made by picking out a mite from a burrow with a needle. Alternatively, scrapings can be looked at in the same way.

Management

The management of scabies falls into two equally important halves:

(1) Getting rid of the patient's own scabies and ensuring that all family and those who have had prolonged contacts are treated, even if they are asymptomatic. This means checking who lives at home and who visits regularly and ensuring the patient knows how to apply the treatment correctly.
(2) Making sure that the patient and contacts do not catch it again which means that all family members and sexual contacts must be treated too, whether they say they are itchy or not (BAD, 2004).

Of the topical scabicides in use (Maliathon, Permethrin and Sulphur), on recent review, Permethrin appears to be the most effective (Strong and Johnstone, 2007). This must be applied correctly in order to be effective.
Procedure:

(1) All those who need treatment should apply it at the same time.
(2) Avoid bathing before application as this increases absorption into the blood and removes the treatment from their site of action on the skin (BNF, 2008).

(3) Treatment should be applied to the whole body, including the scalp, face, neck and ears.
(4) Special care needs to be taken with genitalia, flexures, fingernails, webs of the fingers and toes.
(5) Leave the treatment on for at least 12 hours before washing off.
(6) When hands are washed during this period (or a child's nappy changed), treatment should be reapplied.
(7) Apply two treatments 1 week apart.
(8) Ordinary washing of clothes and bedding is sufficient (BAD, 2004).

Ivermectin, an oral antihelminthic appears to be an effective (off license) treatment (Strong and Johnstone, 2007) and may be useful in the management of crusted scabies and epidemics. Plant derivatives, for example neem, turmeric and tea tree oil, are promising future treatments (Heukelbach and Feldmeier, 2006).

Following effective treatment, itching can take up to 6 weeks to subside unless reinfestation occurs. This allows time for lesions to heal and for eggs and mites to reach maturity (i.e. beyond the longest incubation interval), if treatment fails (Strong and Johnstone, 2007). Scabies nodules can take longer to subside and topical corticosteroids may be indicated.

Lice

Lice are flat, wingless blood-sucking insects that lay their eggs or nits on hairs and clothing. There are two species: body lice (includes head lice) and pubic lice. These are often very stigmatising conditions.

Body lice

The body louse is usually seen in people living in poor social conditions and is spread by infested bedding and clothing. Excoriation is common and lichenification and pigmentary changes may occur. The lice are seen on the clothing, not the person. It can be treated by washing clothing and bedding and topical application of maliathon or permethrin.

Head lice (Pediculosis capitis)

These are a worldwide phenomenon and affect people of all ages but are very common among children with those aged 4–11 years most affected (Wyndham, 2008). The itching usually starts at the side and back of the head and the scratching often results in secondary infection and matted hair. The nits or eggs are often easier to see than the lice (Gawkrodger, 2003). They are more common in girls and in urban areas and spread by head to head contact. For reasons which are unclear, some children experience persistent head lice infestations which last weeks, or even years (Gordon, 2007). For many of these children and their families, this is very problematic and the strain and difficulties which should not be underestimated are well documented by Gordon. The families she studied experienced ostracisation and social isolation and feelings of failure as parents. They sought help from a multitude of services while trying to keep the lice a secret from their communities and well demonstrated the ways in which head lice made them lose their sense of perspective.

Management

This needs to be with the pediculicide to which the lice are most likely to be sensitive and will vary from district to district. Maliathon, permethrin or carbaryl lotion are all commonly used. Shampoos are too weak to be effective so lotion or liquid preparations should be used. Alcoholic preparations are most effective but can be irritant (BNF, 2008).

(1) Apply pediculicide to all areas of the scalp and to all the hairs from their roots to their tips.
(2) Leave on for 12 hours before washing off and repeat after a week to kill any lice which have hatched out after the first application.
(3) If lice are found after the second treatment, then treatment should start again with a different pediculicide.
(4) Alcohol-based lotions can sting but shampoos which are on for a short time are less effective.
(5) Hair should also be combed on a daily basis with the help of a good light and a magnifying glass. Combing (which can be very time consuming) should go on until no living lice have been found for 2 weeks. Using a conditioner to lubricate the hair make may combing easier. The comb should be washed regularly to remove lice and eggs (BAD, 2008).

Pubic lice

Pubic lice results in severe itching with secondary infection and eczema. Maliathon or permethrin should be applied to all the body and any secondary infection treated. Sexual partners also need to be treated.

AIDS and the skin

Acquired immune deficiency syndrome (AIDS) is caused by the HIV which affects immunocompetent cells including CD4 T-cells and macrophages. Dermatological involvement in AIDS has been appreciated since the first recognition of the disease (Bunker and Gotch, 2004). The proportion of patients with skin complications and the number of these manifestations in any one patient increase as HIV progresses and AIDS develops. The incidence and severity of several common dermatological conditions covered in this chapter, for example herpes simplex and herpes zoster, folliculitis, viral warts, mollusca, tinea and scabies, are increased in patients with HIV, often in correlation with their CD4 count. Skin disease may therefore provide the first suspicion of the diagnosis of HIV infection and may also present with unusual signs and symptoms, coexist with other pathologies or be altered by treatment, all of which may make them a challenge to diagnose and manage. As highlighted by Bunker and Gotch (2004), good history-taking and examination is therefore vital.

Conclusion

The success of treatments relies on both nurses and parents, carers and patients working together. As nurses, we need to explore the extent to which patients follow advice about treatments and medications. This means discussion and exploration with patients using open questioning as this is more likely to lead to admission about potential difficulties with adherence. Education is vital to explain patho-mechanisms and medication. The patient's level of knowledge about the disorder needs to be assessed so that gaps can be filled in. Treatment rationale and ramifications of non-adherence need to be discussed and instructions simplified, adjusted or interpreted if necessary (Popovich and McAlhany, 2007) to ensure understanding. Adherence is likely to be better when the patient believes the medication is safe. The tailoring of management to meet individual needs and the simplification of treatment regimens to make them realistic and achievable are also essential. Niggermann (2005) also suggests the use of reminders or practical tips such as the use of calendars and tick boxes to reduce medication omissions. The importance of follow-up which is appropriate and negotiated with the patient will also enhance the relationship of trust which Popovich and McAlhany (2007) suggest improves the level of adherence.

The first step towards a successful outcome in the management of all these infections and infestations is accurate diagnosis but this must be coupled with adherence to management to prevent the risk of further spread and achieve positive outcomes. Education is therefore key.

References

All Parliamentary Group on Skin (APPGS) (2008). *Commissioning of Services for People with Skin Conditions*. London: APPGS.

Braue, A., G. Ross, G. Varigos and H. Kelly (2005). Epidemiology and impact of childhood molluscum contagiosum: A case series and critical review of the literature. *Pediatric Dermatology*, **22**(4): 287–294.

British Association of Dermatologists (BAD) (2004). *Scabies Patient Information Leaflet*. London: British Association of Dermatologists.

British Association of Dermatologists (2006). *Staphylococcal Scalded Skin Syndrome: Patient Information Leaflet*. London: British Association of Dermatologists.

British Association of Dermatologists (2007). *Boils Patient Information Leaflet*. London: British Association of Dermatologists.

British Association of Dermatologists (2008). *Head Lice Patient Information Leaflet*. London: British Association of Dermatologists.

British National Formulary (BNF) (2008). No 56 London: BMJ Publishing.

Brogan, P.A., A. Bose, D. Burgner *et al.* (2002). Kawasaki disease: An evidence based approach to diagnosis, treatment, and proposals for future research. *Archives of Disease in Childhood*, **86**: 286–290.

Broomhead, C. (2007). Fungal infections of the skin and nails. *Practice Nurse*, **33**(9):25–29.

Buchanan, P. (2006). Onychomycosis: Managing patients at risk. *Journal of Community Nursing*, **20**(6): 35–40.

Bunker, C. and F. Gotch (2004). AIDS and the skin. In: Burns, T., Breatnach, S., Cox, N., Grifiths, C. (Eds), *Rook's Textbook of Dermatology* (7th edition), pp. 26.1–26.41. London: Blackwell Science.

Burr, S. (2003). Impetigo. In: Barnes, K. (Ed.), *Paediatrics: A Clinical Guide for Nurse Practitioners*, pp. 70–72. London: Elsevier Science.

Charman, C. and S. Lawton (2006). *Eczema: What Really Works*. London: Robinson.

Clayton, Y.M. (2000). Superficial fungal infections. In: Harper, J., Oranje, A. and Prose, N. (Eds), *Textbook of Paediatric Dermatology*, pp. 447–467. Oxford: Blackwell Science.

Courtenay, M., N. Carey and J. Burke (2007). Independent extended nurse prescribing for patients with skin conditions: A national questionnaire survey. *Journal of Clinical Nursing*, (16): 1247–1255.

Cox, N. (2006). Oedema as a risk factor for multiple episodes of cellulitis/erysipelas of the lower leg: A series with community follow-up. *British Journal of Dermatology*, (155): 947–950.

Crawford, F. and S. Hollis (2007). Topical treatments for fungal infections of the skin and nails of the foot. *Cochrane Database of Systemic Reviews*, (3): Art No: CD001434. DOI:10.1002/14651858. CD001434.pub2.

Docherty, C. (2001). Infections and infestations. In: Hughes, E., Van Onselen, J. (Eds), *Dermatology Nursing: A Practical Guide*. London: Churchill Livingstone.

Gawkrodger, D. (2003). *Dermatology: An Illustrated Colour Text*. London: Churchill Livingstone.

Gibbs, S. and I. Harvey (2006). Topical treatments for cutaneous warts. *Cochrane Database of Systematic Reviews*, (3): Art No: CD001781. DOI:10.1002/14651858.CD01871.pub2.

González, U., T. Seaton, G. Bergus, J. Jacobson and C. Martinez-Monzon (2007). Systemic antifungal therapy for tinea capitis in children. *Cochrane Database of Systemic Reviews*, (4): Art No: CD004685. DOI:10.1002/14651858. CD004685.pub2.

Goodyear, H. (2000). Herpes simplex virus infections. In: Harper, J., Oranje, A., Prose, N. (Eds), *Textbook of Paediatric Dermatology*, pp. 321–328. Oxford: Blackwell Science.

Gordon, S.C. (2007). Shared vulnerability: A theory of caring for children with persistent head lice. *The Journal of School Nursing*, 23(5): 283–292.

Gould, F.K., R. Brindle, P.R. Chadwick *et al.* on behalf of the MRSA Working Party of the British Society for Antimicrobial Chemotherapy (2009). Guidelines (2008) for the prophylaxis and treatment of methicillin-resistant *Staphylococuus aureus* (MRSA) infections in the United Kingdom. *Journal of Antimicrobial Chemotherapy Advance Access*, published12 March 2009.

Graham-Brown, R. and Burns, T. (2006). *Lecture Notes: Dermatology* (9th edition). Oxford: Blackwell Science.

Harnden, A., R. Mayon-White, R. Perera, D. Yeates, M. Goldacre and D. Burgner (2009). Kawasaki disease in England: Ethnicity, deprivation and respiratory pathogens. *The Pediatric Infectious Disease Journal*, 28(1): 21–24.

Hay, R. and M.K. Moore (2004). Mycology. In: Burns, T., Breatnach, S., Cox, N., Grifiths, C. (Eds), *Rook's Textbook of Dermatology* (7th edition), pp. 31.1–31.101. London: Blackwell Science.

Health Protection Agency (2007). *Tinea Capitis in the United Kingdom. A report on its Diagnosis, Management and Prevention*. London: Health Protection Agency.

Heukelbach, J. and H. Feldmeier (2006). Scabies. *The Lancet*, (367) 9524, 1767–1774.

Higgins, E.M., L.C. Fuller and C.H. Smith (2000). Guidelines for the management of tinea capitis. *British Journal of Dermatology*, 143: 53–58.

Kilburn, S., P. Featherstone, B. Higgins, R. Brindle and M. Severs (2003). Interventions for cellulites and erysipelas. (Protocol) *Cochrane Database of Systematic Reviews*, (1): Art No: CD004299. DOI:10.1002/.14651858. CD004299.

Klassen, T.P., L. Hartling, N. Wiebe and E. Belsecl (2005). Acyclovir for treating varicella in otherwise healthy children and adolescents. *Cochrane Database of Systematic Reviews*, (4): Art No: CD002980. DOI: 10.1002/14651858. CD002980.pub3.

Koning, S., A.P. Verhagen, L.W.A. van Suijlekom-Smit, A. Morris, C.C. Butler, J.C. van der Wouden (2003). Interventions for impetigo. *Cochrane Database of Systematic reviews*, (2): Art No: CD003261. DOI:10.1002/14651858.CD003261.pub2.

Loffeld, A., P. Davies, A. Lewis and C. Moss (2005). Seasonal occurrence of impetigo: A retrospective 8-year review (1996–2003). *Clinical and Experimental Dermatology*, 30: 512–514.

Macartney, K. and P. McIntyre (2008). Vaccines for post-exposure prophylaxis against varicella (chickenpox) in children and adults. *Cochrane Database of Systematic Reviews*, 3: Art No: CD001833. DOI:10.1002/14651858. CD001833.pub2.

McCormick, A., D. Fleming and J. Charlton (1995). *Morbidity Statistics from General Practice. Fourth National Study 1991–1992*. London: HMSO.

Nathwani, D., M. Morgan, R.G. Masterton *et al.* (2008). Guidelines for UK practice for the diagnosis and management of methicillin-resistant *Staphylococcus aureus* (MRSA) infections in the community. *Journal of Antimicrobial Chemotherapy*, (61): 976–994.

Niggermann, B. (2005). How can we improve compliance in pediatric pneumology and allergology? *Allergy*, 60(6): 735–738.

Penzer, R. (2005). Common superficial fungal infections of the skin. *Nursing in Practice*, Jul/Aug 31–34.

Popovich, D. and A. McAlhany (2007). Accurately diagnosing commonly misdiagnosed circular rashes. *Pediatric Nursing*, 33(4): 315–320.

Quartey-Papafio, C.M. (1999). Importance of distinguishing between cellulitis and varicose eczema of the leg. *British Medical Journal*, 318: 1672–1673.

Royal College of Nursing/British Dermatological Nursing Group (2008). *Competencies for an Integrated Career and Competency Framework for Dermatological Nursing*, pp. 48–49. London. Royal College of Nursing.

Resnick, S.D. (2000). Staphylococcal and streptococcal skin infections: Pyodermas and toxin-mediated syndromes. In: Harper, J., Oranje, A., Prose, N. (Eds), *Textbook of Paediatric Dermatology*, pp. 369–372. Oxford: Blackwell Science Ltd.

Roberts, D.T., W.D. Taylor and J. Boyle (2003). Guidelines for treatment of onychomycosis. *British Journal of Dermatology*, 148(3): 402–410.

Shuru, D. (2003). Varicella (chickenpox). In: Barnes, K. (Ed.), *Paediatrics: A Clinical Guide for Nurse Practitioners*, pp. 227–229. London: Elsevier Science.

Sterling, J.C., S. Handfield-Jones and P.M. Hudson (2001). Guidelines for the management of cutaneous warts. *British Journal of Dermatology*, 144(1): 4–11.

Strong, M. and P.W. Johnstone (2007). Interventions for treating scabies. *Cochrane Database of Systematic Reviews*, (3): Art No: CD0032 0. DOI:1002/14651858. CD000320. pub2.

Tebruegge, M., M. Kuruvilla and I. Margarson (2006). Does the use of calamine or antihistamine provide symptomatic relief from pruritis in children with varicella zoster infection? *Archives of Disease in Childhood*, 91: 1035–1036.

van der Wouden, J.C., J. Menke, S. Gajadin *et al.* (2006). Interventions for cutaneous molluscum contagiosum. *Cochrane Database of Systemic Reviews*, (2): Art No: CD004767. DOI:10.1002/14651858. CD004767.pub2.

Watson, T. and G.P. de Bruin (2007). Impact of cutaneous disease on the self-concept: An existential – Phenomenological study of men and women with psoriasis. *Dermatology Nursing*, 19(4): 351–364.

Weller, R., J.A.A. Hunter, J. Savin and M. Dahl (2008). *Clinical Dermatology* (4th edition). Oxford: Blackwell Publishing.

Wiffen, P.J., H.J. McQuay, J.E. Edwards and R.A. Moore (2005). Gabapentin for acute and chronic pain. *Cochrane Database of Systematic Reviews*, (3): Art No: CD005452. DOI: 10.1002/14651858. CD005452.

Wyatt, H. (2008). Non-accidental injury in dermatology. *Dermatological Nursing*, 7(4): 30–36.

Wyndham, M. (2008). Picture. *Community Practitioner*, 81(2): 33.

Less common skin conditions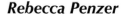

13

Rebecca Penzer

Introduction

It is something of a challenge to select the most common, uncommon skin conditions to include in this chapter. The conditions that have been included here are the ones that someone working in a general setting is most likely to see. Those working in a specialist area are likely to see all of them at some point in time. Also included in this chapter are some conditions which do not fit easily into any of the other chapters and are actually quite common, e.g. rosacea and pityriasis rosea.

The structure of this chapter is to provide an outline of the disease itself; the way it presents and its pathogenesis and then to describe the treatments that are relevant to each condition, along with evidence for selection of the treatment if any is available. Any specific nursing care activities will be included in the section on treatment. This chapter will not repeat the information given in previous chapters about the importance of considering quality of life, concordance and psycho-social impact, although of course all these issues will be pertinent.

Blistering conditions

Blisters can appear in the skin as a result of a number of causes. These include:

- Congenital in which there are faults in the way the layers of skin adhere together;
- Physical in which the skin splits because of some kind of injury, e.g. sheering forces;
- Infections which cause disruption in the layers of the skin (usually the epidermis) which lead to blistering, e.g. impetigo;
- Inflammation in its acute phase can lead to secondary blistering, e.g. eczema;
- Immunobullous disease in which immunologically mediated damage leads to splitting of the layers of skin either between the dermis and the epidermis or between the layers of the epidermis, e.g. bullous pemphigoid (Graham-Brown and Bourke, 1998).

In this section, the focus will be on the more common congenital diseases and the immunobullous diseases.

Epidermolysis bullosa

This describes a group of inherited blistering disorders which generally present early in life, although milder forms of the disease may not present until later in life. The autosomal dominant forms of epidermolysis bullosa (EB) require just one parent to have the faulty EB gene and the autosomal recessive forms require both parents to pass on an EB gene. This genetically determined group of conditions are characterised by the fact that the layers of skin do not adhere to each other normally, leading to splits between the layers of skin. Where these splits

occur will determine the exact type of EB that an individual experiences (see Table 13.1).

Treatment

The treatment for all forms of EB focus on protecting the skin, minimising trauma and reducing the likelihood of infection. A systematic review found that there was no reliable trial evidence for other interventions for treating EB (Langan and Williams, 2009). The more severe forms will also involve ensuring adequate nutritional intake and surgery to manage scarring which can cause 'webbing' to develop between

Table 13.1 Summary of the types of epidermolysis bullosa.

Type of EB	Type of inheritance	Level of cleavage	Subtype	Location of blisters	Course of disease
EB simplex	Autosomal dominant	Within the basal cells of the epidermis	Generalised	Areas of trauma or friction	Intense levels of blistering starting as a neonate, which heal without scarring but can lead to severe incapacity continuing into adulthood.
			Weber–Cockayne	Hands and feet following trauma	As above, although onset may be delayed until adolescence or adulthood.
			Dowling Meara	Generalised severe form. Blisters present at birth, face, trunk and limbs. May involve mouth, GI and respiratory tracts	Very rare. Can be fatal to infants however may subside as the child grows up.
Junctional	Autosomal recessive	Within lamina lucida of the basement membrane zone		Widespread including mouth and pharynx	Eroded areas are widespread and hard to heal. Begin in neonatal period. Child often dies early due to sepsis.
Dystrophic	Autosomal recessive	Subepidermal with loss of anchoring fibrils		Widespread including mouth, pharynx and eyes	Blisters appear either from trauma or spontaneously and heal with scarring. If mouth/pharynx is involved, there can be problems with eating and eye scarring can lead to blindness. Nails and teeth are abnormal and squamous cell carcinomas may develop in atrophic areas.
	Autosomal dominant			Smaller blisters generally appearing on limbs and areas of trauma	Less serious than recessive but scarring does occur and blistering continues throughout life.

fingers and toes. Thus, consideration must be given to soft furnishing, padded with sheepskins and soft clothes that do not rub or scratch. The child must always be handled with great care to minimise the amount of blistering caused by friction and trauma. For those who have the various forms of EB simplex, healing occurs without scarring and although this may take some time it does usually happen. Dystrophic forms of EB, particularly the recessive forms, will scar and require great care to be given to dressings and preventing infections.

The most important feature of any dressings that are used is that they are non-adherent and that they can stay in place for a number of days without requiring changing. Thus a secondary absorbent dressing may need to be placed over the primary non-adherent one. Dressings should not be stuck to the skin but secured with light bandages or cotton tubular dressings. If dressings do become stuck to the skin, it may cause less trauma to remove them whilst soaking in a bath during bathing (Ly and Su, 2008). Pain relief during dressing change is likely to be necessary; the choice of pain relief dependant on the level of pain. For some, Entonox may provide sufficient relief during the dressing change and avoids the problems of drowsiness associated with some pain relief.

Nutritional problems occur most commonly in the more severe forms of EB; junctional, dystrophic recessive and Dowling Meara. From an early age, neonates can develop blisters in their mouths, the lips and on the tongue which make feeding very painful. This may be helped by using teething gel and white soft paraffin on the lips, but oral feeding may in the end prove too difficult. In this instance, a long-term nasogastric tube should be used. Breast feeding is rarely successful as the child's face becomes blistered whilst suckling and rubbing against its mother's breast.

At all ages, EB sufferers are likely to have high calorific requirements due to the calories required for wound healing. This in combination with the difficulty of eating orally can mean that maintaining adequate nutrition is extremely challenging. Gastrostomy feeding may be necessary.

Physiotherapy will be helpful for those with dystrophic recessive EB in order to help minimise the contractions caused by scarring.

EB in all its forms can be a distressing condition, particularly as it occurs so early in life and as there is little effective treatment, only symptom management. It is important that an accurate diagnosis is made early on so that the parents know what to expect by way of disease severity. For those with the recessive form of the condition there is unlikely to have been any previous experience of the disease. It is important that parents have the opportunity to discuss the likelihood of having subsequent children with the disease, with a genetic counsellor. Prenatal diagnosis is possible.

Immunobullous diseases

Bullous pemphigoid

The most common of the immunobullous conditions, bullous pemphigoid predominantly affects the older population usually occurring in the seventh or eighth decade. It affects men and women equally. The split in the skin is subepidermal leading to tense fluid filled blisters in which the roof of the blister is the full thickness of the epidermis (Figure 13.1). The split is

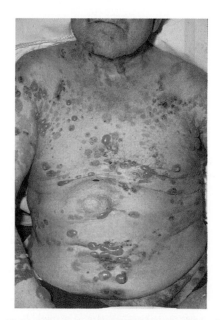

Figure 13.1 Bullous pemphigoid. (Source: Reprinted from Graham-Brown and Burns, 2006.)

triggered by the presence of a specific antibody, its action is directed at the basement membrane complex (probably the hemidesmosomes (see Chapter 2). The blisters often occur in flexures and around 50% of patients have lesions on the mucous membranes, the mouth being most commonly affected (Wojnarowska *et al.*, 2002). Prior to the blisters developing, it is usual for patients to experience an irritating erythematous rash which may look somewhat urticarial. The blisters themselves may be haemorrhagic (blood filled).

Diagnosis is usually confirmed by a biopsy which should be taken from the edge of a new blister. This will show the subepidermal split. Direct immunofluorescence will show the antibodies lining up along the basement membranes of the cells. The disease is self-limiting and blisters will eventually stop forming; however this may take years, so treatment is usually necessary and desirable.

Treatment

Intensity of treatment will depend on the severity of the disease. The overall aim of treatment is to suppress the symptoms of blister formation, pruritis and urticaria, so that quality of life is maintained. This is generally achieved by immunosuppression of some description. Because the patient population is generally elderly, the treatment of symptoms with potent immunosuppression can cause a level of morbidity or even mortality, thus treatments must be closely monitored and there is a significant need for expert nursing care.

For more mild to moderate disease control may be gained by the use of very potent topical steroids (particularly 0.05% clobetasol proprionate) alone. This may be sufficient to gain control and oral therapies may not be needed. A review of the evidence for BP treatment regimes shows that there is little consensus about exact levels of oral treatment (Wojnarowska *et al.*, 2002). However, the evidence does indicate that oral corticosteroids (usually prednisolone) should be used to control new blister formation in severe forms of the disease. 1 mg/kg is the commonly recommended starting dose for extensive disease, although in reality the dosage may not be directly related to patient weight and a starting dose of 60 mg is often used. The quality of evidence of the effectiveness of any of the other oral therapies is low; azathioprine is the most common additional treatment used, but the studies looking at its steroid sparing effects are conflicting (Wojnarowska *et al.*, 2002). However, it may be added into a treatment regime if steroids alone are not halting blister formation. In severe disease, topical therapies are often used alongside the oral therapy.

High doses of steroids in elderly patients are associated with significant levels of morbidity and occasionally mortality. Careful monitoring for glucose in the urine and increased blood pressure should be routine. Monitoring the patient's temperature will help indicate if an infection is developing. Eroded areas should be swabbed and sent for culturing if there are signs of infection.

Helping patients to remain comfortable and managing the blisters are key nursing roles. New blister formation should be logged each day as a method of determining treatment efficacy, i.e. if treatment is working, the number of new blisters developing each day will reduce and eventually stop. New blisters need to be broken using minimal skin trauma. Making a small incision with a blade is more effective than lancing with a needle as the incision is less likely to reseal than a hole. The skin should be left in place in order to form a natural dressing over the dermis. If topical steroids are being applied to the lesions, it is easier to apply the product to a non-adherent dressing and then onto the skin – cream is preferable to an ointment. The dressing should be secured using a light bandage or cotton tubular bandage, not tape. Maintaining skin hygiene is important in view of the large areas of open skin. Daily bathing with an antiseptic emollient may be helpful, although no evidence could be found to support this. Bland petrolatum emollients (e.g. white soft paraffin/liquid paraffin) can be helpful to maintain skin comfort particularly in the old blister sites where the skin tends to be dry.

Treatment is gradually reduced over time and then stopped once it appears that the patient is in total remission. Wojnarowska *et al.* (2002) recommend that treatment is reduced every 1–2 months and also states that the appearance of the occasional lesion should not lead to increase in treatment, rather should be taken as an indication that the condition is not being over treated. It is possible for people to experience relapses after periods of remission at which point treatment may need to be introduced again.

Pemphigus

This describes a group of disorders in which the skin splits at different levels within the epidermis. There is dissolution of the intracellular cement which holds the epidermal keratinocytes together caused by an antibody that acts directly on these intracellular proteins. The epidermal cells then no longer hold together and flaccid, easily broken blisters appear. The most common type of pemphigus (pemphigus vulgaris) is still very rare (probably around 1 in a million), although it is seen more commonly in Ashkenazy Jews and Indians. It tends to affect a younger age group than bullous pemphigoid, striking 50- to 60-year olds.

Because the skin splits within the epidermis, the blisters have very thin roofs to them and the skin becomes extensively eroded very quickly leading to fluid and protein loss and the potential for severe skin infections. In addition to this, the mouth and other mucosal surfaces are commonly affected with the consequent difficulty with eating and drinking. Patients with pemphigus can quickly become very unwell.

Treatment and nursing care are similar to bullous pemphigoid, being based on immunosuppression through high dose oral steroids. The patient is likely to be hospitalised and nursing care should include monitoring for the effects of high steroid doses along with fluid balance and care of the skin erosions (blisters will usually burst themselves as they are so fragile). In addition oral care is likely to be needed.

Connective tissue disorders

In this section, the skin signs related to connective tissue disorders will be considered. Examples of connective tissues diseases that have classic skin signs are systemic lupus erythematosus (SLE), systemic sclerosis, morphea and dermatomyositis. Here SLE and systemic sclerosis will be considered in greater detail.

Systemic lupus erythematosus

Systemic lupus erythematosus is seen most commonly in young women of child bearing age. Its progression is usually through a series of exacerbations followed by periods of remission (Figure 13.2). Systemically it affects many organs as well as the skin, including joints, heart and pericardium, lungs, kidneys, brain and haemopoietic system. The disease is characterised by the development of cytotoxic antibodies and immune complexes (Graham-Brown and Bourke, 1998). The symptoms of SLE are outlined in Box 13.1. (Note that the first four symptoms are also present in cutaneous lupus erythematosus when systemic disease is not present (or only very mildly).

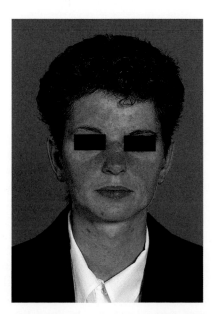

Figure 13.2   Lupus. (Source: Reprinted from Weller *et al.*, 2008.)

Box 13.1   Clinical features of SLE

Erythematous plaque on face but also on neck, ears or scalp;
Follicular plugging;
Scarring in the plaques which can lead to permanent hair loss when on the scalp;
Mouth, nasal epithelium and conjunctiva may also be affected;
Photosensitivity (more marked in SLE);
Raynaud's phenomenon;
Diffuse patchy hair loss;
'Butterfly patch' across the face, more accurately described as a blotchy, evanescent, erythematous rash which is more widely distributed than just across nose and cheeks (Graham-Brown and Bourke, 1998);
Vasculitis.

Box 13.2   Clinical features of systemic sclerosis

Tight shiny face;
Loss of facial wrinkles;
Beaked nose;
Narrowing of the mouth with perioral furrowing;
Facial telangiectasia;
Raynaud's phenomenon;
Tightening of the skin on digits creating progressive contractures;
Painful ulcers at ends of fingers which can progress to resorption of underlying terminal phalanges;
Calcinosis.

Treatment for SLE

Early treatment of plaques with potent topical steroids is important to minimise scarring. Advice about avoiding sun exposure should also be given. Otherwise, the mainstay of treatment for SLE is immunosuppressive comprising of oral steroids and/or azathioprine.

Systemic sclerosis

An autoimmune disease of unknown cause, systemic sclerosis is 3–4 times more common in women than in men and usually starts between the ages of 30–40 (although later in men) (New Zealand Dermatological Society Incorporated, 2009). It is a multisystem disease in which vasculopathy of small arteries produce symptoms affecting the gastrointestinal (GI) tract, lungs, kidneys, heart, liver, nervous and musculoskeletal systems (Graham-Brown and Burns, 2006). The typical skin symptoms are created by 'thickening of the skin'; there is also destruction of the hair follicles and sweat glands. Box 13.2 lists these symptoms. Note that a milder form of the

condition is called CREST. When there is no systemic disease but skin sclerosis is present this is known as morphea.

Treatment for systemic sclerosis

No treatment has been shown to be effective for treating systemic sclerosis.

Drug reactions

Drug-related eruptions of the skin may be caused by a substance which has been used systemically or one that has been applied topically. The level of severity of a drug reaction will vary; however, in most cases, the only way to resolve the eruption is to remove the individual from the medication that has caused the problem. In this section, a number of different types of drug-induced skin eruptions will be considered. For each type, the drugs that are most likely to cause the reaction are listed in the relevant boxes, please note (these are not necessarily comprehensive. It is worth remembering that if an individual is sensitive to a particular drug, they may also react to different drugs that are chemically similar. The skin can respond adversely in

---

Box 13.3 Common drugs that can cause fixed drug reactions

Phenolphthalein	Paracetamol
Tetracyclines	Chlordiazepoxide
Sulphonamides	Non-steroidal
Quinine	anti-inflammatories

Box 13.4 Categories of drugs that can cause toxic erythema

Antibiotics	Barbituates
Antihypertensives	Hydantoins
Non-steroidal anti-inflammatories	

---

a wide, varied way to drugs. Whilst morbilliform type reactions are common, the skin may respond in a number of other ways, e.g. taking on vasculitic or acneiform appearance (Graham-Brown and Bourke, 1998).

Fixed drug reactions

As the name suggests, fixed drug reactions are oval-shaped lesions that are either solitary or multiple, and sometimes have a blistered centre. They occur quickly after taking the sensitising drug (within a few hours) and will reoccur, usually in the same place, each time the drug is taken see Box 13.3. They leave behind a hyperpigmented area of skin. The lesions can occur anywhere on the body but frequently appear on mucosal surfaces including lips and genitalia.

Toxic erythema

The skin may respond adversely in a number of different ways; toxic erythema describes the most common morbilliform presentations where there are symmetrical erythematous macules and papules, larger more confluent patches or urticated plaques. These initial presentations may progress into a more severe picture, e.g. drug hypersensitivity syndrome (DHS) (see later) or toxic epidermal necrolysis. Patients with a suppressed immune system, for example those who have the human immunodeficiency virus (HIV), are more susceptible to drug reactions of this type (Box 13.4).

Drug hypersensitivity syndrome

This is a serious type of drug reaction which has an 8% mortality rate (New Zealand Dermatological Society Incorporated, 2009). It generally occurs 1–8 weeks after the medication is commenced and has three key symptoms: fever, skin rash and organ involvement which generally occur in that order. The rash starts with papules and pustules against a background of erythema and may progress to erythroderma and/or a general exfoliative picture. The degree to which the organs are being affected should be monitored through blood tests assessing liver function and eosinophilia. The cause of DHS is unclear; there is some thought that it is caused by a defect in the liver which affects the way it metabolises certain drugs or that it is related to a co-infection with herpes virus 6. What is more certain is that there is a genetic component to DHS and thus relatives should be counselled (Box 13.5).

Drug-induced skin pigmentation

There are a wide range of skin pigmentations caused by drugs; indeed it is thought that 10–20% of all cases of acquired skin pigmentation are related to drugs (New Zealand Dermatological Society Incorporated, 2009). Although the pigmentation is usually benign, it can become socially unacceptable and may have a significant psychological impact on the patient. In most instances, stopping the drug will mean that the skin colour returns to normal; however, this may take some time and in some instances becomes permanent.

Box 13.5 Drugs that can cause DHS

Abacavir	Diltiazem	NSAIA
Allopurinol	Gold salts	Phenobarbitone
Atenolol	Isoniazid	Phenytoin
Azathioprine	Lamotrigine	Sulfasalazine
Captopril	Mexiletine	Sulphonamides
Carbamazepine	Minocycline	Trimethoprim
Clomipramine	Nevirapine	
Dapsone	Oxicam	

Pigmentation in the skin may occur for a number of reasons. These include:

- Accumulation of certain heavy metals in the dermis following dermal vessel damage. Sufficient accumulation of the heavy metal will cause pigment change without any associated increase in the level of melanin.
- Drug–pigment complexes might be formed with melanin in the skin, exposure to sunlight can trigger this reaction.
- Other drugs will trigger the accumulation of melanin as a non-specific post-inflammatory change. This may be worsened by exposure to sunlight.
- Some drugs can cause pigmentation by directly accumulating and/or reacting with substances in the skin.

Table 13.2 taken from www.dermnetnz.org outlines the clinical features associated with the drugs that are most likely to cause pigmentation.

Treatment involves stopping the drug involved if the pigmentation is causing distress. However, as can be seen from Table 13.2, most pigmentary changes are aggravated (and often triggered) by exposure to the sun. Therefore advice about sun protection is critical to reducing the problems associated with pigmentary changes.

Drug-induced photosensitisation

Photosensitisation reactions can be divided into two broad groups: those that are phototoxic and those that are photoallergic with the former being more common.

Drugs that may cause photosensitisation are listed in Box 13.6.

Phototoxic sensitisation describes a direct damage to skin tissue caused by the light activating the photosensitising substance. The reaction can occur at virtually any time post-exposure to the photosensitising substance and light, from immediately to hours afterwards. Its appearance is usually that of sunburn (it may be accompanied by vesicles and blisters); however, amiodarone and sunlight turn the skin a blue-green colour in sensitive individuals. The reaction only occurs in the sun-exposed sites. In addition nail changes may be seen with the nails lifting from the nail bed (onycholysis). For those with darker skin colours, this may be the only sign of the drug-induced photosensitisation.

Photoallergic sensitisation is usually caused by topical applications and is a cell-mediated immune response in which the antigen is the light activated, photosensitising agent. It is characterised by an eczematous type, itchy reaction that can spread to anywhere on the body and will appear 24–72 hours after the exposure to the photosensitising substance and sunlight.

Treatment involves avoiding where possible the medications that lead to photosensitisation. However, in many instances, the therapeutic value of the drugs will outweigh the photosensitisation risks and the patient should be given information and support to protect their skin from the sun using sunscreens, clothing and avoidance.

Table 13.2   Drugs that can cause pigmentary changes.

Drug/drug group	Clinical features
Antipsychotics (chlor-promazine and related phenothiazines)	• Bluish-grey pigmentation, especially in sun-exposed areas. • Pigmentation is cumulative and some areas may develop a purplish tint. • Pigmentation of the conjunctiva in the eye may also occur, along with cataracts and corneal opacities.
Phenytoin	• 10% of patients develop pigmentation of the face and neck resembling chloasma (clearly defined, roughly symmetrical dark brown patches). • Fades after a few months when drug has been stopped.
Antimalarials	• About 25% of patients receiving chloroquine or hydroxychloroquine for several years develop bluish-grey pigmentation on face, neck and sometimes lower legs and forearms. • Continuous long-term use may lead to blue-black patches, especially in sun-exposed areas. • Nail beds and corneal and retinal changes may also develop.
Cytotoxic drugs	• Busulfan, cyclophosphamide, bleomycin and adriamycin have all produced hyperpigmentation to some degree. • Banded or diffuse pigmentation of nails often occurs.
Amiodarone	• Blue-grey pigmentation in sun-exposed areas (face and hands). • Photosensitivity occurs in 30–57% of patients whilst 1–10% show skin pigmentation. • Skin pigmentation is reversible but may take up to 1 year for complete resolution after the drug has been stopped.

Source: New Zealand Dermatological Society Incorporated (2009).

Box 13.6   **Drugs that can cause photosensitisation**

Amiodarone	Tetracyclines
Chlorpromazine	Thiazides
Nalidixic acid	Quinine
Sulphonamides	

Lichen planus

In the USA, lichen planus (LP) has been reported to affect 1% of new patients seen at health care clinics, with most patients being between the ages of 30 and 60, although it can affect any age. There does not seem to be any gender differences. LP can be described as a cell-mediated immune response of unknown origin. The response may be provoked by a viral infection (and there may be a particular association with hepatitis C), by a drug or by a stressful event (Chuang and Stitle, 2008).

Lichen planus represents a wide range of clinical manifestations which are described below. However, the disease is characterised by a number of histological features:

■ Marked liquefaction (conversion to liquid) of the basal layer;
■ Expansion of the granular cell layer;
■ Dense subepidermal infiltrate, predominantly of T-lymphocytes.

Clinically, patients may present with disease limited to one or two areas of skin, more uncommonly the presentation may be extensive affecting both skin and mucous membranes (Figure 13.3). It is not uncommon for mucous membranes to be affected without any symptoms on the skin. In 85% of cases, the lesions will clear from the skin in 18 months time (New Zealand Dermatological Society Incorporated, 2009) but where disease is more extensive and affecting the mucous membranes it can take considerably longer. In around 10% of patients there will also be nail changes.

Classic presentation

The lesions are shiny flat-topped papules which vary in size from being pin-prick to more than a centimetre. The shape of the lesion is often described as polygonal and they may be distributed closely together or widely spread, in linear formation or in rings. They are purplish in colour (known as violaceous) and there are often grey or white lines and dots scattered over the surface; these are known as Wickham's striae. The most common locations for the lesions are wrists, lower back and ankles; however, they can occur anywhere on the body. For some people, scalp papules appear which may progress to atrophic

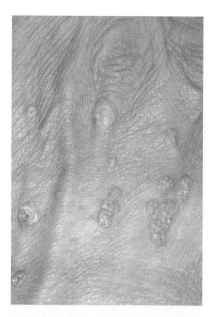

Figure 13.3 Lichen planus. (Source: Reprinted from Graham-Brown and Burns, 2006.)

cicatrical alopecia. Mucous membrane involvement is common; lesions are usually found on the bucal mucosa and tongue, although they can affect conjunctivae, the larynx, the tonsils, the bladder, the vulva, the GI tract and the anus. The presentation is white or grey streaks forming a reticular pattern against a violaceous background. They may become ulcerative; this is linked to an increased risk of malignant transformation, particularly in men.

Symptoms related to the skin lesions vary from nothing to severe pruritis. Scale may also be associated with LP and it tends to be the thicker, scalier areas which are most itchy. As already mentioned the lesions usually clear within 18 months, but during that time some lesions will disappear and other new ones appear. Hyperpigmentation can occur where the lesions have been and this seems to be more common in darker skin colours. On the mucous membranes, lesions can be accompanied with a stinging sensation; they may become painful should the lesions deteriorate and become erosive.

Nail changes in LP occur because of nail plate thinning; this results in longitudinal grooving and ridges. Other nail changes may include subungual hyperkeratosis, onycholysis and longitudinal melanonychia. Rarely the nails may disappear altogether.

Hypertrophic LP

It has already been mentioned that the lesions can become thickened; in extreme cases, this is known as hypertrophic LP and is characterised by extreme pruritis. It usually occurs on the lower limbs particularly around the ankles. These lesions are chronic in nature and can take years to clear. When they do, scarring and hyperpigmentation can remain.

Erosive LP

This type of LP affects mucosal surfaces, usually the mouth and genitals. It is painful and usually chronic in nature. It may be associated with classical cutaneous LP or it can occur alone. The main clinical features of oral erosive LP are large, painful ulcers which heal with scarring. Healing may take weeks. The lesions can occur on the sides of the tongue, insides of the cheeks, on the gums or inside the lips. It mainly affects adults, usually women and children are rarely affected.

Genital erosive LP in women can cause extensive changes to the mucosa and structure of the genitals. The labia minora and entrance to the vagina can become red and raw; more drastically the clitoral hood can disappear and the labia minora stick to each other or the labia majora. The subsequent scarring may cause the labia majora to close over the vagina. If LP affects the inside of the vagina, it may bleed easily on contact and there is a mucky discharge. Genital erosive LP is much less common in men; it causes redness and tenderness of the glans. These changes can be extremely painful particularly when passing urine or having sexual intercourse. The latter may become impossible for women who have considerable structural changes to their genitals.

Bullous LP

This is a rare condition, blisters are seen forming either within the LP papules or alone.

Actinic LP

Lesions of LP are induced by exposure to sunlight.

Treatment for LP

The mainstay of treatments for LP are topical steroids. The cutaneous form will need to be treated with potent or very potent topical products, usually for a 4- to 6-week course. The resolving lesions will flatten to be the same as the rest of the skin surface; it is important to monitor this as the sign of clearance as some pigmentation may remain. If the disease persists, intermittent courses of topical steroids will be needed. For more severe disease, particularly erosive and hypertrophic variants,

oral immunosuppressive therapy may be required. This may be oral steroids, ciclosporin or methotrexate.

For those with oral and genital disease, good hygiene measures should be maintained. Soaps should be avoided when washing the genital area; a soap substitute such as aqueous cream may be used instead. A petrolatum emollient ointment may be helpful to provide some relief from general discomfort. Applying topical steroids in the oral cavity will be enhanced by an inhaler spray or pastes. A number of small studies reviewed by Ruzicka *et al.* indicate that topical calcineurin inhibitors, specifically topical tacrolimus, are helpful for erosive genital and oral LP (Ruzicka *et al.*, 2003). Specifically a 2008 study considered 10 patients with erosive oral LP, 7 of whom had no lesions after 30 days of pimecrolimus compared to 2 with no lesions in the control group. A further 30 days of treatment cleared the lesions in the patients who did not respond in the first 30 days (Volz *et al.*, 2008). This is, however, using the treatment off license.

Pityriasis rosea

This rash of unknown origin can last up to 12 weeks and then resolves spontaneously. It usually affects teenagers and young adults. It may be slightly itchy and scaly but is otherwise asymptomatic. It is sometimes preceded by a generalised viral infection.

The presentation of pityriasis rosea develops over time starting with a single oval patch called a herald patch. This is usually 2–5 cm in diameter and precedes the rest of the rash by up to 20 days. Characteristically, it has a slightly scaly trailing edge; this describes the edge just inside the patch. After the herald patch the rest of the lesions, which are similar although usually smaller, appear mainly over the trunk but also affecting the arms and legs. The distribution of these lesions is often compared to a fir tree, in that they follow the lines of the ribs around the trunk. Lesions do not usually appear on the face.

Nursing care will centre around helping to reassure the patient that what they have is self-limiting and non-contagious. Patients may have been wrongly diagnosed with either psoriasis or tinea corporis and it should be clarified that pityriasis rosea is not related to either of these conditions. Good skin care such as washing with a soap substitute and using a topical emollient may be helpful especially if the skin is itchy. For particularly itchy skin, a brief course of topical steroids (moderate potency) may provide some relief. However, it is unlikely to make any difference to the course of the condition.

Primary cutaneous T-cell lymphomas

Lymphomas are tumours of the lymph nodes and lymphatic system. When the tumour occurs in the skin with no sign of involvement elsewhere in the body, they are known as primary cutaneous lymphomas; of these 65% are T-cell type. The incidence of primary cutaneous lymphomas is about 0.4 per 100,000 people per year and of these approximately two-thirds are T-cell in origin (Whittaker *et al.*, 2003). There appears to be a higher incidence in men. There are a number of types of T-cell lymphoma which can be generally categorised into indolent (or low grade, slow growing) types or the more aggressive lymphomas. These are listed in Table 13.3; however, in this section only the most common T-cell lymphoma, mycosis fungoides (MF) (accounting for 50% of all primary cutaneous lymphomas), is considered in any detail.

Clinical staging for T-cell lymphoma

Box 13.7 outlines how the disease develops in different parts of the body, T indicating the skin, N lymph nodes, M visceral involvement and B haematological involvement.

Once the clinical level of involvement has been established, this can be summarised using the grading system outlined in Box 13.8.

Table 13.3   Types of primary cutaneous T-cell lymphoma.

Indolent	Aggressive
Mycosis fungoides (MF)	Sezary syndrome
MF variants	Adult T-cell
• Fulliculotrophic	leukaemia/lymphoma
• Pagetoid reticulosis	
• Granulomatus slack skin	
Primary cutaneous CD30⁺ lymphoproliferative disorders	Extranodal NK/T-cell lymphoma, nasal type
Subcutaneous panniculitis-like T-cell lymphomas	Primary cutaneous peripheral T-cell
Primary cutaneous CD4⁺ small/medium pleomorphic T-cell lymphoma	

Box 13.7   Summary of clinical changes seen in T-cell lymphoma

T1: Patches or plaques <10% body surface area

T2: Patches of plaques > 10% body surface area

T3: Tumours

T4: Erythroderma

N0: No palpable nodes

N1: 1 palpable node without histological involvement (dermatopathic)

N2: Non-palpable nodes with histological involvement

N3: Palpable nodes with histological involvement

M0: No visceral disease

M1: Visceral disease

B1: No haematological involvement

B2: Sezary count >5% of total peripheral blood lymphocytes

Source: Whittaker et al. (2003).

Box 13.8   Burn and Lambert grading system

Stage IA: T1 N0
Stage IB: T2 N0
Stage IIA: T1/2 N1
Stage IIB: T3 N0/1
Stage III: T4 N0/1
Stage IVA: T any N 2/3
Stage IVB: T any N any M1

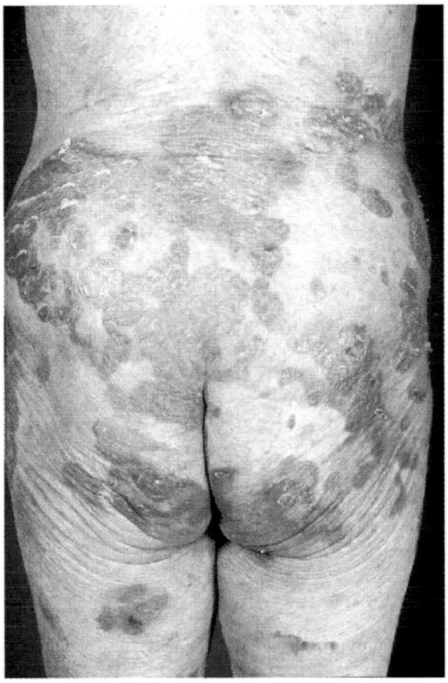

Figure 13.4   Mycoses fungoides.

Mycosis fungoides

Diagnosis of MF is made through an elliptical biopsy, particularly in the early stages it can be difficult to distinguish from other chronic skin conditions such as psoriasis or discoid eczema. The initial patch stage of the disease occurs when lymphocytes infiltrate the skin causing the patches or lumps to appear. As this is a disease which progresses very slowly, it may take years before the individual moves into the next phase of the disease (Figure 13.4). Table 13.4 is reproduced from the British Association of Dermatologist guidelines and indicates the survival rates for different stages of the disease (Whittaker *et al.*, 2003). As the disease progresses the skin signs change too, moving from patches to thickened plaques and eventually on to skin tumours. Although the prognosis is generally good and treatment can control symptoms, abnormal cells can eventually infiltrate other organs including blood, lymph nodes, heart, liver, lungs and spleen (New Zealand Dermatological Society Incorporated, 2009). It may not be necessary to involve the multidisciplinary team in the care of someone who has very early MF, but throughout

Table 13.4   Survival rates for cutaneous T-cell lymphoma.

	IA	IB	IIA	IIB	III	IVA	IVB
OS at 5 years (%)	96–100	73–86	49–73	40–65	40–57	15–40	0–15
OS at 10 years (%)	84–100	58–67	45–49	20–39	20–40	5–20	0–5
DSS at 5 years (%)	100	96	68	80		40	0
DSS at 10 years (%)	97–98	83	68	42		20	0
Disease progression at 5 years (%)	4	21	65	32		70	100
Disease progression at 10 years (%)	10	39	65	60		70	100

Source: Whittaker *et al.* (2003).
OS – overall survival
DSS – disease specific survival

the later stages the input from specialist cancer services is vital.

Treatments

Early stage MF (IA to IIA) can be treated conservatively with emollients and moderate potency topical steroids. However, dependant on the extent of skin signs and the thickness of the plaques, phototherapy (in the form of PUVA) and radiotherapy may need to be introduced. Resistant cases may need the addition of α-interferon to PUVA therapy. Patients with more advanced disease (IIB and above) will need to have systemic therapy which may include chemotherapy, immunotherapy or extracorporeal photophoresis (Whittaker *et al.*, 2003). Novel retinoids are being developed for use in MF with the hope that there will be fewer toxicities associated with these forms of treatment.

As has already been mentioned, prognosis is good in the early stages of MF. However, as the disease progresses to later stages, treatment may become palliative and a key focus of care is to maintain comfort and as much quality of life as possible. If ulcerated lesions are present, these will require nursing intervention and consideration given to pain relief.

Rosacea

Although often considered alongside acne (and indeed has been called 'acne rosacea') rosacea is, in fact, a distinct condition with features that set it apart from acne. It usually affects the older age group of 30- to 60-year olds and women are three times more likely than men to get it, although men tend to get it more severely. Rosacea is characterised by facial flushing and pustule formation (Figure 13.5). Unlike acne there are no whiteheads or blackheads and the pustules tend to be domed in shape rather than pointed. The skin is generally sensitive and facial oedema can occur. More severe cases can affect the eyes. The course of the disease is unpredictable, with periods of remission followed by relapse lasting for variable lengths of time.

Four subtypes of rosacea exist (Layton, 2008).

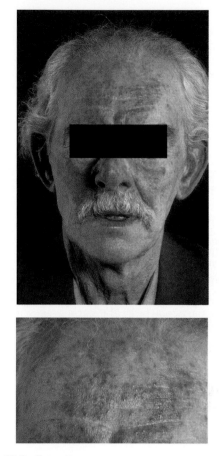

Figure 13.5   Rosacea.

Erythematotelangiectatic rosacea

As the name suggests, this type of rosacea is characterised by facial redness in the central zone often accompanied by telangiectasia (superficial blood vessels) and the patient usually experiences stinging and soreness. There may be other types of rosacea that accompany this subtype.

Papulopustular rosacea

Again facial redness is in evidence along with stinging and soreness but also accompanied by pustules. The skin may be extremely sensitive to topical products which generally aggravate the stinging sensations. Occasionally other parts of the body besides the face may be affected such as the chest, ears and in bald men the scalp. When these other areas are affected, it tends to indicate that the condition will be resistant to treatment.

Phymatous rosacea

This type of rosacea is much more common in men and may exist without any other signs of the disease. Excessive growth of sebaceous glands and connective tissues leads to an enlarged, mis-shapen nose which is often linked (wrongly) to excessive drinking. Rhinophyma may start with pustules and redness in its early stages.

Occular rosacea

Eye symptoms include grittiness, redness and soreness, conjunctivitis or blepharitis may occur. As a result, vision may be blurred and there can be an increased sensitivity to light. In around 5% of cases, there may be more severe damage to the eyes. It should be noted that ocular problems may occur long before there are any skin symptoms.

Whilst rosacea is a relatively common condition affecting around 10% of the population, there is little clarity about its pathophysiology. It is generally agreed that there is genetic predisposition which is aggravated by environmental factors with around 70% of cases reporting worsening when exposed to UV. Box 13.9 outlines some of the trigger factors that can worsen rosacea. The facial flushing may be caused by damage to the blood vessels which lead to vessel dilatation. There might be some association with a hair follicle mite called *Demodex folliculorum* as there is an increased incidence of these in rosacea papules in some people (New Zealand Dermatological Society Incorporated, 2009). It is well recognised that topical steroids aggravate rosacea and should not be used as part of the treatment. Other oil-based skin applications can also make the condition worse.

Treatment

General advice for patients with rosacea centre around trying to keep the facial skin cool and avoiding the trigger factors listed earlier. For

---

> **Box 13.9   Trigger factors for rosacea**
>
> Heat: from ambient temperature, spicy food, hot drinks, hot showers bath
>   UV exposure
>   Topical steroids
>   Oil-based moisturisers and make-up products
>   Alcohol

---

some direct cooling of the skin using an ice pack or fan can be helpful. The rest of this section looks at the various treatments that are available for treating rosacea.

Rosacea can either be treated using oral antibiotics or topical therapies. A Cochrane review revealed that the level of evidence for these treatments were generally poor, but that topical metronidazole or azelaic acid were both effective with less evidence showing efficacy of the oral metronidazole or tetracyclines (van Zuuren *et al.*, 2005).

Topical azelaic acid

When topical azelaic acid applications are used, the face should be gently cleansed and then the topical application applied to the dried skin. As a general guide, one finger tip unit (FTU) per two palms worth of area affected is a good guideline, but it is advisable to follow manufacturer's recommendations as different brands will vary slightly. For example Finacea recommends 1 FTU for the face and Skinoren 2 FTU. (Further details about specific products can be found from the Electronic Medicines Compendium – www.emc.medicines.org.uk). The treatment should be applied twice daily and gently massaged into the face. After use the individual should be instructed to wash their hands. The patient should expect to see significant improvement in 4–8 weeks, although it can be used over a prolonged period of many months if necessary.

The most common side effect is skin soreness and irritation and this can be minimised by reducing the amount of treatment used each day (to just once daily), before gradually building up to the recommended dosages. Because the products are irritating, care should be taken to avoid contact with the eyes and other mucous membranes. Should contact occur the areas should be washed with large amounts of water. There is little evidence for any ill effects that would mean the products needed to be stopped during pregnancy or breast feeding; however, this should be discussed for each individual case.

Topical antibiotics

There are a number of different brands of topical metronidazole, some of which come in a gel formulation and others in cream. Again, the Electronic Medicines Compendium will give specific advice about the use of each product. In general the method of application is similar to that of azelaic acid. The face should be gently cleansed and dried before an application of a thin layer of the product is gently massaged into the face. It should be used twice daily, but unlike azelaic acid should not be used constantly for more than 9 weeks. Because metronidazole becomes less effective when exposed to UV light, individuals should be warned not to go out in the sunshine whilst using the product.

It can act as an irritant and one of the side effects is skin burning and soreness. It may make the eyes water if it is applied too closely or gets into the eye by mistake. For some there are other undesirable effects which include a metallic taste in the mouth, tingling or numbness of the extremities, nausea and exacerbation of the rosacea. It is recommended that metronidazole should be discontinued in pregnancy and whilst breast feeding.

Oral antibiotics

If oral antibiotics are prescribed, they are usually for a relatively prolonged course of around 6–12 weeks, the dose depending on disease severity. Metronidazole should be swallowed with water before or after a meal whereas the tetracyclines should be taken on an empty stomach to aid absorption.

Whilst the above treatments should be effective to some degree, none of them are curative. Once they have been discontinued, it is quite likely that the rosacea will recur.

Other treatments

There are a number of other treatments which have limited evidence related to their efficacy but which might be helpful in some cases.

- *Anti-inflammatories*: It has already been stated that topical steroids will aggravate rosacea; however, some have found the topical calcineurin inhibitors (tacrolimus and pimecrolimus) helpful. Oral non-steroidal anti-inflammatories such as diclofenac might also be helpful in reducing facial redness, but it is important to be aware of the potential serious side effects (e.g. peptic ulceration).
- *Isotretinoin*: This drug was discussed extensively in the chapter on acne and its potential side effects discussed at length. It may be helpful particularly for those who do not respond to antibiotics; however, a low dose over a prolonged period of time is likely to be needed.
- *Clonidine*: This is an example of an alpha 2 receptor antagonist which may reduce vascular dilatation which leads to the facial flushing. Side effects are usually mild but may include low heart rate and blood pressure, dry eyes, blurred vision and gastrointestinal disturbance.
- *Vascular laser*: May be used to treat telangiectasia successfully. Other methods if lasers are not available include sclerotherapy (injections of strong saline solution), diathermy or cautery. Intense pulsed light has been shown in a small study to have significant impact on the erythema and telangiectasia, an effect which was maintained at 6 months (Papageorgiou *et al.*, 2008).
- *Surgery*: This may be necessary for people with rhinophyma in order to reshape the nose.

Urticaria

Urticaria describes a group of conditions in which itchy weals and red patches occur in the skin. They affect both children and adults. The weals are caused by the release of histamine or other chemicals from mast cells. These in turn increase the permeability of small blood vessels which leak into the skin causing localised swelling (Figure 13.6). Urticaria can be short lived or long term and appear in small patches or large areas, map-like, across the body. In some instances, urticaria is accompanied by angioedema in which there is deeper swelling often of hands, eyelids or lips, but can occur anywhere.

There are many different classifications of urticaria. Table 13.5 is taken from guidelines from the British Association of Dermatologists (Grattan and Humphreys, 2007).

Acute urticaria

Acute urticaria can be classified further as either allergic or non-allergic. Allergic is less common and may be an allergy to an ingested substance, e.g. a food or medicine, through a sting or through contact with a substance such as latex. Usually the allergic response will be mild requiring no emergency care; however sometimes the allergy may result in anaphylactic shock requiring emergency care and an injection of adrenaline.

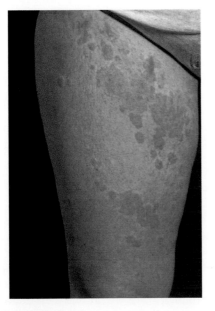

Figure 13.6 Urticaria.

Table 13.5 Different types of urticaria.

Overall clinical description of urticaria	Subtypes
Ordinary	Acute (up to 6 weeks continuous activity) Chronic (6 weeks or more of continuous activity) Episodic (acute, intermittent or recurrent activity)
Physical (reproducibly induced by the same stimulus)	Mechanical (e.g. delayed pressure, symptomatic dermographism, vibratory angioedema) Thermal (e.g. cholinergic, cold contact, localised heat) Others (e.g. aquagenic, solar, exercise induced)
Angiodema without weals	Idiopathic Drug induced (e.g. ACE inhibitors) C1 esterase-inhibitor deficiency
Contact urticaria (with allergens or chemicals)	
Urticarial vasculitis (as defined by a skin biopsy)	
Autoinflammatory syndromes	Hereditary (e.g. cryopyrin-associated periodic syndromes) Acquired (e.g. Schnitzler syndrome)

Non-allergic causes of acute urticaria are much more common and include:

- Infections such as sinusitis, helicobacter, viral hepatitis;
- Serum sickness due to blood transfusions, viral illness or certain drugs (this is accompanied by other symptoms including sickness, fever, joint pain and swollen lymph glands);
- Certain medicines such as morphine (and other opiates), codeine and radiocontrast agents can cause a non-allergic release of

mast cell granules such as histamine. Aspirin and other non-steroidal anti-inflammatories can also produce urticaria but through the production of leukotrienes which are potent mediators of immediate hypersensitivity reactions and inflammation;

■ Non-allergic food reactions can be caused by salicylates in fruit (which are highest in berry and dried fruits but occur in most fruits), azo food dye benzoate preservatives (New Zealand Dermatological Society Incorporated, 2009).

Chronic urticaria

In some instances, chronic urticaria is due to autoimmune disease and may be related to other autoimmune conditions such as thyroid or coeliac disease. In these cases autoantibodies will be found. In other cases there are no circulating autoantibodies and it is a more difficult condition to determine a cause for, often impossible. This type of urticaria is known as chronic idiopathic urticaria.

Physical urticaria

Five minutes following physical contact, the skin produces a weal that will last 15–30 minutes. Some people experience just the physical type of urticaria and others have it in combination with a more chronic type. The cause is unknown.

Dermographism

This literally describes skin writing and the individual experiences weals wherever the skin is touched be this through stroking the skin, touching it on furniture or the gentle pressure of clothes. The weals are usually itchy and aggravated when scratched, they can be worse when the individual is warm or upset.

Thermal

Certain temperature ranges can cause urticarial reactions. For example cholinergic describes the tiny red dots that appear on the skin following sweating, these can be very itchy. Cold contact urticaria usually strikes when cold skin is warming up after being exposed to cold outdoor temperatures. When the weals are widespread it can cause fainting attacks. Localised heat and solar urticaria are less common but describe the development of weals following exposure to said stimuli.

Contact urticaria

This is caused by physical contact either through the skin or mucous membranes, with a substance leading to either an allergic or non-allergic response. An IgE elicited response may be caused by a range of substances including white flour, latex, cosmetics or fish. A non-allergic reaction is caused by contact with substances such as nettles, certain insects (e.g. a hairy caterpillar). Weals may be limited to the contact area or may become more widespread.

Investigations

On the whole, diagnosis is usually made through clinical observation. Particularly for ordinary urticaria there is usually no need to perform any specific investigatory tests. However in acute and episodic cases allergic responses may be verified using skin prick tests and CAP fluoroimmunoassay tests on blood. If patients with chronic ordinary urticaria are not responding to antihistamines, it may be helpful to determine whether there are other autoimmune conditions present, e.g. check thyroid function. Long-standing urticaria that is not responding to treatment may be biopsied to identify whether there is a vasculitis present (Gittins, 2008).

Treatments

Primarily treatment revolves around antihistamine use and most people with urticaria do respond to these. However, some people do not respond and a few get worse. It is considered good practice to give people a choice of two non-sedating antihistamines to see which one they respond best to and it may be necessary to prescribe in doses which exceed the manufacturer's recommendations (Grattan and Humphreys, 2007). In acute type urticaria, oral steroids might be used for a short course and there is some evidence to show that ciclosporin can be helpful for those who are non-responsive to antihistamines (Grattan and Humphreys, 2007).

General advice to patients should also include avoiding things that appear to trigger the urticaria, e.g. fruits which contain salicylates. Aspirin is also likely to be problematic for those sensitive to salicylates and this should be avoided as should non-steroidal anti-inflammatories. General measures which may be helpful include keeping the skin cool (e.g. applying ice packs) and avoiding alcohol which is a vasodilator and make the skin feel hotter. Urticaria can be difficult to manage successfully and patients are likely to need ongoing support.

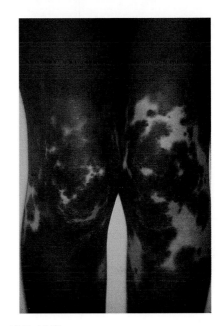

Figure 13.7   Vitiligo.

Vitiligo

Vitiligo may be thought of as an uncommon condition, but in fact around 1% of the population has it. Vitiligo is characterised by areas of skin that lose their pigment (Figure 13.7). For reasons that are not entirely clear, melanocytes, which are the pigment making cells, are destroyed. It is not certain what triggers this, although it may be related to an injury such as sunburn or to psychological stress. There are three possible theories as to why the melanocytes behave in this way.

(1) Abnormally functioning nerve cells injure the melanocytes;
(2) There is an autoimmune response in which the body's own immune system attacks the melanocytes as they are viewed as foreign bodies;
(3) The melanocytes destroy themselves.

Whatever the mechanism may be, areas of totally depigmented skin are created, often symmetrical in nature, in which there are few other symptoms (e.g. no scaling or inflammation). Occasionally vitiligo will be segmental in nature with asymmetric patches occurring on just one part of the body.

When the disease is seen in children, there is a much greater likelihood of spontaneous repigmentation than in adults. Repigmentation starts around the hair follicle and then spreads across the patch until the spots coalesce. For adults the disease may be progressive with more and more areas of skin becoming depigmented, for others the patches are more static. Many will notice cycles in which there are periods of fairly rapid pigment loss, followed by periods of stability, followed by further loss of pigment, etc. Vitiligo is clearly more obvious in skin types 4 and above. But for all skin types it can have a serious impact on the individual's psychological well-being. Individuals also have to take a great deal of care when out in the sun, as the areas of depigmentation are much more prone to burning than the rest of the skin.

Pigment loss is not limited to the skin; for some people there is also pigment loss from the hair leading to white or grey head hair, eyebrows, eyelashes or body hair.

Treatment

Whilst there are a number of treatments available which may be of some help in the short term, there is very little evidence for their long-term efficacy or safety (Whitton *et al.*, 2006). Potent topical steroids can sometimes induce repigmentation and although it is not a licensed use the calcineurin inhibitors have shown some effect especially in areas such as the face where potent topical steroids may be particularly damaging. PUVA can also lead to repigmentation, although this may need to be long term. A couple of studies have suggested that PUVA in combination with calcipotriol may be effective, but the long-term results have not been evaluated. A 2008 guideline summarises the treatments for vitiligo along with the level of evidence associated with them (Gawkrodger *et al.*, 2008).

Camouflage

Using skin camouflage products can help to provide a uniformity to skin tone and colour which hides the depigmentation. There is a wide range of colours within the product palette and the camouflage practitioner will mix no more than three of these together to make a skin tone colour that suits the patient (Davies, 2007). Once cover creams have been applied, they are fixed with either a spray or powder which means they become fully waterproof. This allows the individual to leave the camouflage products on for up to a week and continue to wash as normal. In order to remove the product, skin cleansers are used.

Patients who are diagnosed with vitiligo may need significant levels of psychological support. Whilst treatment options are limited, it is not helpful to say there is nothing that can be done. For some, repigmentation may occur with treatments, but it is important to be realistic about the fact that these changes are unlikely to be permanent. More importantly patients need to know that they are not alone and the National Vitiligo Society (http://www.vitiligosociety.org.uk/) may be able to provide invaluable support. Skin camouflage is always an option, some may choose to see a practitioner privately; however, a referral from the GP should be an option.

Conclusion

There are many hundreds of differential diagnoses in dermatology. This section has looked at:

(a) Those conditions that are commonly seen but yet do not fit neatly into any of the other chapters, e.g. rosacea and pityriasis rosea;
(b) Those common, uncommon conditions such as bullous pemphigoid and vitiligo.

Careful assessment of skin signs and symptoms is required to ensure correct diagnosis. This will increasingly become a nursing role as nurse practitioners and nurse prescribers become more common place.

References

Chuang, T. and L. Stitle (2008). Lichen Planus. Retrieved 3 April 2009, from http://emedicine.medscape.com/article/1123213-overview.

Davies, V. (2007). The use of camouflage in skin conditions. *Dermatological Nursing*, **6**(4): 16–20.

Gawkrodger, D., A. Ormerod *et al.* (2008). Guideline for the diagnosis and management of vitiligo. *British Journal of Dermatology*, **159**(5): 1051–1076.

Gittins, S. (2008). Recognition and management of urticarial vasculitis. *Dermatological Nursing*, **7**(4): 20–27.

Graham-Brown, R. and J.F. Bourke (1998). *Mosby's Color Atlas and Text of Dermatology*. London: Mosby.

Graham-Brown, R. and T. Burns (2006). *Lecture Notes: Dermatology* (9th edition). Oxford: Blackwell publishing.

Grattan, C. and F. Humphreys (2007). Guidelines for the assessment and management of urticaria in adults and children. *British Journal of Dermatology*, **157**(6): 1116–1123.

Langan, S. and H. Williams (2009). A systematic review of randomised controlled trials of treatment for inherited forms of epidermolysis bullosa. *Clinical and Experimental Dermatology*, **34**(1): 20–25.

Layton, A. (2008). Clinical aspects and treatment of rosacea. *Dermatological Nursing*, **7**(2): 26–29.

Ly, L. and J. Su (2008). Dressings used in epidermolysis blister wounds: A review. *Journal of Wound Care*, **17**(11): 482, 484–486.

New Zealand Dermatological Society Incorporated (2009). DermnetNZ. Retrieved 25 March 2009, from www.dermnetnz.org.

Papageorgiou, P., W. Clayton *et al.* (2008). Treatment of rosacea with intensed pulsed light: Significant improvement and long lasting results. *British Journal of Dermatology*, **159**(3): 628–632.

Ruzicka, T., T. Assmann *et al.* (2003). Potential future dermatological indications for tacrolimus ointment. *European Journal of Dermatology*, **13**(4): 331–342.

van Zuuren, E., M. Graber *et al.* (2005). Interventions for rosacea. *Cochrane Database of Sytematic Reviews*, (3). htt://www. cochrane.org/reviews/en/ab003262.html accessed 8/12/09.

Volz, T., U. Caroli *et al.* (2008). Pimecrolimus cream 1% in erosive oral lichen planus – A prospective randomised double-blind vehicle-controlled study. *British Journal of Dermatology*, **159**(4): 936–941.

Weller, R., J.A.A. Hunter, J. Savin and M. Dahl (2008). *Clinical Dermatology* (4th edition). Oxford: Blackwell Publishing.

Whittaker, S., J. Marsden *et al.* (2003). Joint British Association of Dermatologists and UK Cutaneous Lymphoma Group guidelines for the management of primary cutaneous T-cell lymphomas. *British Journal of Dermatology*, **149**(6): 1095–1107.

Whitton, M., D. Ashcroft *et al.* (2006). Interventions for vitiligo. *Cochrane Database of Sytematic Reviews*, (1). htt://www. cochrane.org/reviews/en/ab003263.html accessed 8/12/09.

Wojnarowska, F., G. Kirtschig *et al.* (2002). Guidelines for the management of bullous pemphigoid. *British Journal of Dermatology*, **147**(2): 214–221.

Appendices

Appendix 1 – The psoriasis area severity index (PASI)

This version of the PASI tool reproduced by kind permission of Shering-Plough Ltd (UK), copyright reserved.

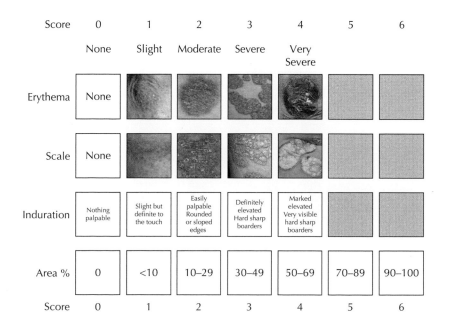

Score	0	1	2	3	4	5	6
	None	Slight	Moderate	Severe	Very Severe		
Erythema	None						
Scale	None						
Induration	Nothing palpable	Slight but definite to the touch	Easily palpable Rounded or sloped edges	Definitely elevated Hard sharp boarders	Marked elevated Very visible hard sharp boarders		
Area %	0	<10	10–29	30–49	50–69	70–89	90–100
Score	0	1	2	3	4	5	6

Date | Patient name | Hospital number

	Head	Upper limbs	Trunk	Lower limbs
Erythema (E)				
Induration (I)				
Scaling (S)				
Sum (E+I+S)				
Area score				
Sum × Area				
	×0.1	×0.2	×0.3	×0.4

____ + ____ + ____ + ____ = ____

Total PASI score

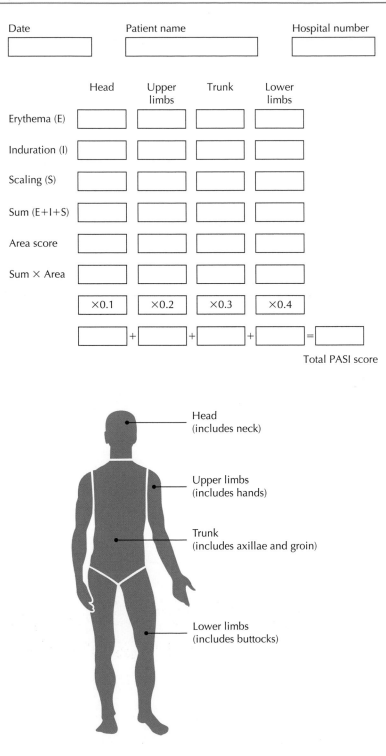

Head
(includes neck)

Upper limbs
(includes hands)

Trunk
(includes axillae and groin)

Lower limbs
(includes buttocks)

Appendix 2 – The SCORAD index

Permission kindly received from Dr Stalder on behalf of the European Task Force on Atopic Dermatitis.

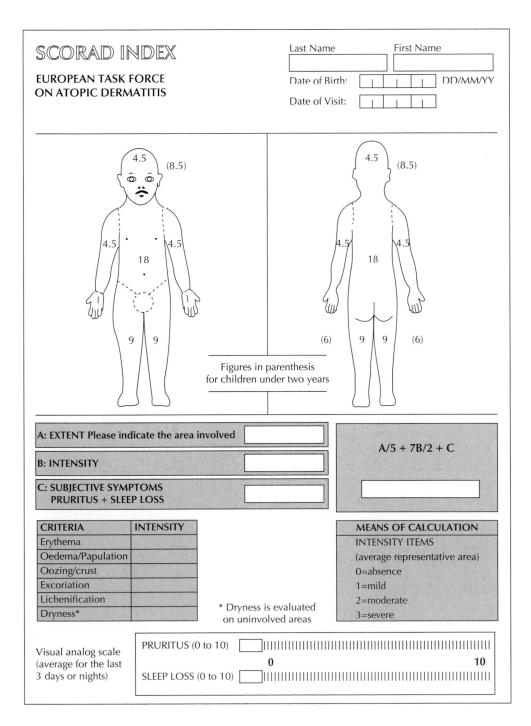

SCORAD INDEX

EUROPEAN TASK FORCE
ON ATOPIC DERMATITIS

Last Name

First Name

Date of Birth: | | | | DD/MM/YY

Date of Visit: | | | |

4.5 (8.5)

4.5 4.5

18

9 9

4.5 (8.5)

4.5 4.5

18

(6) 9 9 (6)

Figures in parenthesis
for children under two years

A: EXTENT Please indicate the area involved

B: INTENSITY

C: SUBJECTIVE SYMPTOMS
PRURITUS + SLEEP LOSS

A/5 + 7B/2 + C

CRITERIA	INTENSITY
Erythema	
Oedema/Papulation	
Oozing/crust	
Excoriation	
Lichenification	
Dryness*	

* Dryness is evaluated
on uninvolved areas

MEANS OF CALCULATION

INTENSITY ITEMS
(average representative area)
0=absence
1=mild
2=moderate
3=severe

Visual analog scale
(average for the last
3 days or nights)

PRURITUS (0 to 10) |||||||||||||||||||||||||||||||||||||||||||||||
0   10

SLEEP LOSS (0 to 10) |||||||||||||||||||||||||||||||||||||||||||||||

Appendix 3 – Examples of emollients with excipients

Less greasy for dry skin	Most greasy for very dry skin	
Lotions	**Creams and gels**	**Ointments**
	Balneum plus (contains urea and anti-pruritic) (*benzyl alcohol, polysorbates*)	Unguentum M (*cetostearyl alcohol, polysorbate, propylene glycol, sorbic acid*)
Eucerin lotion (10% urea) (*benzyl alcohol, isopropyl palmitate*)	Double base	50% white soft paraffin 50% liquid paraffin
E45 lotion (*cetyl alcohol, hydroxybenzoate*)	E45 cream (*cetyl alcohol, hydroxybenzoate, isopropyl palmitate*)	White soft paraffin
Dermol 500 lotion (contains antiseptic) (*cetostearyl alcohol*)	Eucerin cream (10% urea) (*benzyl alcohol, isopropyl palmitate, wool fat*)	Emulsifying ointment (*cetostearyl alcohol*)
Aveeno (*benzyl alcohol, cetyl alcohol, isopropyl palmitate*)	Diprobase cream (*cetostearyl alcohol, chlorocresol*)	Yellow soft paraffin
	Dermol cream (contains antiseptic) (*cetostearyl alcohol*)	Diprobase ointment
Vaseline Dermacare	Lipobase (*cetostearyl alcohol, hydroxybenzoate*)	Hydrous ointment (*phenoxyethanol*)
	Oilatum (*benzyl alcohol, cetylstearyl alcohol*)	Epaderm (*cetostearyl alcohol*)
	Ultrabase (*fragrance, hydroxybenzoate, disodium edentate, stearyl alcohol*)	Hydromol ointment (*cetostearyl alcohol*)
	Zerobase (*cetostearyl alcohol, chlorocresol*)	Aquaphor
	Aquadrate (contains urea)	
	Decubal (*cetyl alcohol, hydroxybenzoate*)	
	Calmurid (contains urea)	
	Nutraplus (contains urea) (*hydroxybenzoate, propylene glycol*)	
	Cetraben (*cetostearyl alcohol, hydroxybenzoate*)	
	Hydromol cream (*cetostearyl alcohol, hydroxybenzoate*)	
	Sensicare emollient (*cetostearyl alcohol*)	
	Aqueous cream (soap substitute) (*phenoxyethanol, cetostearyl alcohol*)	

Index